Dr Tim PRIEST

Birmingham Heartlands + Solihull NHS Trust

2002
YEAR BOOK OF
ANESTHESIOLOGY AND
PAIN MANAGEMENT™

The 2002 Year Book Series

Year Book of Allergy, Asthma, and Clinical Immunology™: Drs Rosenwasser, Boguniewicz, Milgrom, Routes, and Spahn

Year Book of Anesthesiology and Pain Management™: Drs Chestnut, Abram, Black, Lang, Roizen, Trankina, and Wood

Year Book of Cardiology®: Drs Schlant, Gersh, Graham, Kaplan, and Waldo

Year Book of Critical Care Medicine®: Drs Dellinger, Parrillo, Balk, Bleck, Carcillo, and Royster

Year Book of Dentistry®: Drs Zakariasen, Boghosian, Dederich, Hatcher, Horswell, and McIntyre

Year Book of Dermatology and Dermatologic Surgery™: Drs Thiers and Lang

Year Book of Diagnostic Radiology®: Drs Osborn, Birdwell, Dalinka, Groskin, Maynard, Oestreich, Pentecost, and Ros

Year Book of Emergency Medicine®: Drs Burdick, Cone, Cydulka, Hamilton, Loiselle, and Niemann

Year Book of Endocrinology®: Drs Mazzaferri, Fitzpatrick, Horton, Kannan, Kennedy, Kreisberg, Meikle, Molitch, Osei, Poehlman, and Rogol

Year Book of Family Practice®: Drs Bowman, Dexter, Gilchrist, Morrison, Neill, and Scherger

Year Book of Gastroenterology™: Drs Lichtenstein, Ginsberg, Katzka, Kochman, Morris, Nunes, Rosato, and Stein

Year Book of Hand Surgery®: Drs Berger and Ladd

Year Book of Medicine®: Drs Barkin, Frishman, Jett, Klahr, Loehrer, and Mazzaferri

Year Book of Neonatal and Perinatal Medicine®: Drs Fanaroff, Maisels, and Stevenson

Year Book of Neurology and Neurosurgery®: Drs Bradley, Gibbs, and Verma

Year Book of Nuclear Medicine®: Drs Gottschalk, Blaufox, Coleman, Strauss, and Zubal

Year Book of Obstetrics, Gynecology, and Women's Health®: Drs Mishell, Kirschbaum, and Miller

Year Book of Oncology®: Drs Loehrer, Eisenberg, Glatstein, Gordon, Johnson, Pratt, and Thigpen

Year Book of Ophthalmology®: Drs Wilson, Cohen, Eagle, Grossman, Laibson, Maguire, Nelson, Penne, Rapuano, Sergott, Shields, Spaeth, Tipperman, Ms Gosfield, and Ms Salmon

Year Book of Orthopedics®: Drs Morrey, Beauchamp, Peterson, Swiontkowski, Trigg, and Yaszemski

Year Book of Otolaryngology-Head and Neck Surgery®: Drs Paparella, Holt, Keefe, and Otto

Year Book of Pathology and Laboratory Medicine®: Drs Raab, Bejarano, Bissell, Silverman, and Stanley

Year Book of Pediatrics®: Dr Stockman

Year Book of Plastic and Aesthetic Surgery™: Drs Miller, Bartlett, Garner, McKinney, Ruberg, Salisbury, and Smith

Year Book of Psychiatry and Applied Mental Health®: Drs Talbott, Ballenger, Frances, Jensen, Markowitz, Meltzer, and Simpson

Year Book of Pulmonary Disease®: Drs Jett, Hunt, Maurer, Peters, Phillips, and Ryu

Year Book of Rheumatology, Arthritis, and Musculoskeletal Disease™: Drs Panush, Hadler, Hellmann, Lahita, Lane, and Le Roy

Year Book of Sports Medicine®: Drs Shephard, Alexander, Cantu, Kohrt, Nieman, and Shrier

Year Book of Surgery®: Drs Copeland, Bland, Cerfolio, Daly, Deitch, Eberlein, Howard, Luce, and Seeger

Year Book of Urology®: Drs Andriole and Coplen

Year Book of Vascular Surgery®: Dr Porter

2002

The Year Book of
ANESTHESIOLOGY
AND PAIN
MANAGEMENT™

Editor-in-Chief
David H. Chestnut, MD

Associate Editors
Stephen E. Abram, MD
Susan Black, MD
John D. Lang, Jr, MD
Michael F. Roizen, MD
Mark F. Trankina, MD
Margaret Wood, MD, FRCA

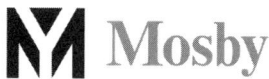 Mosby

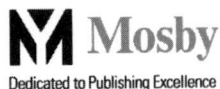
Dedicated to Publishing Excellence

Vice President, Continuity Publishing: Glen P. Campbell
Senior Manager, Continuity Production: Idelle L. Winer
Production Editor: Jason Gonulsen
Composition Specialist: Betty Dockins
Senior Illustrations and Permissions Specialist: Chidi C. Ukabam

Printed in the United States of America
Composition by Thomas Technology Solutions, Inc.
Printing/binding by Sheridan Books, Inc.

Editorial Office:
Mosby, Inc.
11830 Westline Industrial Drive
St. Louis, MO 63146
Customer Service: hhspcs@harcourt.com

International Standard Serial Number: 1073-5437
International Standard Book Number: 0-323-01565-4

Editorial Board

Table of Contents

Journals Represented

Mosby and its editors survey approximately 500 journals for its abstract and commentary publications. From these journals, the editors select the articles to be abstracted. Journals represented in this YEAR BOOK are listed below.

Acta Anaesthesiologica Scandinavica
American Journal of Cardiology
American Journal of Gastroenterology
American Journal of Obstetrics and Gynecology
American Journal of Respiratory and Critical Care Medicine
American Journal of Surgery
Anaesthesia and Intensive Care
Anesthesia and Analgesia
Anesthesiology
Annals of Internal Medicine
Annals of Surgery
Annals of Thoracic Surgery
Annals of Vascular Surgery
Archives of Physical Medicine and Rehabilitation
Archives of Surgery
British Journal of Anaesthesia
British Journal of Obstetrics and Gynaecology
British Journal of Surgery
British Medical Journal
Canadian Journal of Anesthesia
Chest
Circulation
Clinical Chemistry
Clinical Pharmacology and Therapeutics
Critical Care Medicine
European Journal of Anaesthesiology
European Journal of Pain
European Journal of Vascular and Endovascular Surgery
European Respiratory Journal
Intensive Care Medicine
Journal of Bone and Joint Surgery (American Volume)
Journal of Cardiothoracic and Vascular Anesthesia
Journal of Clinical Anesthesia
Journal of Critical Care
Journal of General Internal Medicine
Journal of Hand Surgery (British)
Journal of Maternal-Fetal Medicine
Journal of Neurosurgery
Journal of Neurosurgery: Spine
Journal of Pain and Symptom Management
Journal of Pharmacology and Experimental Therapeutics
Journal of Rheumatology
Journal of Surgical Research
Journal of Thoracic and Cardiovascular Surgery
Journal of Vascular Surgery
Journal of the American College of Surgeons
Journal of the American Medical Association

Lancet
Mayo Clinic Proceedings
Nature
New England Journal of Medicine
Obstetrics and Gynecology
Pain
Pediatric Neurology
Pediatrics
Regional Anesthesia and Pain Medicine
Southern Medical Journal
Spine
Stroke
Surgery
Veterinary Human Toxicology

STANDARD ABBREVIATIONS

The following terms are abbreviated in this edition: acquired immunodeficiency syndrome (AIDS), cardiopulmonary resuscitation (CPR), central nervous system (CNS), cerebrospinal fluid (CSF), computed tomography (CT), deoxyribonucleic acid (DNA), electrocardiography (ECG), health maintenance organization (HMO), human immunodeficiency virus (HIV), intensive care unit (ICU), intramuscular (IM), intravenous (IV), magnetic resonance (MR) imaging (MRI), ribonucleic acid (RNA), ultrasound (US), and ultraviolet (UV).

NOTE

The YEAR BOOK OF ANESTHESIOLOGY AND PAIN MANAGEMENT™ is a literature survey service providing abstracts of articles published in the professional literature. Every effort is made to ensure the accuracy of the information presented in these pages. Neither the editors nor the publisher of the YEAR BOOK OF ANESTHESIOLOGY AND PAIN MANAGEMENT™ can be responsible for errors in the original materials. The editors' comments are their own opinions. Mention of specific products within this publication does not constitute endorsement.

To facilitate the use of the YEAR BOOK OF ANESTHESIOLOGY AND PAIN MANAGEMENT™ as a reference tool, all illustrations and tables included in this publication are now identified as they appear in the original article. This change is meant to help the reader recognize that any illustration or table appearing in the YEAR BOOK OF ANESTHESIOLOGY AND PAIN MANAGEMENT™ may be only one of many in the original article. For this reason, figure and table numbers will often appear to be out of sequence within the YEAR BOOK OF ANESTHESIOLOGY AND PAIN MANAGEMENT™.

Introduction

It is an honor and a privilege for me to assume the responsibilities of Editor-in-Chief of the 2002 YEAR BOOK OF ANESTHESIOLOGY AND PAIN MANAGEMENT. The previous Editor-in-Chief, John H. Tinker, MD, has been one of my mentors during the last 18 years. In 1984, Dr Tinker and Dr Roy Pitkin (who was Professor and Head of the Department of Obstetrics and Gynecology) recruited me to join the faculty of the University of Iowa College of Medicine. For 10 years, Dr Tinker helped prepare me for my present position as Chair of the Department of Anesthesiology at the University of Alabama at Birmingham (UAB). In 1994—the year that I assumed my present position as Chair of Anesthesiology at UAB—Dr Tinker invited me to join the Editorial Board for the 2002 YEAR BOOK OF ANESTHESIOLOGY AND PAIN MANAGEMENT. It has been a pleasure to work with him in this capacity these last 8 years.

I am grateful that 3 of our longstanding (and popular) editors have agreed to continue to serve on the Editorial Board. Michael F. Roizen, MD, recently resigned as Chair of Anesthesia and Critical Care at the University of Chicago to become Dean of the College of Medicine at SUNY Upstate Medical University in Syracuse. Stephen E. Abram, MD, and Margaret Wood, MD, FRCA, continue in their positions as Chairs of Anesthesiology at the University of New Mexico School of Medicine and the College of Physicians and Surgeons of Columbia University, respectively. I am grateful for their ongoing commitment to the YEAR BOOK.

I am pleased to welcome 3 UAB Anesthesiology Faculty to the Editorial Board. Susan Black, MD, is Professor of Anesthesiology and Associate Director of the Neuroanesthesia Section in our Department. Dr Black will primarily review articles related to neuroanesthesia and pediatric anesthesia. John D. Lang, Jr, MD, is Associate Professor of Anesthesiology and Surgery at UAB. Dr Lang is an attending physician in the UAB Hospital Surgery ICU, and he also serves as Director of the Pre-Anesthesia Assessment Clinic at UAB. Dr Lang will primarily review articles related to critical care and perioperative medicine. Finally, Mark F. Trankina, MD, Associate Professor of Anesthesiology at UAB, has also joined the Editorial Board. Dr Trankina provides anesthesia for cardiothoracic surgery in both adults and children. Dr Trankina will primarily review articles related to cardiothoracic anesthesia and transesophageal echocardiography.

It is a pleasure for me to work with such a distinguished group of editors. These editors are outstanding physicians and scholars that I know and trust, and I am confident that you will find their insight to be informative and helpful. Service on the YEAR BOOK Editorial Board is a labor of love—and also a great tool for continuing medical education, *both* for the editors and the readers. I hope that you enjoy reading our selections and accompanying comments as much as we have enjoyed preparing them for you.

David H. Chestnut, MD

1 Studies of Outcomes, Risks, Costs, and Benefits

Assessment Instruments Used During Anaesthetic Simulation: Review of Published Studies
Byrne AJ, Greaves JD (Morriston Hosp, Swansea, UK; Royal Victoria Infirmary, Newcastle upon Tyne, UK)
Br J Anaesth 86:445-450, 2001   1–1

Background.—Complex simulations of anesthesia are now possible, which facilitate the assessment of anesthetists' performance without the use of real patients. In the past, the assessment instruments used to measure performance in anesthesia simulation have been harshly criticized for poor design, which limited their utility. Five aspects of the reported assessments used in the evaluation of a simulator-based assessment system were examined. These aspects are the type of simulator, the type of simulation, the efficacy of the assessment, the performance aspects to be assessed, and the assessment instruments applied in conjunction with the simulation.

Methods.—A literature search was conducted with the MEDLINE and EMBASE databases to identify articles published between 1980 and 2000 that described assessment of performance during simulated anesthesia.

Results.—Thirteen articles were identified; however, only 4 of these articles were designed to investigate the validity or reliability of the assessment systems. All the studies involved the assessment of anesthetist performance during a simulated general anesthetic, during which critical incidents were presented. None of the studies directly assessed propositional knowledge. However, all the studies included some assessment of procedural knowledge. Psychomotor skills were not specifically assessed in any of the investigations. Scoring in many of the studies was done by videotape review. Psychological tests have been used in the operating room to measure the performance of anesthetists, but there were no reports of this type of assessment. Only 4 studies were primarily designed to investigate the validity and reliability of assessment performed in the simulator.

None of the studies attempted to prove the content validity of their assessments.

Conclusions.—Efficacy of the assessment systems used to evaluate performance during anesthesia simulation has not been established. Thus, it would be premature to introduce simulator-based tests for certification or recertification of anesthetists.

▶ This excellent article shows that the efficacy of methods for assessment of performance during anesthesia simulation and crisis management simulation has not been appropriately determined. The authors believe that the introduction of simulation-based tests for certification or recertification is premature. One interesting point that would have been good to see in this article is a comparison with a simulation assessment considered to work— such as airplane pilot simulation. We don't see that analysis here. What testing do such airplane simulators use, and what testing is shown to prove reliability of simulators and the usefulness of those airplane simulators? Once again, as with many good studies and articles, we are left with more questions than answers.

M. F. Roizen, MD

Statistical Analysis by Monte-Carlo Simulation of the Impact of Administrative and Medical Delays in Discharge From the Postanesthesia Care Unit on Total Patient Care Hours
Dexter F, Penning DH, Traub RD (Univ of Iowa, Iowa City; Univ of Toronto; North Dakota State Univ, Fargo)
Anesth Analg 92:1222-1225, 2001   1–2

Introduction.—A reduction of length of stay (LOS) in the postanesthesia care unit (PACU) could reduce nursing costs, which account for the majority of PACU costs. One cause of prolonged PACU LOS is the lack of an available hospital room, delaying PACU discharge. An economic case study considered the following question: "If patients never again had to wait for admission to a ward from the PACU, what effect would this have on total PACU LOS?"

Methods.—The use of computer simulation to estimate the impact of an administrative delay on total PACU LOS was reviewed. Analysis was performed using the times of admission and discharge of all patients cared for in the PACU between April 1, 1999 and March 30, 2000. The phase I PACU considered was in a tertiary, academic surgical suite with a mixture of outpatient, inpatient, and same-day admit cases. In the analysis, the probability distribution for the chance that a patient will be delayed was identified, PACU LOS were fitted to 3-parameter log normal distributions, 2 simulated LOS were generated, and a patient arrival was generated.

Discussion.—A total of 100,000 simulations were performed. For the PACU described in the case study, total PACU time would have been decreased by <5%, even if all administrative delays were eliminated. This is very unlikely to produce decreased PACU staffing costs. A PACU manager can focus on uncommon but prolonged delays or common but brief delays. Neither, however, may be important financially. Computer simulation can be used to estimate the impact of delays in PACU discharge on total PACU hours and whether reduction of delays would have a significant financial impact.

▶ I wish I could understand this article, because it may have an important impact in environments where operating and recovery rooms are limited. The authors pose the question well: If a patient never again had to wait for admission to a ward from the PACU, what effect would this have on total PACU LOS? The authors analyze this and conclude that this type of simulation had value for determining how much effort one should put to this problem.

My bias on this issue is to say that the frustration occurring because of such delays and the consequent morale changes that occur mean that we should eliminate any delays that can practically be eliminated, but Dexter and colleagues may know better.

M. F. Roizen, MD

The Impact on Revenue of Increasing Patient Volume at Surgical Suites With Relatively High Operating Room Utilization

Dexter F, Macario A, Lubarsky DA (Univ of Iowa, Iowa City; Stanford Univ, Calif; Duke Univ, Durham, NC)
Anesth Analg 92:1215-1221, 2001   1–3

Introduction.—Some hospitals in the United States are trying to lose less money by performing more cases. The present analysis applies specifically to surgical suites that limit the hours that the operating room (OR) staff are available to care for elective surgery cases. Staffing costs are thus fixed, and hospitals can maximize utilization of the surgical suites. The term "utilization" means "adjusted utilization" as defined by the Association of Anesthesia Clinical Directors. Thus a utilization of 90% corresponds to patients being in an OR for 75% to 80% of staffed OR hours. Computer simulation was used to determine the revenue impact of using a 15% reduced fee-for-service contract to increase the volume of referred patients by 11% at a surgical suite with 90% utilization.

Methods.—Operating room utilization was calculated after simulating the creation and scheduling of thousands of cases. The baseline computer simulations had 7 assumptions that were modified by considering 6 separate scenarios. The variable costs considered were those that change in direct proportion to workload, such as disposable supplies, not OR labor.

Results.—According to computer simulations, for a surgical suite with a 90% (adjusted) utilization, an increase in the volume of referred patients by the amount expected to fill the surgical suite (100%/90%) would increase utilization by less than 1% for a hospital surgical suite and 4% for an ambulatory surgical suite. A 15% reduction in payment for the new patients would not increase revenue for the hospital surgical suite. In fact, this strategy might lead to a decrease in revenue with the additional patients displacing other more lucrative patients from OR time. An ambulatory surgery center might achieve a small financial benefit from the strategy. Results would be different for surgical suites with an initial lower utilization, increasing utilization by 6%.

Conclusion.—For hospitals with a relatively high (90%) adjusted OR utilization, increased patient volume is likely to result in a decrease in contribution margin. Scheduling the hospital surgical suite is inherently different from other aspects of hospital scheduling.

▶ This is a wonderful study showing that when patient care is discounted and there is a high volume of utilization, net revenues to the institution decrease. One of the subsegments in this article is the implication for academic medical centers. It is clearly hard to increase OR volume beyond 90% and that's the critical point examined in this article. For those of you in management who are concerned with OR volumes and discounts, and are pressured by the administration or deans to do one thing or the other to increase volume, study this article carefully; it is an important contribution.

M. F. Roizen, MD

What Do Outpatients Value Most in Their Anesthesia Care?
Fung D, Cohen M (Univ of Toronto; North Bay Gen Hosp, Ont, Canada)
Can J Anesth 48:12-19, 2001   1–4

Background.—It is important to obtain feedback from patients to gain insight into the quality of clinical practice and hospital programs. Until recently, most of the large surveys designed to elicit patient evaluation of anesthesia programs have relied on multi-item questionnaires developed without the direct input of patients. Surveys constructed by anesthesiologists tend to ask patients to report what they perceived or felt, but the questions may not reflect on what patients themselves want in the anesthesia experience. An approach that first attempted to determine what patients value or prefer in their care before formulating a multi-item questionnaire to determine whether these preferences had been met would have greater validity. This study builds on an earlier investigation that attempted to construct a comprehensive list of those features of outpatient anesthesia that were most important to patients. A new group of surgical outpatients were asked to rank items drawn from this list and also asked an expert panel of anesthesiologists to predict the rankings that patients placed on the different elements.

Methods.—A mailback questionnaire with 36 items was given postoperatively to 45 surgical outpatients and to 15 expert anesthesiologists. The patients and anesthesiologists were asked to indicate the 3 highest ranking items from each of 4 lists of 9 items, which represented preoperative, intraoperative, predischarge, and postdischarge outpatient anesthesia care.

Results.—All the anesthesiologists and 30 outpatients returned questionnaires. Elements representing information and communication were ranked highest by outpatients in all 4 phases of care, and physical conditions tended to be least valued. In contrast, although anesthesiologists were able to correctly predict what patients would value in the predischarge and postdischarge phases of care, they undervalued the importance of communication and information to patients in the preoperative and intraoperative phases of care.

Conclusions.—These findings underscore the importance that patients place on effective communication and the provision of adequate information in all phases of anesthesia care, including preoperative and intraoperative care.

▶ This is a particularly interesting study to me because it says that preoperative evaluation has an added benefit that most people don't realize—that of communication with the patient. I understand this because most patient complaints about preoperative evaluation are that they didn't spend enough time with physicians or they were not given thorough explanations. I commend this study; it is an outstanding study that expresses the fact that preoperative concerns, discussions in the operating room, and clear discharge discussions are very important to patients.

M. F. Roizen, MD

Measurement of Individual Clinical Productivity in an Academic Anesthesiology Department
Abouleish AE, Zornow MH, Levy RS, et al (Univ of Texas, Galveston)
Anesthesiology 93:1509-1516, 2000   1–5

Background.—One important issue facing anesthesiology departments, whether in private or academic settings, is the ability to measure individual clinical productivity, work performed, or contributions to the clinical mission. In the private sector these measurements have become the basis of compensation, particularly profit distribution. In the academic setting, measurement of clinical productivity in anesthesiology departments is being demanded by medical school administrators and budget committees who may not understand the fundamental factors that determine the work output of anesthesiologists in comparison with other specialties. The practice and billing of anesthesia service make it difficult to quantify individual productivity. Several methods of measuring individual productivity by using billing and scheduling data for the clinical activities of faculty members of an anesthesiology department at a university medical center were evaluated.

Methods.—The methods for measuring individual productivity included normalized clinical days per year (nCD/y), time units per operating room day worked (TU/OR day), normalized time units per year (nTU/y), total American Society of Anesthesiologists (ASA) units per OR day (tASA/OR day), and normalized total ASA units per year (ntASA/y). Billing and scheduling data were collected and analyzed for the 1998 fiscal year. All clinical sites and all clinical faculty anesthesiologists were included unless they spent less than 20% of their time in the fiscal year providing clinical care. Outliers, which were defined as faculty with productivity greater or less than 1 SD from the mean, were examined in detail.

Results.—nCD/y identified faculty who worked more than their clinical full-time equivalent would have predicted. TU/OR day and tASA/OR day were most successful in identifying apparently low-productivity faculty as those who worked a large portion of their time in obstetric anesthesia or an ambulatory surgicenter. The tASA/OR method identified specialty anesthesiologists as apparently high-productivity faculty. The nTU/y and ntASA/y methods were products of the per-OR day measurement and nCD/y.

Conclusions.—Each of the reporting methods was indicative of certain types of productivity more than other types. The most appropriate measure or combination of measures of productivity can be identified by defining the type of service most important to reward. The nCD/y method was found to be the most useful in determining individual productivity because it measures an anesthesiologist's contribution to daily staffing, includes all clinical sites, is independent of nonanesthesia factors, and can be easily collected and determined.

▶ For those involved in putting anesthesia productivity systems into place, especially those who include research, pain clinics, and ICUs, this is a first step. An overall taxing mechanism is needed no matter what is in place to make up for call time and obstetrics or pediatrics, where the units may have a necessity to be less full than others. This article gives a good view of the differences between different systems and measures of clinical productivity.

M. F. Roizen, MD

The Role of Anesthesiologists in Canadian Undergraduate Medical Education
Brull R, Bradley JW (Univ of Toronto)
Can J Anesth 48:147-152, 2001   1–6

Background.—Anesthesiologists, with their broad-based knowledge and technical skill, are a significant resource for undergraduate medical education and are well qualified to teach physiology, pharmacology, resuscitation, pain management, perioperative assessment, and technological medicine. Many anesthesiologists are also well suited to teach medical ethics, including consent, allocation of scarce resources, and end-of-life decision making. Anesthesiologists also play a critical role in a variety of hospital settings, including the operating room, postanesthesia care unit,

ICU, preadmission clinic, obstetric ward, and pain clinic, all of which provide excellent teaching environments for problem-based learning (PBL). The recent shift by medical schools in North America to the small-group PBL model has increased the demand for teaching faculty, which presents an ideal opportunity for anesthesiologists to participate in a variety of teaching roles within the reformed undergraduate curricula. The current role of anesthesiologists in undergraduate medical education in Canada was investigated.

Methods.—A questionnaire comprising 93 items was mailed to the undergraduate course chairs/coordinators for anesthesia at all 16 Canadian medical schools.

Results.—Among all faculty anesthesiologists in Canada, 1.7% teach preclerkship lectures, 4.9% teach seminars, and 4.9% teach PBL tutorials. These anesthesiologists teach an average of 3.3 hours of preclerkship lectures and 12.8 hours of preclerkship seminars at each medical school, and the topics most often taught are pharmacology and perioperative patient assessment. Thirteen schools have mandated an anesthesia rotation during clerkship, with an average duration of 9.6 days. There was some variety in the clerkship teaching methods, with 10 schools providing seminars, 8 schools using videos, 6 schools using computers, 6 schools using an airway skills laboratory, and 4 schools using an anesthesia simulator. In the clerkship anesthesia seminars, the most commonly taught subjects are airway management and fluid therapy.

Conclusions.—Very few faculty anesthesiologists in Canada participate in undergraduate medical education at the preclerkship level, and there is a great deal of variation in the amount and the format of teaching in the undergraduate curricula, particularly at the preclerkship level. However, it appears that the anesthesiologists in Canada are taking on a more important role in teaching at the clerkship level. It would appear that either medical schools in Canada are overlooking the potential advantages to undergraduate medical education that anesthesiologists offer at the preclerkship level, or that many anesthesiologists are reluctant to take on teaching responsibilities at this level.

▶ It is interesting that of the 16 medical schools studied, not many afforded huge amounts of time for education to their medical students in their first 2 years. Yet 13 of the 16 had rotations in their third and fourth year. One wishes that more preoperative pain therapy and ICU therapy, as well as pharmacology, were taught by anesthesiologists. Is this a hazard of the private practice model that is used largely in Canadian institutions? Or do I not understand the model?

M. F. Roizen, MD

Preparedness for Clinical Practice: Reports of Graduating Residents at Academic Health Centers

Blumenthal D, Gokhale M, Campbell EG, et al (Harvard Med School, Boston)
JAMA 286:1027-1034, 2001   1–7

Introduction.—There is a need for ongoing monitoring of residents' preparedness for practice at completion of their graduate medical education. A national sample of residents in their final year of education were surveyed to gather benchmark data regarding self-reported preparedness of residents to undertake a wide variety of tasks common to their specialties.

Methods.—A 1998 stratified random sample of residents from 8 specialties (internal medicine, pediatrics, family practice, obstetrics/gynecology, psychiatry, general surgery, orthopedic surgery, and anesthesia) from academic health centers in the United States were assessed. The primary outcome measures were residents' reports of their preparedness to perform clinical and nonclinical tasks relevant to their specialties. There were a total of 2626 respondents (65% response rate).

Results.—Residents in all specialties rated themselves as prepared to manage most of the common conditions they would experience in their clinical career. More than 10% of residents in each specialty reported they felt unprepared to address 1 or more tasks relevant to their disciplines, including caring for patients with human immunodeficiency virus/acquired immunodeficiency syndrome or substance abuse (family practice) or nursing home patients (internal medicine); performance of spinal surgery (orthopedic surgery) or abdominal aortic aneurysm repair (general surgery); and management of chronic pain (anesthesiology).

Conclusion.—Overall, residents in their final year of education at academic health centers rated their clinical preparedness as high. There are opportunities for improvement in preparing residents for clinical practice.

▶ All program directors in anesthesiology continuously update the curriculum for their residents to make sure that residents are prepared to enter either academic or private practice. This survey is a self-assessment by residents on how they feel they were prepared for clinical practice. In anesthesia, more than 90% of anesthesia residents believe themselves prepared to administer regional anesthesia, day surgery anesthesia, complex subspecialty anesthesia and so on, but 32% of anesthesiology residents felt unprepared to manage chronic pain. Academic health centers have worked hard to maintain their educational role in the face of financial and clinical pressure; it appears from this report that they have done a good but not perfect job.

M. Wood, MD, FRCA

A Comparative Study of General Anesthesia, Intravenous Regional Anesthesia, and Axillary Block for Outpatient Hand Surgery: Clinical Outcome and Cost Analysis

Chan VWS, Peng PWH, Kaszas Z, et al (Univ of Toronto)
Anesth Analg 93:1181-1184, 2001   1–8

Background.—These Canadian authors prospectively compared clinical outcomes, time efficiency, and hospital costs associated with 3 means of providing anesthesia for outpatient hand surgery: general anesthesia (GA), IV regional anesthesia (IVRA), and brachial plexus block (BPB).

Methods.—The research subjects were 126 patients undergoing elective outpatient hand surgery. Patients undergoing carpal tunnel release, ganglion excision, or bilateral hand surgery were excluded. The patient decided whether to undergo GA (n = 39; 62% men; mean age, 39 years) or regional anesthesia; for the latter, the anesthesiologist decided whether to use IVRA (n = 45; 58% men; mean age, 39 years) or BPB (n = 42; 69% men; mean age, 41 years). Postoperatively, patients spent a minimum of 30 minutes in the postanesthesia care unit (PACU) and were discharged from the PACU and the day surgery unit (DSU) according to standardized criteria. Demographic and clinical data were recorded in detail, and data regarding the direct expenses incurred by the hospital were obtained.

Results.—The 3 patient groups did not differ significantly in demographics, type of surgery, or operative time. Two patients in the IVRA group and 3 patients in the BPB group had to be converted to GA. The duration of anesthesia was significantly longer in the BPB group, primarily because anesthesia induction took longer in that group than in the GA and BPB groups. Postoperatively, significantly more patients in the GA group required opioid analgesics for pain than in the IVRA or BPB groups (85% vs 51% or 43%). Patients in the GA group were also significantly more likely to experience nausea and vomiting requiring medication (62% vs 18% for IVRA and 12% for BPB). Patients in the IVRA group had the most rapid recovery from anesthesia and the shortest time to discharge from the PACU, the DSU, and the hospital. Accordingly, the total hospital costs were significantly less in the IVRA group than in the GA or BPB groups ($214 vs $300 or $317).

Conclusions.—In patients undergoing outpatient hand surgery, regional anesthesia causes less nausea and vomiting postoperatively than GA and is associated with quicker postanesthesia recovery. IVRA, in particular, was associated with the shortest PACU, DSU, and overall hospital stays and with the lowest direct hospital costs. In some cases, tourniquet pain with IVRA may require switching to GA; the addition of an opioid or nonsteroidal anti-inflammatory drug to the local anesthetic can preempt tourniquet pain.

▶ This is a study of interest to both anesthesiologists and hospital administrators!

M. Wood, MD, FRCA

Mortality Among Patients Admitted to Hospitals on Weekends as Compared With Weekdays

Bell CM, Redelmeier DA (Univ of Toronto)
N Engl J Med 345:663-668, 2001
1–9

Background.—In most acute care hospitals, the level of staffing is lower on weekends than on weekdays. Accordingly, some studies have suggested that in-hospital mortality rates are higher on weekends than on weekdays. Data from all acute care hospitals in Ontario, Canada over a 10-year period were examined to compare mortality rates between patients admitted on weekends and those admitted on weekdays.

Methods.—Between 1988 and 1997, 3,789,917 patients were seen at the emergency department of an acute care hospital in Ontario, Canada and were admitted. Medical records were examined to determine whether they were admitted on a weekend (from midnight Friday to midnight Sunday) or on a weekday and whether the patient died in hospital. Other data collected included age, sex, Charlson score for comorbidity, and diagnosis. Three diagnoses were prespecified as being most likely to accentuate the consequences of lower staffing levels on weekends. These "positive conditions" were ruptured abdominal aortic aneurysm, acute epiglottis, and pulmonary embolism. In addition, 3 diagnoses were prespecified as being unlikely to be associated with differences in mortality rates between weekend and weekday admissions. These "control conditions" were myocardial infarction, acute intracerebral hemorrhage, and acute hip fracture. Finally, the 100 most common causes of death (responsible for 91% of all deaths) were identified, and differences in mortality rates between patients admitted on weekends and those admitted on weekdays were examined.

Results.—For patients with 1 of the 3 positive conditions, mortality rates were significantly higher for those admitted on a weekend than for those admitted on a weekday (Table 2). The differences in mortality rates persisted even after adjustment for age, sex, and comorbidities. For patients with 1 of the 3 control conditions, however, mortality rates did not differ significantly between weekend and weekday admissions. In 23 conditions of the 100 most common causes of death, admission on a weekend was associated with significantly higher mortality rates than admission on a weekday (Table 3). These differences in mortality rates also persisted after adjustment for age, sex, and comorbidities. Conversely, in none of these 100 conditions was a weekend admission associated with significantly lower mortality rates compared with a weekday admission. Median odds ratios for death among patients admitted on a weekend did not differ significantly for men versus women, for teaching versus nonteaching hospitals, for patients who arrived by ambulance versus those who did not, or for patients who underwent surgery versus those who did not.

TABLE 2.—In-Hospital Mortality According to the Day of Admission*

Condition	No. of Admissions	Weekday Admission	Weekend Admission	Odds Ratio (95% CI) Unadjusted	Odds Ratio (95% CI) Adjusted†
		Mortality Rate Percent			
Positive‡					
Ruptured abdominal aortic aneurysm (ICD-9 codes 4413 and 4414)	5,454	36	42§	1.32	1.28 (1.13-1.46)
Acute epiglottitis (ICD-9 code 4643)	1,139	0.3	1.7¶	5.47	5.28 (1.01-27.50)
Pulmonary embolism (ICD-9 code 4151)	11,686	11	13‖	1.25	1.19 (1.03-1.36)
Control∗∗					
Myocardial infarction (ICD-9 code 410)	160,220	15	15	1.02	1.03 (1.00-1.06)
Intracerebral hemorrhage (ICD-9 code 431)	10,987	44	44	1.01	1.01 (0.93-1.11)
Acute hip fracture (ICD-9 code 820)	59,670	7	6	0.95	0.97 (0.90-1.04)

*Odds ratios are for death among patients admitted on a weekend as compared with those admitted on a weekday.
†Adjustment was made for age, sex, and the score on the Charlson comorbidity index.
‡Positive conditions were those hypothesized to be associated with a higher mortality rate among patients admitted on weekends than among those admitted on weekdays.
§$P < .001$ for the comparison with weekday admission.
¶$P = .04$ for the comparison with weekday admission.
‖$P = .009$ for the comparison with weekday admission.
∗∗Control conditions were those hypothesized to be associated with similar mortality rates for weekend and weekday admissions.
Abbreviation: ICD-9, International Classification of Diseases, Ninth Revision.
(Reprinted by permission of *The New England Journal of Medicine,* from Bell CM, Redelmeier DA: Mortality among patients admitted to hospitals on weekends as compared with weekdays. *N Engl J Med* 345:663-668, 2001. Copyright 2001, Massachusetts Medical Society. All rights reserved.)

Conclusions.—In this 10-year study of almost 3.8 million emergency hospital admissions, the risk of in-hospital mortality was significantly higher for patients admitted on a weekend than for those admitted on a weekday. In particular, mortality rates for 3 complex disorders associated with a high mortality rate outside the critical care setting (ie, ruptured abdominal aortic aneurysm, acute epiglottis, and pulmonary embolism) were significantly higher among patients admitted on a weekend. Mortality rates for patients admitted on weekends remained significantly higher even after adjustment for comorbid conditions, which argues against the claim that patients who are admitted on weekends are more sick than those admitted on weekdays. A more likely explanation is that the increased mortality on weekends is related to reduced weekend staffing. Perhaps maintaining a more consistent level of care throughout the week would reduce the mortality rates associated with emergency admission on the weekend.

TABLE 3.—Conditions for Which Weekend Admission Was Associated With Significantly Higher Mortality Than Was Weekday Admission*

Condition	No. of Admissions	Mortality Rate Weekday Admission Percent	Mortality Rate Weekend Admission Percent	Odds Ratio (95% CI)† Unadjusted	Odds Ratio (95% CI)† Adjusted‡
Cancer of the trachea, bronchus, or lung	27,013	44	48	1.18	1.19 (1.12-1.25)
Secondary cancer of the respiratory or digestive tract	13,249	37	39	1.11	1.13 (1.04-1.23)
Chronic ischemic heart disease	52,900	8.7	9.3	1.08	1.06 (0.99-1.14)
Cardiac dysrhythmia	76,907	5.4	6.1	1.14	1.17 (1.09-1.25)
Unspecified condition requiring after care	5,912	43	64	1.36	1.28 (1.12-1.46)
Colon cancer	11,966	25	28	1.19	1.15 (1.04-1.27)
Secondary cancer at other specified sites	12,616	23	26	1.19	1.18 (1.07-1.30)
Aortic aneurysm	7,636	37	43	1.27	1.24 (1.11-1.39)
Pancreatic cancer	5,723	41	44	1.15	1.19 (1.05-1.36)
Breast cancer in women	5,192	39	48	1.47	1.37 (1.19-1.56)
General cardiovascular symptoms	7,074	28	32	1.22	1.35 (1.19-1.54)
Prostate cancer	8,369	22	25	1.25	1.21 (1.06-1.37)
Stomach cancer	4,583	36	41	1.25	1.26 (1.09-1.46)
Cancer of the rectosigmoid or anus	5,018	27	31	1.22	1.23 (1.05-1.43)
Acute pulmonary heart disease	11,920	11	13	1.25	1.20 (1.05-1.38)
Cancer of the brain	5,586	19	24	1.30	1.29 (1.11-1.50)
Cancer of the liver or intrahepatic bile ducts	2,291	45	51	1.31	1.38 (1.13-1.69)
Renal failure	3,339	30	36	1.34	1.31 (1.09-1.58)
Myeloma or immunoproliferative cancer	3,203	25	30	1.26	1.26 (1.04-1.52)
Intracranial hemorrhage (unspecified)	3,525	18	22	1.23	1.21 (0.98-1.48)
Intestinal disorder (unspecified)	10,351	4.8	6.0	1.25	1.28 (1.04-1.56)
Cardiac-conduction disorder	8,081	3.3	5.3	1.63	1.72 (1.33-2.21)
Leukemia (unspecified cell type)	779	33	43	1.52	1.60 (1.11-2.31)

*Conditions are listed in descending order according to the total number of associated deaths. The mortality rates and odds ratios for the entire list of the 100 conditions are available as Supplementary Appendix 1 with the full text of this article at http://www.nejm.org.

†Odds ratios are for death among patients admitted on a weekend as compared with those admitted on a weekday. $P < .05$ for all unadjusted odds ratios.

‡Adjustment was made for age, sex, and the score on the Charlson comorbidity index.

(Reprinted by permission of *The New England Journal of Medicine*, from Bell CM, Redelmeier DA: Mortality among patients admitted to hospitals on weekends as compared with weekdays. *N Engl J Med* 345:663-668, 2001. Copyright 2001, Massachusetts Medical Society. All rights reserved.)

▶ This is an important descriptive study with a finding that clearly requires further work. A large number of patients (ie, 3,789,917 admissions) were analyzed. I selected this article because there are anesthetic implications: specified diseases were studied that are of interest to our specialty because we might be involved in their treatment, namely, acute epiglottitis and acute hip fracture.

M. Wood, MD, FRCA

2 Preoperative Evaluation

Myoclonus Secondary to the Concurrent Use of Trazodone and Fluox-etine

Darko W, Guharoy R, Rose F, et al (Upstate Med Univ, Syracuse, NY)

Vet Hum Toxicol 43:214-215, 2001   2–1

Introduction.—Myoclonus in individuals taking antidepressants has been linked to increased serotonin activity resulting from inhibition of the cytochrome P450 enzyme system. The case of a patient who had myoclonus while receiving therapeutic doses of trazodone and fluoxetine is reported.

> *Case Report.*—A 39-year-old man with a history of HIV infection, depression, and pneumonia had fever, fatigue, and productive yellowish cough for 2 weeks. He was treated with kevofloxacin, lamivudine/zidovudine, dapsone, nevirapine, trimethoprim, and zolpidem and also received trazodone (50 mg daily) 2 months before admission. He had bilateral coarse tremors of both hands that disappeared with rest, pneumocystis carinii pneumonia, and tuberculosis. Zolpidem was replaced with fluoxetine (20 mg daily) 3 days after admission, and the trazodone dose was increased to 100 mg on day 4. His tremors increased, and trazodone and fluoxetine were discontinued on day 10. The tremors disappeared 7 days later.

Discussion.—The myoclonus was dose dependent and associated with the degree of serotonin inhibition. Myoclonus can appear without other signs of toxicity.

Conclusion.—Patients receiving antidepressant medications can have drug-induced myoclonus as a result of increased serotonin activity.

Discontinuation of the Bleeding Time Test Without Detectable Adverse Clinical Impact

Lehman CM, Blaylock RC, Alexander DP, et al (Univ of Utah, Salt Lake City; ARUP Labs Inc, Salt Lake City, Utah)
Clin Chem 47:1204-1211, 2001   2–2

Objective.—Whether bleeding time (BT) tests aid in the diagnosis of platelet dysfunction disorders and predict the risk of abnormal bleeding is unsupported by clinical evidence. Clinical outcomes after discontinuation of the BT test at one tertiary-care university medical center were reported.

Methods.—The BT test was discontinued in January 1999. Platelet transfusions to patients with normal platelet counts, the average number of nonirradiated, nonleukocyte-reduced apheresis and pooled platelet units transfused, and the number of doses of 1-deamino-8-D-arginine vasopressin (DDAVP) administered before and after discontinuation of the BT test were compared.

Results.—The ordering frequency of platelet-aggregation tests was unchanged during the 5 months after the BT test was discontinued. With respect to total platelet-aggregation studies, total patients receiving DDAVP, and uremic patients receiving DDAVP, there was no difference in clinical practice behavior before and after discontinuing the BT test. A before-and-after comparison of renal biopsy patient variables showed no changes. An analysis of patients in the Major Surgery Risk Pool revealed that discontinuation of the BT test did not lead to an increased risk in bleeding complications. There were significantly more biopsies of renal allografts after discontinuation than before discontinuation, and results showed a significantly larger average decrease in hematocrit for allografts versus native kidneys. There was no increase in overall use of DDAVP after discontinuation of the BT test.

Conclusion.—Discontinuation of the BT test did not have any clinically significant, negative effects at this institution.

▶ If the test does not have any benefit, discontinuing its use should not have any adverse effect, and that's what these authors found. It's comforting to know that the analysis of this test showed it to have no benefit beforehand.

M. F. Roizen, MD

The Accuracy of Coagulation Tests During Spinal Fusion and Instrumentation

Horlocker TT, Nuttall GA, Dekutoski MB, et al (Mayo Clinic, Rochester, Minn)
Anesth Analg 93:33-38, 2001   2–3

Objective.—Patients undergoing spinal fusion and instrumentation who require massive transfusion are at increased risk of developing a perioperative coagulopathy caused by dilution of coagulation factors and platelets, fibrinolysis, or both. Although coagulation studies are important for determining which patients are at risk for significant bleeding, the coagulation test values that are normal or abnormal have not been defined for this patient population. The sensitivity, specificity, and accuracy of different coagulation tests were retrospectively evaluated, and the cutoff values were determined for guiding transfusion therapy.

Methods.—Records of 244 patients (43% male), aged 1 to 83 years, who underwent spinal fusion with or without instrumentation between January 1994 and July 1995 were reviewed for preexisting coagulopathy, preoperative administration of anticoagulant medication, chronic steroid use, preoperative hemoglobin levels, results of anticoagulation tests, surgical indication, surgical approach, and number of levels fused. Wilcoxon's ranked sum test was used to determine the correlation between increased surgical bleeding and estimated blood loss, perioperative transfusion requirements, and changes in bleeding parameters. The sensitivity, specificity, and positive and negative predictive values of the international normalized ratio (INR), prothrombin time (PT), and activated partial thromboplastin time (aPTT) were determined with the receiver operating characteristic curve.

Results.—Excessive bleeding during surgery was noted in 39 patients (16.0%) and was more likely to occur in patients with preoperative coagulopathy. Tumor surgery and an increased number of posterior levels fused were associated with excessive bleeding. Preoperative administration of warfarin, heparin, aspirin, or other nonsteroidal anti-inflammatory medications did not increase the risk of excessive bleeding. Patients with increased bleeding had larger blood losses, received significantly more intraoperative autotransfusion and allogenic red blood cells, and required more platelets and fresh frozen plasma intraoperatively and postoperatively. The sensitivities of the INR, PT, and aPTT were 94%, 90%, and 85%, respectively. The respective specificities were 88%, 64%, and 64%. The relative accuracies were 0.9 at a value of 1.4 for INR, 0.73 at a value of 13.5 seconds for PT, and 0.71 at a value of 30.9 seconds for aPTT. Thromboelastogram values were only marginally useful. Age and sex did not predict bleeding.

Conclusion.—INR, PT, and aPTT can be used to distinguish patients at increased risk for bleeding during spinal fusion.

▶ Wow, the INR has a pretty darn good predictive value with a cutoff level of 1.4. It's unusual to see something with a sensitivity (or positivity in disease) of 94% and a specificity (or negativity in health) of 88%. This is pretty darn impressive in deciding whether a patient is going to have excessive bleeding. Of course, one could look in the field. I don't know if that was examined in this study.

M. F. Roizen, MD

An Abnormal Dipyridamole Thallium/Sestamibi Fails to Predict Long-term Cardiac Events in Vascular Surgery Patients

de Virgilio C, Wall DB, Ephraim L, et al (Harbor-UCLA Med Ctr, Torrance, Calif)

Ann Vasc Surg 15:267-271, 2001   2–4

Objective.—The ability of dipyridamole-thallium (DTHAL) and sestamibi (DMIBI) to predict adverse perioperative cardiac events has recently been called into question. There is even less information regarding the long-term predictive value of the test. Whether the DTHAL/DMIBI test could predict adverse cardiac events or mortality on long-term follow-up in moderate-risk patients undergoing elective vascular surgery was prospectively evaluated at a major vascular surgery center.

Methods.—Adverse cardiac events, including myocardial infarction, congestive heart failure, ventricular tachycardia, unstable angina, cardiac arrest, and cardiac death, more than 30 days after major vascular surgery were recorded for 75 patients (average age, 65 years; 76% male) with at least one Eagle clinical risk factor. Patients were followed up for an average of 15.5 months.

Results.—The average number of clinical risk factors was 1.8. There were 35 (47%) patients with a normal DTHAL/DMIBI, 26 (35%) with reversible ischemia, and 14 (18%) with a fixed defect. During follow-up, 12 (16%) patients had adverse cardiac events including 9 patients with congestive heart failure, 2 with unstable angina, and 1 with myocardial infarction. Eight patients (11%) died, 2 from cardiac events. The adverse cardiac event rate was 11.5% for patients with reversible ischemia and 18.4% for other patients (odds ratio, 0.58). The sensitivity, specificity, and positive and negative predictive values for adverse cardiac events in patients with reversible ischemia were 25%, 63%, 12%, and 82%, respectively. The cardiac event rates for patients with and without abnormal DTHAL/DMIBI were similar (17.5% vs 14.3%). The respective overall mortality rates for patients with and without reversible ischemia were 7.7% and 12.2% (odds ratio, 0.60). The respective mortality rates for patients with normal versus abnormal DTHAL/DMIBI results were 11.4% and 10%.

Conclusion.—There is no association between reversible ischemia or DTHAL/DMIBI test results and long-term postoperative cardiac events in patients who have had major vascular surgery.

▶ The controversy over whether to screen and how to screen especially in vascular surgery patients continues. I don't think this study is definitive enough to answer it, but it does make me think that use of these as routine screening tests for vascular surgery might not be wise.

M. F. Roizen, MD

Alcohol Withdrawal After Open Aortic Surgery

Illig KA, Eagleton M, Kaufman D, et al (Univ of Rochester, NY)
Ann Vasc Surg 15:332-337, 2001   2–5

Objective.—Although major surgery can precipitate alcohol withdrawal, there appears to be a particularly high incidence of withdrawal after aortic operations. The incidence and effect of alcohol withdrawal after aortic operations were retrospectively investigated.

Methods.—A chart review of all 75 patients undergoing elective open aortic surgery for repair of abdominal aortic aneurysms (n = 44) or aortoiliac occlusive disease (n = 31) during 1997 identified those with possible alcohol withdrawal–like syndrome (AWLS). AWLS was defined as prolonged agitation or confusion and response to conventional treatment for withdrawal. Patients with AWLS surviving more than 48 hours were compared with patients undergoing carotid endarterectomy (n = 260), lower extremity bypass (n = 128), and total colectomy (n = 50).

Results.—Aortic surgery patients had significantly higher total fluid intake (7643 mL) and blood loss (2475 mL) than all other patients. AWLS was diagnosed in 7 (12%) aortic surgery patients and 1 (2%) total colectomy patient. None of these patients died. Compared with other patients, aortic surgery patients with AWLS had a significantly longer stay in intensive care (13 vs 4 days), more days receiving mechanical ventilation (10 vs 2 days), more days receiving nonoral feedings (11 vs 6 days), and a longer hospital stay (23 vs 10 days). Patients with AWLS tended to have poorer hepatic function than did other patients. The most common symptoms of AWLS were disorientation, anxiety, agitation, and hyperdynamic vital signs that increased on postoperative days 1 to 3 despite withdrawal treatment.

Conclusion.—AWLS is much more common after open aortic surgery than after other types of surgery and significantly increases postoperative hospital stay and morbidity. Better methods of identifying these patients need to be developed.

▶ Is alcohol withdrawal more likely because patients who are having open aortic surgery are more likely to drink, or is it just the longer postoperative period? I think what this study does tell us is that when a patient will require more than 1 day of hospitalizion after surgery, we need to ask about the frequency of alcohol use to be forewarned about the risk of alcohol withdrawal.

M. F. Roizen, MD

Arterial Graft Occlusion After Pelvic Surgery in the Lithotomy Position
Thornton MP, Thornton MR, Hormis AP, et al (Northern Gen Hosp, Sheffield, England)
Eur J Vasc Endovasc Surg 21:564-566, 2001   2–6

Background.—Ischemia of the lower limbs can occur during surgical procedures that require prolonged elevation of the legs and can lead to the development of a compartment syndrome after surgery. Pelvic surgery offers special risks because of the position required and the length of the procedure. A case was reported in which the limb ischemia that occurred was believed to result from a compartment syndrome, but the cause was found to be a crushed iliac stent.

> *Case Study.*—Man, 54, had restorative proctocolectomy for ulcerative colitis. Five years before he had undergone a left-to-right iliofemoral bypass with a polytetrafluoroethylene graft for severe intermittent claudication, and 2 years later he required stenting of a left external iliac artery stenosis to relieve recurrent claudication. The Lloyd-Davies position was assumed for 7 hours during the colorectal surgery, and the patient's feet were cool with absent pulses at the conclusion of the procedure. Based on complaints of severe bilateral calf pain, further examination revealed compartment pressures of 110 mm Hg (left) and 68 mm Hg (right). Ischemia remained after bilateral fasciotomies, so duplex scanning was performed, revealing monophasic flow in both common femoral arteries suggestive of thrombosis of the iliofemoral bypass and the donor left iliac artery. Graft and donor left external iliac artery occlusion was confirmed, and a left axillo-bifemoral bypass with a rifampicin gelatin-soaked graft was performed. Discomfort recurred in 4 weeks, with an inflamed lower abdomen and pyrexia; pus was draining from the left groin wound. Drainage and antibiotic irrigation were carried out, but the graft was infected and had to be removed. In performing vascular reconstruction, the Palmaz stent from the left external iliac artery was noted to be crushed, most probably during the colorectal operation.

Conclusions.—Palmaz stents are not placed in arteries subject to compression, but the risk in pelvic placement is minimal, making this case unusual. These stents are difficult to detect on palpation or during surgery, requiring duplex scanning for proper identification. If stents are suspected because of previous vascular disease, patients who require surgery performed in the lithotomy position should be scanned so care can be taken to protect the stents. In addition, the procedure itself should be kept to the minimum required time.

▶ This is a very interesting case report because it talks about complications of stents that all of us who are involved in positioning patients during anesthesia and surgery should know about.

M. F. Roizen, MD

Preoperative Assessment of Primary Varicose Veins: A Duplex Study of Venous Incompetence
Jutley RS, Cadle I, Cross KS (Aberdeen Royal Infirmary, Scotland)
Eur J Vasc Endovasc Surg 21:370-373, 2001   2–7

Background.—The recurrence rate after surgery for primary uncomplicated varicose veins has been reported to be as high as 65%. In most cases the recurrences are associated with inappropriate or inadequate primary surgery. The preoperative assessment of primary varicose veins has traditionally included a clinical examination with the Trendelenburg test. However, this has been shown to be an unreliable test, with clinical uncertainty rates as high as 40%, depending on which superficial vein is assessed. Clinical accuracy has been improved with the recent introduction of the adjunctive use of continuous-wave hand-held Doppler (HHD) evaluation. However, there are still problems with inaccuracy in the use of HHD because of the inability to identify with confidence the vessel being insonated. The gold standard is color-flow duplex scanning, which in the United Kingdom is reserved for specialist vascular units or for patients in which complex disease, such as recurrence, is suspected. A reduction in recurrence rates for varicose veins would result in major savings for the United Kingdom's National Health Service. The value of preoperative duplex scanning in primary uncomplicated varicose vein surgery was investigated.

Methods.—This was a retrospective study of an existing prospectively collected database of patients seen in a noninvasive vascular laboratory between June 1998 and September 1999 for duplex scanning of primary uncomplicated varicose veins. Vascular laboratory case notes were assessed, and significant anatomic variations that would have been difficult to detect clinically with or without the use of HHD were noted. Correlations with clinical findings were also evaluated.

Results.—A total of 176 patients and 223 limbs were assessed, and 77 limbs (30%) had a competent saphenofemoral junction. Pure saphenofemoral reflux was found in 61 (27%) limbs, and 53 (24%) limbs had significant anatomic variations. Short saphenous vein incompetence was found in 42 (19%) limbs, and 67% of these were not suspected on clinical examination.

Conclusions.—These findings suggest that preoperative duplex scanning is indicated in any patient with uncomplicated primary varicose veins in whom venous surgery is being considered. The use of preoperative duplex scanning in these patients could positively affect recurrence rates and lower costs.

▶ I'm often asked by family and friends to give referrals for varicose vein operations. I have been hesitant to do so because of the high recurrence rates. This study explains why. Unless you perform color-flow duplex scanning, you are unlikely to find the 24% of patients who have significant anatomic variations that are otherwise unknown preoperatively. Thus, the message here is preoperative evaluation with color-flow duplex scanning should be the gold standard for this operation.

M. F. Roizen, MD

Electrocardiographic Exercise Stress Testing for Cardiac Risk Assessment in Patients Undergoing Noncardiac Surgery
Gauss A, Röhm H-J, Schäuffelen A, et al (Univ of Ulm, Germany)
Anesthesiology 94:38-46, 2001   2–8

Background.—Whether exercise ECGs are useful in predicting perioperative cardiac risk is a matter of debate. The predictive value of exercise ECGs, resting ECGs, and clinical variables in predicting perioperative cardiac complications was examined in a prospective study.

Methods.—The subjects were 185 patients (147 men and 38 women; median age, 67 years) undergoing elective noncardiac surgery requiring general anesthesia. All patients were at intermediate risk for cardiac complications because of confirmed or suspected coronary artery disease. Most patients (149, or 81%) were undergoing vascular surgery, while the remainder (36, or 19%) were undergoing abdominal surgery. Resting ECGs were obtained and exercise stress testing was performed at a median of 1 day before surgery.

Ambulatory Holter monitoring was begun before surgery and continued until 2 days after surgery. During surgery, patients were monitored by echocardiography; a 12-lead ECG; and measurements of serum creatinine kinase, creatine kinase isoenzyme MB, cardiac troponin-T, and creatinine levels. ECGs and laboratory measurements were also performed daily for 5 days after surgery. The incidence of cardiac death, myocardial infarction, minor myocardial cell injury, unstable angina pectoris, congestive heart failure, and ventricular tachyarrhythmias during surgery was monitored, and potential risk factors for a perioperative cardiac complication were identified by logistic regression analyses.

Results.—Preoperative ECG results were abnormal in 40 patients (22%), and the preoperative exercise ECG showed ST-segment depression of 0.1 mV or greater in 56 patients (30%). Only 24% of patients achieved 85% of their predicted heart rate. Of the 185 patients, 16 (8.6%) had an intraoperative cardiac complication; 6 had perioperative myocardial infarction and 10 had myocardial cell injury. Multivariate analyses identified the following significant independent predictors of adverse cardiac events:

Preoperative Cardiac Risk Assessment
(n = 185)

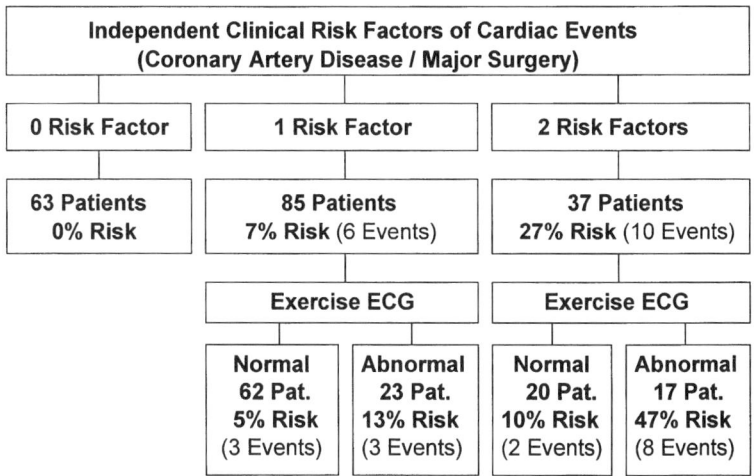

FIGURE 1.—Risk stratification using in retrospect the 2 independent clinical risk factors followed by further differentiation of the findings of the exercise ECG. *Abbreviation: Pat.*, Patients. (Courtesy of Gauss A, Röhm H-J, Schäuffelen A, et al: Electrocardiographic exercise stress testing for cardiac risk assessment in patients undergoing noncardiac surgery. *Anesthesiology* 94:38-46, 2001. Copyright, American Society of Anesthesiologists, Inc. Used with permission of Lippincott-Raven Publishers.)

definite coronary artery disease (odds ratio [OR], 8.8), evidence of ST-segment depression of 0.1 mV or greater on exercise ECG (OR, 5.2), major surgery (OR, 4.7), and reduced left ventricular performance (OR, 2.0). Risk stratification was improved by combining clinical findings and exercise ECG results (Fig 1). Of the 63 patients who had neither major surgery nor vascular surgery, none had a cardiac complication. Of the 85 patients with 1 of the 2 major clinical risk factors, 7% had a cardiac complication. Of the 37 patients who had both major clinical risk factors, 27% had a cardiac complication. Within this last group, the risk of cardiac complications in the 20 patients with normal exercise ECG results was 10%, while that in the 17 patients with abnormal exercise ECG results was 47%.

Conclusion.—In intermediate-risk patients undergoing elective noncardiac surgery, preoperative exercise stress testing that reveals an ST-segment depression of 0.1 mV or greater is an independent predictor of the risk of perioperative cardiac complications. Among patients undergoing major surgery or vascular surgery, preoperative stress testing can further improve risk stratification.

▶ This study is important for anesthesiologists as it looks prospectively at exercise stress testing for high-risk noncardiac surgery. The amazing thing in this study is that these patients were able to undergo exercise stress testing, even though 80% were having anesthesia for vascular surgery. In 39% of patients having a positive stress test as determined by a ST-segment depression of greater than 0.1 mV, surgery was continued. Fourteen patients ended up with a major postoperative coronary event. The authors concluded after demonstrating statistically that the occurrence of a ST-segment depression of 0.1 mV or more in a preoperative exercise stress is a statistically significant independent predictor of preoperative cardiac events. This predictive value occurred even though 76% of the patients were not able to reach 85% of their maximal predicted heart rate and 80% of the patients received vascular surgery.

Perhaps the most interesting analysis of the article shows that you can separate patients by 2 clinical risk factors: (1) Do they have known coronary artery disease? and (2) Are they undergoing vascular surgery? If neither of these applied, they had no coronary disease event risk according to this study. If they had 1 or 2 of these, they were further segregated by exercise ECG. Those with both and positive exercise ECG results had a 47% risk of a major cardiac event afterward. Those with only 1 risk factor had a 13% risk. The 47% and the 13% risks are both more than 2 times higher than the risk of those without changes in their ST-segment on exercise ECG. My take-home from this study: If I were going to undergo vascular surgery and I had not already had an exercise ECG test, I would undergo exercise ECG testing and if results were positive, angiography and stent placement.

M. F. Roizen, MD

Diffuse Brachial Plexopathy After Interscalene Blockade in a Patient Receiving Cisplatin Chemotherapy: The Pharmacologic Double Crush Syndrome
Hebl JR, Horlocker TT, Pritchard DJ (Mayo Clinic and Found, Rochester, Minn)
Anesth Analg 92:249-251, 2001   2–9

Introduction.—Cisplatin, an alkylating chemotherapeutic drug used to treat a variety of cancers, has the potential for toxic side effects including renal dysfunction, acoustic nerve damage, and sensory peripheral neuropathy. Even years after discontinuation of treatment, cisplatin neuropathy is irreversible in a large proportion of patients. No published reports have examined the safety of regional anesthesia in patients exposed to cisplatin. In the case presented here, severe, diffuse brachial plexopathy developed after interscalene blockade in a patient receiving cisplatin therapy.

> *Case Report.*—A girl, 14, with newly diagnosed osteogenic sarcoma, was scheduled for proximal humeral resection and reconstruction. The patient had just completed 15 weeks of a combination chemotherapy regimen that included a cumulative cisplatin dose of 840 mg/m^2. The regimen had not produced cardiac or neurologic toxicities. Surgery was preceded by an interscalene blockade in which bupivacaine 25 mL 0.5% with 1:200,000 epinephrine was injected. All appeared normal until the second post-

operative day when neurologic examination demonstrated severe sensory and motor dysfunction within the ulnar, median, and radial nerve distributions. The patient was unable to flex or extend her fingers or wrist. Electromyography revealed diffuse brachial plexus injury and axonotmesis. Chemotherapy continued postoperatively for an additional 27 weeks. Early signs of partial neurologic recovery were apparent 4 months later, and the patient could flex and extend her fingers and detect light touch. Complete sensory loss, however, persisted within the radial distribution. Eighteen months after surgery there was still distinct weakness within the musculature supplied by the median nerve, and 2-point discrimination was reduced within the ulnar, median, and radial nerve distributions.

Discussion.—Perioperative nerve injuries, long recognized as a complication of regional anesthesia, are associated with needle trauma, local anesthetic toxicity, and other surgical and patient factors. Previous or current cisplatin therapy may also be a contributing factor. In this patient, whose cumulative dose of cisplatin was large, subclinical neuropathy was probably present before regional anesthesia was administered and contributed to a "double crush" syndrome.

▶ Crush syndrome is the application of 1 or more contributing factors to nerve injury such as a metabolic derangement causing a previously dysfunctional but clinically asymptomatic nerve. Cisplatin exposes the patient to a dose-dependent peripheral neuropathy, which generally occurs after a cumulative dose of 300 mg/m². The incidence of peripheral neuropathy approaches 85% in patients receiving doses larger than 300 mg/m². The authors believe that we should not perform peripheral nerve blocks in such patients. Although this is a case report, it has an excellent mechanistic explanation of such injuries.

M. F. Roizen, MD

Outcome of Thoracoabdominal Aortic Operations Using Deep Hypothermia and Distal Exsanguination
Carrel TP, Berdat PA, Robe J, et al (Univ Hosp Berne, Switzerland)
Ann Thorac Surg 69:692-695, 2000   2–10

Introduction.—Significant perioperative morbidity, with ischemic damage of the spinal cord and malperfusion of the abdominal organs, may occur during surgery of the descending and thoracoabdominal aorta. The protective techniques of moderate hypothermic left heart bypass and cardiopulmonary bypass (CPB) using deep hypothermic circulatory arrest were compared in 2 series of patients who underwent an operation between 1982 and 1998.
Methods.—Group 1 included 90 patients with moderate hypothermic left heart bypass and cross-clamped aorta. The 38 group 2 patients un-

derwent deep hypothermic CPB and a period of circulatory arrest during confection of the proximal anastomosis; the distal anastomosis was performed during distal exsanguination and proximal reperfusion. Preoperative demographic and cardiovascular risk factors were similar in groups 1 and 2, except that a higher percentage of group 2 patients had a previous aortic operation and a higher percentage of group 1 had Marfan syndrome.

Results.—Early (30-day) mortality was significantly higher in group 1 (16.6%) than in group 2 (5.2%). Paraplegia occurred in 8 group 1 patients (8.8%), but in only 1 patient from group 2 (2.6%). The 2 groups did not differ in the incidence of significant complications (myocardial infarction, cardiac arrhythmia, pulmonary dysfunction, and renal failure), except that re-exploration for bleeding occurred only in group 1 (11% of patients). Multivariate analysis identified rupture and acute type B dissection as predictors of early mortality in group 1; no predictive factors of adverse outcome were found in group 2.

Discussion.—Spinal cord injury is a devastating complication of operation of the descending and thoracoabdominal aorta. Both mechanical and pharmacologic methods have been used to protect the spinal cord during ischemia. In this series of patients, deep hypothermia combined with distal exsanguination significantly improved outcome after such operations. This technique allowed easy confection of proximal and distal anastomoses without significantly prolonging surgery.

▶ This is a controversial article showing that deep hypothermia and circulatory arrest resulted in a better outcome than did moderate hypothermia and aortic cross-clamp for descending thoracoabdominal aortic reconstruction. Obviously, success is dependent on local factors, and these surgeons must be excellent to accomplish the results they had. I've always thought that many outcome studies (like politics) are local, and surgical skill has been local. But those of us now watching robotic surgery are beginning to question if all surgery is indeed still local. So the question remains, are the results of this study applicable to your institution?

M. F. Roizen, MD

Epidural Analgesia and Arterial Reconstructive Surgery to the Leg: Effects on Fibrinolysis and Platelet Degranulation
Bew SA, Bryant AE, Desborough JP, et al (St George's Hosp Med School, Cranmer Terrace, London; Leeds General Infirmary, England; Epsom Gen Hosp, Surrey, England)
Br J Anaesth 86:230-235, 2001   2–11

Introduction.—Studies of patients undergoing arterial reconstructive surgery to the leg have found that the choice of anesthetic has no influence on overall morbidity or mortality. There is some evidence, however, that epidural analgesia improves the success rate of the graft. Epidural analgesia may prevent the usual cortisol response to surgery, which results in an increase in plasminogen activator inhibitor-1 (PAI-1) and adverse effects on fibrinolysis. This issue was examined in a study of 30 patients scheduled for arterial reconstructive surgery to the leg.

Methods.—Patients were randomized to receive either general anesthesia (GA) or general anesthesia plus epidural analgesia (GAE). Postoperative analgesia was provided by morphine infusion in the GA group and epidural analgesia in the GAE group. Blood samples collected at 0, 2, 4, 6, 12, and 24 hours, and at 2, 3, and 5 days were analyzed for cortisol, PAI-1, interleukin-6 (IL-6), and beta thromboglobulin (βTG, a marker for platelet degranulation). Patients were observed for 30 days for graft-related and systemic complications.

Results.—The GA and GAE groups were comparable in preoperative characteristics, previous vascular surgery, current medication, reason for surgery, type of graft, and duration of surgery. Perioperative management, including fluid preload and intraoperative fluid management, were also similar. Graft-related and systemic complications were uncommon in both GA and GAE groups, and the 2 groups showed no significant changes in cortisol, PAI-1, or βTG. In both groups, IL-6 values increased significantly after 4 hours and remained elevated until day 3.

Conclusion.—The addition of epidural analgesia to general anesthesia in patients undergoing arterial reconstruction to the leg appeared to have no effect on graft-related and systemic complications. No changes in cortisol, PAI-1, IL-6, or βTG were observed.

▶ This study confirms my biases and thus, I love it. I've been fortunate to work at places where the surgeons were so good, and the complication rate was so low after either general or epidural anesthesia that you could not compare outcome in routine aortic reconstruction. We had to use suprarenal aortic reconstruction to find differences. This study reports similar findings, which forces me to conclude (courtesy of Linda Rice, MD) that "great surgery does not require great anesthesia, it just deserves it; whereas, a poor surgeon requires great anesthesia." Is it possible that only when you have poor technical surgery that you will see the benefits of the choice of epidural analgesia to outcome after peripheral vascular reconstruction?

M. F. Roizen, MD

Measuring Patient Satisfaction With Anaesthesia: Perioperative Questionnaire Versus Standardised Face-to-Face Interview
Bauer M, Böhrer H, Aichele G, et al (Univ of Heidelberg, Germany)
Acta Anaesthesiol Scand 45:65-72, 2001   2–12

Background.—Patient satisfaction is an essential component of quality management, and measuring patient satisfaction has become increasingly important in anesthesia. Assessment of patient satisfaction with anesthesia improves the quality of care, improves and strengthens the relationship between the patient and the anesthesiologist, and can be used as a marketing tool in customer orientation. However, adequately determining the level of patient satisfaction can be difficult. A variety of tools, such as postoperative visits and patient questionnaires, may be used to assess patient satisfaction with anesthesia. This study had two aims: (1) to quantify the degree of patient satisfaction with anesthesia and thus allow a comparison with future quality control studies, and (2) to compare the effectiveness of the questionnaire technique with standardized face-to-face interviewing in measuring patient satisfaction.

Methods.—A total of 700 patients were prospectively studied on the second postoperative day, with patients randomly assigned to either complete a written questionnaire or answer the same questions in a face-to-face interview. The questionnaire was divided into parts that investigated anesthesia-related discomfort on a 3-point scale and general satisfaction with anesthesia care on a 4-point scale.

Results.—The response rate was 84%. The most frequent sensations reported in responses to questions on anesthesia-related discomfort were drowsiness (>75%), pain at the surgical site (>55%), and thirst (>50%). Responses to questions regarding overall satisfaction indicated a high degree of satisfaction (>90%). There were only minor differences between the questionnaire and face-to-face interview techniques in responses to questions regarding anesthesia-related discomfort; however, patients in the interviews consistently responded more critically than those who completed questionnaires regarding overall satisfaction with anesthesia.

Conclusions.—Patient satisfaction with anesthesia may be more accurately assessed with the standardized interview than with the questionnaire. Areas in which quality improvements are possible include emergence from anesthesia, postoperative pain therapy, and the treatment of postoperative nausea and vomiting.

▶ For those of us who are concerned with truth and true criticism, the standardized interview may be better than the questionnaire for assessing patient satisfaction. Those who want good satisfaction ratings will use a check-off questionnaire. This is an eye-opening study and a very clever one as well.

M. F. Roizen, MD

Preoperative Treatment With Recombinant Human Growth Hormone Prevents Ischemia Reperfusion-Induced Diaphragmatic Dysfunction
Moneley D, Barry MC, McLaughlin R, et al (Royal College of Surgeons, Dublin; Beaumont Hosp, Dublin)
J Surg Res 97:81-84, 2001   2–13

Background.—The primary source of morbidity and mortality after elective aortic surgery is cardiovascular complications. Thus far, research has focused on lung parenchymal damage after reperfusion injury, but injury to the mechanical ventilatory mechanism may also have a role in respiratory dysfunction. In previous studies it was demonstrated that systemic ischemia reperfusion (IR) injury produces respiratory muscle dysfunction at 24 and 48 hours, a finding that has been confirmed in clinical studies of patients undergoing elective abdominal aortic surgery. In these patients, preoperative treatment with recombinant human growth hormone (rhGH) prevented the expected deterioration in postoperative respiratory dysfunction. The effects of aortic clamping and revascularization on diaphragmatic muscle function in a small animal model and the role of preoperative treatment with rhGH in the prevention of diaphragmatic muscle dysfunction were investigated.

Methods.—A total of 18 male Sprague-Dawley rats were randomly assigned to 3 groups. A control group underwent laparotomy only. The IR group underwent laparotomy with infrarenal cross-clamping for 30 minutes followed by revascularization of the lower torso for 2 hours. The IR + rhGH group was treated with rhGH for 5 days before laparotomy and aortic cross-clamping followed by lower torso revascularization for 2 hours. Diaphragmatic function was assessed in all rats ex vivo with electrical field stimulation in a tissue bath.

Results.—A significant impairment of diaphragmatic twitch was evident 2 hours after IR injury (control, 242.01 + 38.45 g; IR, 108.55 + 7.15 g). Pretreatment with rhGH prevented this impairment. IR injury also significantly impaired tetanic function, and this impairment was also prevented by pretreatment with rhGH.

Conclusions.—These findings suggest a role for the preoperative administration of rhGH in the prevention of the impairment of diaphragmatic function associated with infrarenal aortic cross-clamping and revascularization.

▶ Don't get excited yet, but maybe we have found a use for rhGH in adults. rhGH does not delay aging, increase libido, or open blocked arteries; if anything, it increases risk of tumor growth. But in this study of rats rhGH did a remarkable thing: it reversed diaphragmatic dysfunction. The authors state that this study was stimulated after they noticed rhGH did so in human beings undergoing abdominal aneurysm repair, and it possibly did so because if its anabolic effects. Is this a new and great use for rhGH? Only time will tell, but these are very impressive data.

M. F. Roizen, MD

The Prevalence and Predictors of the Use of Alternative Medicine in Presurgical Patients in Five California Hospitals

Leung JM, Dzankic S, Manku K, et al (Univ of California, San Francisco; John Muir Med Ctr, Walnut Creek, Calif; Kaiser Permanente Med Ctr, San Francisco; et al)
Anesth Analg 93:1062-1068, 2001   2–14

Background.—The popularity and use of over-the-counter alternative medicines, such as herbal medicine, has been increasing in recent years. Many consumers in the United States are seeking greater autonomy in the management of a variety of health issues, including the management or prevention of chronic disease, enhancing overall well-being and cognitive function, and increasing longevity. Unlike prescription medication, herbal medicines and other dietary supplements are not subject to the rigorous premarketing testing of safety and efficacy. Thus, the mechanisms of action, toxicity, dose-response relationship, and potential drug interactions for these alternative medicines may not be known. The prevalence of the use of alternative medicines in the United States is unknown but is thought to be widespread. The prevalence and predictors of the use of alternative medicine supplements were measured in presurgical patients in 5 hospitals in California.

Methods.—Use of these supplements was measured through a self-administered questionnaire in a total of 2560 patients aged 18 years or older. All the patients were awaiting elective noncardiac surgery at 5 hospitals in the San Francisco area.

Results.—The use of alternative medicines was acknowledged by slightly more than 39% of these patients, with herbal medicines being the most frequently used type of alternative supplement (67%). Among patients who used alternative medicine supplements, 44% did not consult their primary physician regarding the use of these products, and 56% did not inform their anesthesiologists before surgery about their use of alternative medicines. On multivariable logistic regression, the variables associated with the preoperative use of herbal medicine included female gender, age from 35 to 49 years, higher income levels, white race, higher education level, sleep problems, the presence of joint or back pain, the presence of allergies, a history of addiction, and a history of general surgery. However, patients with a history of diabetes mellitus and those with a history of use of antithrombotic medications were less likely to use herbal medicines.

Conclusions.—The use of alternative medicine supplements, particularly herbal medicines, is widespread among surgical patients. The documentation of the use of these products in patients is critical to determining potential drug or anesthesia interactions during surgery.

▶ This is an interesting study that highlights the increased use of alternative medicine supplements by patients who undergo surgery. Although a large percentage of alternative medicine products includes vitamins and minerals, other products are common. Anesthesiologists should be on their guard to ask about use of these products; there is a potential for drug interactions during the perioperative period.

M. Wood, MD, FRCA

Usefulness of Transthoracic Echocardiography as a Tool for Risk Stratification of Patients Undergoing Major Noncardiac Surgery
Rohde LE, Polanczyk CA, Goldman L, et al (Partners Community HealthCare Inc, Boston; Harvard Med School, Boston; Univ of California, San Francisco)
Am J Cardiol 87:505-509, 2001   2–15

Background.—In patients undergoing noncardiac surgery, the most common causes of death are cardiovascular complications. Although multivariable indices for predicting the risk of major cardiac complications have been developed based on clinical data and have been validated, many clinicians perform noninvasive cardiac tests, including echocardiography, to refine clinical assessments of risk. In previous studies, the prognostic significance of left ventricular (LV) function at rest and hypertrophy before noncardiac surgery has been studied, but it is unclear whether these tests augment the information available from routine clinical evaluation. Transthoracic echocardiography (TTE) is frequently performed before noncardiac surgery, but it is not clear whether TTE is sufficiently predictive of perioperative cardiac complications. The incremental information provided by TTE was evaluated after consideration of clinical data for prediction of cardiac complications after noncardiac surgery.

Methods.—A total of 570 patients who were evaluated with TTE before undergoing major noncardiac surgery at a university hospital were studied. Preoperative clinical data and clinical outcomes were prospectively collected according to a structured protocol. The TTE data included LV function, hypertrophy indices, and Doppler measurements.

Results.—Univariate analyses identified an association of preoperative systolic dysfunction with postoperative myocardial infarction, cardiogenic pulmonary edema, and major cardiac complications. Moderate-to-severe hypertrophy of the LV, moderate-to-severe mitral regurgitation, and an increased aortic valve gradient were also found to be associated with major cardiac events. Logistic regression analysis demonstrated that models with echocardiographic variables were significantly more effective in predicting major cardiac complications compared with models that included only clinical variables. Significant information was obtained from echocardiographic data in patients who were at increased risk for cardiac complications according to clinical criteria, but this was not the case in otherwise low-risk patients.

Conclusions.—In selected patients, the use of preoperative TTE before noncardiac surgery can provide important independent data regarding the risk of postoperative cardiac complications.

▶ TTE is increasingly used as a preoperative test by cardiologists, especially in high-risk patients, and cardiac catheterization is being used to a much lesser extent. The information can be helpful to anesthesiologists in predicting which patients may be at risk for cardiac events and providing a logical basis to predict ICU utilization.

M. Wood, MD, FRCA

3 Anesthesia-Related Pharmacology and Toxicology

The Effect of Ketorolac and Sevoflurane Anesthesia on Renal Glomerular and Tubular Function

Laisalmi M, Teppo A-M, Koivusalo A-M, et al (Helsinki Univ Central Hosp)

Anesth Analg 93:1210-1213, 2001   3–1

Background.—Ketorolac, a nonsteroidal anti-inflammatory drug, impairs renal blood flow. Ketorolac acts by nonselectively inhibiting the function of cyclooxygenase enzymes and the synthesis of renal vasodilating postaglandins. Serum inorganic fluoride released during the metabolism of sevoflurane may be increased to levels associated with nephrotoxicity, and there have been reports of renal tubular dysfunction in patients anesthetized with sevoflurane. In a previous study, the authors assessed the renal effects of sevoflurane anesthesia and ketorolac by using conventional measures of renal function. In this study, they assessed the renal effects of this combination by using new, more sensitive markers of renal glomerular and tubular function.

Methods.—The double-blinded, placebo-controlled study enrolled 30 women who were American Society of Anesthesiologists physical status I and II and undergoing elective breast surgery. The women were assigned to receive either ketorolac 30 mg (ketorolac group) or saline (control) at premedication, at the end of anesthesia, and 6 hours after anesthesia maintained with sevoflurane.

Results.—The ketorolac group had peak levels of serum fluoride of 30.1 $\mu mol/L$ at 2 hours after the end of anesthesia, compared with 33.3 $\mu mol/L$ in the control group. Urine α_1-microglobulin indexed to urine creatinine was increased from 2 hours after induction of anesthesia to the first postoperative day in the ketorolac group but not in the control group. In both groups, urine glutathione-S-transferase (GST)-α indexed to urine creatinine (GST-α/creatinine) and GST-π/creatinine were increased at 2 hours after anesthesia and then returned to baseline values. No changes were noted between the groups in serum cystatin C and urine kallikrein or urine output per hour.

Conclusions.—The perioperative administration of ketorolac did not produce glomerular or tubular dysfunction in healthy, well-hydrated patients who were anesthetized with sevoflurane.

▶ It is well recognized that ketorolac can inhibit the synthesis of prostaglandins responsible for renovasodilation, and in some cases impair renal blood flow with deleterious effects. Such toxicity in the perioperative setting might be of concern if sevoflurane was also administered. This randomized, controlled trial used biochemical-sensitive markers of renal glomerular and tubular function. However, it should be pointed out that the clinical relevance of these markers is unknown. In any event, ketorolac, when administered to patients who receive appropriate volume hydration and are anesthetized with sevoflurane, does not appear to produce renal glomerular or tubular dysfunction.

M. Wood, MD, FRCA

The Pharmacokinetics of Dexmedetomidine in Volunteers With Severe Renal Impairment
De Wolf AM, Fragen RJ, Avram MJ, et al (Northwestern Univ, Chicago)
Anesth Analg 93:1205-1209, 2001   3–2

Background.—Dexmedetomidine, a selective α_2-adrenergic agonist, has sedative and analgesic properties, and its use reduces anesthetic requirements. Dexmedetomidine is cleared primarily by hepatic metabolism; little renal clearance occurs in healthy individuals. Whether the drug's pharmacokinetics would change in patients with severe renal impairment was investigated.

Methods.—The research subjects were 5 adults with severe renal disease (24-hour creatinine clearance <30 mL/min; 4 men and 1 woman; mean age, 49 years) and 5 control subjects with normal renal functioning matched for age, sex, weight, and smoking status. For 2 weeks before the study, research subjects stopped taking any medications that could interfere with the study's results. After an overnight fast, research subjects reported to the clinic in the morning, and baseline vital signs and venous blood samples were obtained. Then, all research subjects received an infusion of 0.6 µg/kg dexmedetomidine over 10 minutes. Venous blood samples were drawn at regular times up to 12 hours after the infusion and were assayed for plasma dexmedetomidine. Concentration versus time data were examined via a 2-compartment pharmacokinetic model. In addition, patients estimated the degree of sedation at various times before, during, and after the dexmedetomidine infusion via a 100-mm visual analog scale.

Results.—The dexmedetomidine plasma concentration–time relationship was similar in the patients and in the control subjects. The only pharmacokinetic variable that differed significantly between the 2 groups was the elimination half-life: it was significantly shorter in the patients than in the control subjects (113.4 vs 136.5 min, respectively). The safety profile of dexmedetomidine was similar in both patients and control subjects: the hemodynamic and respiratory responses were similar in the 2 groups, and no patient experienced an adverse event. Sedation scores were also similar between the 2 groups, except that sedation was significantly prolonged in the patients (mean VAS score at 1 hour, 49.2 vs 26.2).

Conclusions.—Dexmedetomidine pharmacokinetics in patients with severe renal disease are only slightly different from those in healthy control subjects. The only pharmacokinetic variable that differed significantly between the 2 groups was the elimination half-life, which was shorter in the patients. Patients also had a longer duration of sedation, possibly because of lower plasma protein binding. Thus, to avoid excessive sedation, the dexmedetomidine dose should be reduced in patients with severe renal disease.

▶ Dexmedetomidine is a selective α_2-adrenergic agonist that is increasingly being used in the ICU for postoperative sedation. The use of this drug in high-risk patients or in those with concomitant disease requires further definition. This study describes the disposition of dexmedetomidine in volunteers with severe renal disease. Marked differences in kinetics were not noted; however, the patients with renal disease seemed to be sedated for a longer period of time. This has been attributed to changes in protein binding.

M. Wood, MD, FRCA

Pharmacokinetics and Metabolism of Intravenous Midazolam in Preterm Infants
de Wildt SN, Kearns GL, Hop WCJ, et al (Erasmus Med Ctr Rotterdam, The Netherlands; Univ of Missouri, Kansas City; Purdue Univ, West Lafayette, Ind; et al)
Clin Pharmacol Ther 70:525-531, 2001   3–3

Background.—Midazolam, a benzodiazepine, is finding expanded use in neonatal intensive care units. We studied the pharmacokinetics and metabolism of midazolam after a single intravenous dose in preterm infants.

Methods.—The pharmacokinetics of midazolam and its hydroxylated metabolite (1-OH-midazolam) after a single 0.1 mg/kg intravenous dose of midazolam were determined in 24 preterm infants (gestational age, 26-34 weeks; postnatal age, 3-11 days) (Fig 1). Blood samples were obtained before drug administration and at 0.5, 1, 2, 4, 6, 12, and 24 hours after the start of the infusion. Midazolam and 1-OH-midazolam concentrations were determined by use of gas chromatography–mass spectrometry.

Results.—Total body clearance, apparent volume of distribution, and plasma half-life of midazolam were (median [range]): 1.8 (0.7-6.7) ml/kg

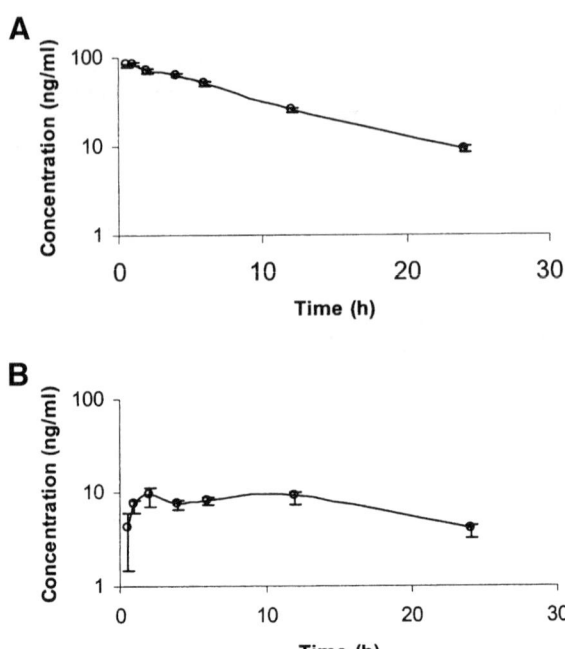

FIGURE 1.—Intravenous midazolam (**A**) and 1-OH-midazolam; (**B**) disposition in preterm infants. Midazolam (n = 24) and 1-OH-midazolam (n = 13) concentration vs time log curve after a single intravenous dose (0.1 mg/kg) to preterm infants. Each *dot* represents mean ± SEM concentration. (Courtesy of de Wildt SN, Kearns GL, Hop WCJ, et al: Pharmacokinetics and metabolism of intravenous midazolam in preterm infants. *Clin Pharmacol Ther* 70:525-531, 2001.)

per minute, 1.1 (0.4-4.2) L/kg, and 6.3 (2.6-17.7) hours, respectively. In 19 of 24 preterm infants, 1-OH-midazolam concentrations could be detected: 1-OH-midazolam (1-OH-M) maximal concentration of drug in plasma (C_{max}), time to reach C_{max} (T_{max}), and 1-OH-M/M area under the concentration-time curve from time zero to the last sampling time point (AUC_{0-t}) ratio were [median (range)]: 8.2 (<0.5-68.2) ng/ml, 6 (1-12) hours, and 0.09 (<0.001-1), respectively. Midazolam plasma clearance was increased in those infants who had indomethacin (INN, indometacin) exposure (Fig 2).

Discussion.—Consequent to immature hepatic cytochrome P450 3A4 (CYP3A4) activity, midazolam clearance and 1-OH-midazolam concentrations are reduced markedly in preterm infants as compared to concentrations in previous reports from studies in older children and adults. Indomethacin exposure and its apparent impact on midazolam clearance support alteration of drug disposition produced by a patent ductus arteriosus or by the direct effects of indomethacin on hemodynamic or renal function.

▶ Neonates in the ICU are increasingly receiving midazolam and fentanyl to provide sedation if they require mechanical ventilation or are to undergo

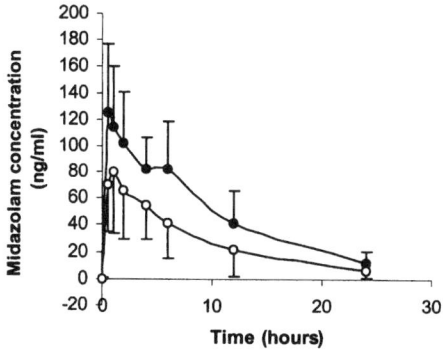

FIGURE 2.—Effect of postnatal indomethacin exposure on midazolam disposition in preterm infants. Midazolam concentration vs time curve after single intravenous dose (0.1 mg/kg) to preterm infants with (n = 11, *open circles*) and without (n = 13, *solid circles*) postnatal indomethacin exposure. Each *dot* represents mean ± SD concentration at each time point. (Courtesy of de Wildt SN, Kearns GL, Hop WCJ, et al: Pharmacokinetics and metabolism of intravenous midazolam in preterm infants. *Clin Pharmacol Ther* 70:525-531, 2001.)

painful invasive procedures. While many believe that the increased use of sedation for small infants in the ICU is an advance, the variability of the pharmacokinetics of midazolam in this group of patients is great. This is an important and detailed study that will allow the more rational administration of drug doses in these small infants.

M. Wood, MD, FRCA

Selective Postoperative Inhibition of Gastrointestinal Opioid Receptors

Taguchi A, Sharma N, Saleem RM, et al (Washington Univ, St Louis; Univ of Louisville, Ky; Univ of Vienna; et al)
N Engl J Med 345:935-940, 2001   3–4

Background.—Almost all patients who undergo major abdominal surgery have transient impairment of bowel motility. Postoperative ileus delays the return of normal gastrointestinal function and the resumption of oral intake, both of which are significant predictors of the length of hospitalization. Opioids taken to control postoperative pain contribute to the delayed recovery of gastrointestinal function. Whether the investigational drug ADL 8-2698 (Adolor, Exton, Pa), a selective opioid antagonist with little oral absorption that does not readily cross the blood–brain barrier, would reduce the severity of ileus after major abdominal surgery was examined.

Methods.—The research subjects were 78 patients undergoing partial colectomy (n = 15) or total abdominal hysterectomy (n = 63). None of the patients had taken corticosteroids or immunosuppressive drugs for 2 weeks or longer before surgery, and none had taken opioid analgesics for 4 weeks or longer before surgery. Two hours before surgery, patients were randomly assigned in equal numbers (26 per group) to receive 1 capsule containing either 1 mg ADL 8-2698 (88% women; mean age, 56 years), 6

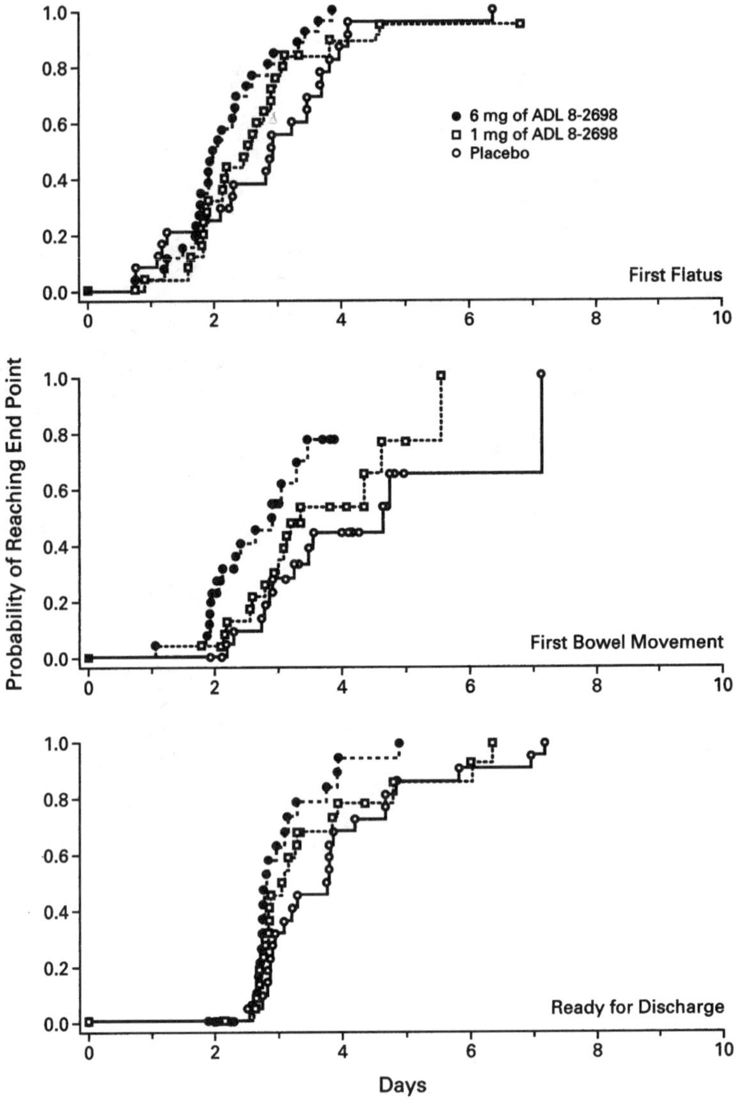

FIGURE 1.—Kaplan-Meier estimates of the primary efficacy outcomes of time to the first passage of flatus, time to the first bowel movement, and time until the patient was ready for discharge. (Reprinted by permission of *The New England Journal of Medicine*, from Taguchi A, Sharma N, Saleem RM, et al: Selective postoperative inhibition of gastrointestinal opioid receptors. *N Engl J Med* 345:935-940, 2001. Copyright 2001, Massachusetts Medical Society. All rights reserved.)

TABLE 3.—Proportional Hazards for the Primary and Secondary Outcomes for Each Treatment Group Adjusted for Type of Surgery*

Outcome	1 mg of ADL 8-2698 vs. Placebo		6 mg of ADL 8-2698 vs. Placebo		6 mg of ADL 8-2698 vs. 1 mg of ADL 8-2698		Overall P Value
	Risk Ratio (95% CI)	P Value	Risk Ratio (95% CI)	P Value	Risk Ratio (95% CI)	P Value	
Time to passage of first flatus	1.2 (0.6-2.2)	0.59	2.5 (1.4-4.7)	0.004	2.1 (1.2-3.9)	0.02	0.007
Time to first bowel movement	1.2 (0.5-2.6)	0.69	2.9 (1.3-6.6)	0.01	2.5 (1.1-5.3)	0.02	0.02
Time to first liquids	1.5 (0.8-2.6)	0.21	1.9 (1.0-3.4)	0.04	1.3 (0.7-2.3)	0.39	0.11
Time to first solids	1.3 (0.7-2.5)	0.38	3.7 (2.0-7.2)	<0.001	2.8 (1.5-5.3)	0.001	<0.001
Time until ready for discharge	1.2 (0.6-2.2)	0.48	2.4 (1.3-4.7)	0.003	2.0 (1.0-4.9)	0.04	0.008
Time until actual discharge	1.4 (0.8-2.6)	0.24	4.3 (2.2-8.2)	<0.001	3.0 (1.7-5.4)	<0.001	<0.001

Note: P values are for the comparison between the specified groups.
*There were 26 patients in each group.
(Reprinted by permission of *The New England Journal of Medicine*, from Taguchi A, Sharma N, Saleem RM, et al: Selective postoperative inhibition of gastrointestinal opioid receptors. *N Engl J Med* 345:935-940, 2001. Copyright 2001, Massachusetts Medical Society. All rights reserved.)

mg ADL 8-2698 (92% women; mean age, 49 years), or placebo (88% women; mean age, 56 years). Patients continued taking a capsule twice a day until the first bowel movement occurred or until discharge from the hospital. All patients received postoperative opioids for pain relief, but none received nonsteroidal anti-inflammatory drugs. Primary outcomes (ie, time to first passage of flatus, time to first bowel movement, and time until ready for hospital discharge) and secondary outcomes (ie, times to first ingestion of liquids and first ingestion of solids, time to actual hospital discharge, and nausea, cramping, itching, and pain scores) were compared between the 3 groups.

Results.—Patients receiving 1 mg ADL 8-2698 had better outcomes than did the placebo group, but between-group differences were not significant. However, compared with the placebo group, patients receiving 6 mg ADL 8-2698 had significantly faster recovery of GI function (Fig 1). This included a significantly shorter median time to the first passage of flatus (49 vs 70 hours), time to the first bowel movement (70 vs 111 hours), and time until the patient was ready for discharge (68 vs 91 hours). The ingestion of first solids and actual hospital discharge also occurred significantly sooner in the 6-mg group. Cumulative morphine sulfate doses and maximal pain, itching, and abdominal cramping scores were similar among the 3 groups. Maximal nausea scores, however, were significantly better in the 6-mg group than in the 1-mg ADL 8-2698 or the placebo groups (mean scores, 18 vs 38; 38 on a 100-point visual analog scale), and none of the patients receiving the 6-mg dose experienced vomiting, compared with about 25% of patients in each of the other 2 groups. The superior efficacy of the 6-mg dose over the 1-mg dose and placebo was still evident after correcting for the type of surgery (Table 3).

Conclusions.—A 6-mg dose of ADL 8-2698 antagonized the activation of GI opioid receptors after major abdominal surgery without inhibiting the analgesic effects of opioids. Recovery of bowel function and a return to solid foods were faster with the 6-mg dose, and the duration of hospitalization was shorter. Furthermore, 6 mg ADL 8-2698 was associated with less nausea and vomiting than in the other 2 groups. Whether the drug would be as efficacious in patients undergoing other types of surgery or in patients treated with epidurally administered local anesthetics remains to be determined.

▶ This study demonstrated the effects of a novel opioid antagonist on postoperative gastrointestinal function and length of hospitalization. The article is also accompanied by an interesting editorial.[1]

M. Wood, MD, FRCA

Reference

1. Steinbrook RA: An opioid antagonist for postoperative ileus (editorial). *N Engl J Med* 345:988-989, 2001.

S(+)-Ketamine for Rectal Premedication in Children
Marhofer P, Freitag H, Höchtl A, et al (Univ of Vienna)
Anesth Analg 92:62-65, 2001   3–5

Background.—Children about to undergo anesthesia are often premedicated to reduce preoperative stress and facilitate induction of inhaled anesthesia. Rectal administration of drugs is a mode of premedication that may be better tolerated by children than other routes. Midazolam is the drug used most often for the premedication of infants and children. Midazolam provides good sedation, anxiolytic and amnestic effects, and fewer side effects. However, the coadministration of racemic ketamine for rectal premedication in children has been described as more effective than midazolam alone for preoperative sedation and anxiolytic potencies. In Europe, racemic ketamine is being replaced by its enantiomer S(+)-ketamine, which has double anesthetic effects in comparison with racemic ketamine. Among the other advantages of S(+)-ketamine in comparison with racemic ketamine are fewer psychomimetic side effects, less salivation, and less loading of substance. The efficacies of rectally administered S(+)-ketamine with and without midazolam, and midazolam alone for premedication in children were compared.

Methods.—A total of 62 children with American Society of Anesthesiologists physical status I and II undergoing elective surgery were studied. The children weighed from 3 to 20 kg. Children in group S (n = 20) were rectally premedicated with 1.5 mg/kg preservative-free S(+)-ketamine. Children in group S/M (n = 22) were rectally premedicated with a combination of 0.75 mg/kg preservative-free S(+)-ketamine and 0.75 mg/kg midazolam. Children in group M (n = 20) were rectally premedicated with

0.75 mg/kg midazolam. Preoperative efficacy of anesthesia was assessed during a period of 20 minutes by means of a 5-point scale ranging from awake (1) to asleep (5). A 4-point scale was used to grade tolerance during anesthesia induction from very good (1) to bad (4).

Results.—A sufficient level of anesthesia was obtained in 86% of children rectally premedicated with midazolam/S(+)-ketamine, compared with 75% of children in the midazolam-only group and 30% in the S(+)-ketamine group. Side effects were rare. The mask acceptance scores were comparable for all 3 groups, but there was a 25% rate of complications during anesthesia induction via face mask in the S(+)-ketamine group.

Conclusions.—S(+)-ketamine, 1.5 mg/kg for rectal premedication in children, provides a poor anesthetic effect and a frequent incidence of side effects during induction of anesthesia via face mask compared with a combination of midazolam/S(+)-ketamine and midazolam alone.

S(+)-Ketamine Increases Muscle Sympathetic Activity and Maintains the Neural Response to Hypotensive Challenges in Humans
Kienbaum P, Heuter T, Pavlakovic G, et al (Universität GH Essen, Germany)
Anesthesiology 94:252-258, 2001   3–6

Background.—The S(+)-isomer of ketamine has recently been approved for clinical use in Europe. Significant pharmacokinetic differences between the isomers were not observed, but S(+)-ketamine was found to exert analgesic and hypnotic effects that were double those observed in the racemic mixture. In addition, nearly every study to date has reported shorter recovery times from anesthesia when the S(+)-isomer is used. It does not appear that the increase in catecholamine plasma concentrations and the cardiovascular response pattern observed in response to S(+)-ketamine differ from those reported in response to the racemic mixture; however, experiments in animal models suggest that the S(+)-isomer inhibits both neuronal and extraneuronal uptake of catecholamines, whereas the R(−)-isomer does not alter extraneural uptake. The hypothesis that S(+)-ketamine alters muscle sympathetic activity (MSA) and muscle sympathetic response to a hypotensive challenge was tested.

Methods.—Microneurography was used to record MSA in the peroneal nerve of 6 healthy volunteers before and during anesthesia with S(+)-ketamine (670 µg/kg intravenously followed by 15 µg · kg^{-1} · min^{-1}). Catecholamine and ketamine plasma concentrations, heart rate, and arterial blood pressure were measured. MSA responses to a hypotensive challenge were assessed by the injection of sodium nitroprusside before and during anesthesia with S(+)-ketamine. The increased arterial pressure observed during anesthesia with S(+)-ketamine was then adjusted to preanesthetic values with infusion of sodium nitroprusside.

Results.—There was a significant increase in MSA burst frequency and incidence with anesthesia with S(+)-ketamine. Anesthesia with S(+)-ketamine was also associated with a 2-fold increase in the plasma concentration of norepinephrine, which paralleled the increase in MSA. Significant increases in heart rate and arterial blood pressure were also noted. When the increased arterial pressure prompted by S(+)-ketamine was decreased to awake values with sodium nitroprusside, further increases in MSA were noted. Throughout anesthesia with S(+)-ketamine, the increased response of MSA to hypotensive challenge was fully maintained.

Conclusions.—Efferent sympathetic outflow to muscle is increased by S(+)-ketamine, and the increase in MSA is maintained in response to arterial hypotension despite increased MSA and arterial pressure during S(+)-ketamine anesthesia.

▶ I selected these 2 articles to alert anesthesiologists that racemic ketamine may be replaced by a single enantiomer S(+)-ketamine, with, we hope, fewer side effects.

M. Wood, MD, FRCA

Gender Differences in the Pharmacokinetics of Propofol in Elderly Patients During and After Continuous Infusion
Vuyk J, Oostwouder CJ, Vletter AA, et al (Leiden Univ, The Netherlands)
Br J Anaesth 86:183-188, 2001   3–7

Background.—The changes that accompany aging can affect men and women differently. Among the areas involved are the pharmacodynamics of anesthetic agents. As more elderly patients undergo surgery and are exposed to anesthesia, specifically propofol, the dosing regimen requires refinement to account for the effects of aging. Male and female elderly patients were given total intravenous anesthesia for general surgery and the concentration-time relationship of propofol during and after termination of the continuous infusion was assessed.

TABLE 2.—The Accuracy (Median Performance Error; MDPE) and Precision (Median Absolute Performance Error; MDAPE) and Interquartile Ranges of the Measured Versus Predicted Propofol Concentrations on the Basis of the Complex Pharmacokinetic Parameter Set of This Study and on the Basis of Those Predicted With the Use of the Pharmacokinetic Parameter Sets by Dyck and Shafer, Schnider and Colleagues and Schüttler and Colleagues

	MDPE (25-75%)	MDAPE (25-75%)
This study	1 (−5 to 13%)	18 (14-22%)
Dyck and Shafer	18 (−5 to 26%)	33 (29-37%)
Schnider and colleagues	20 (9-33%)	27 (20-35%)
Schüttler and colleagues	−38 (−53 to −29%)	40 (32-53%)

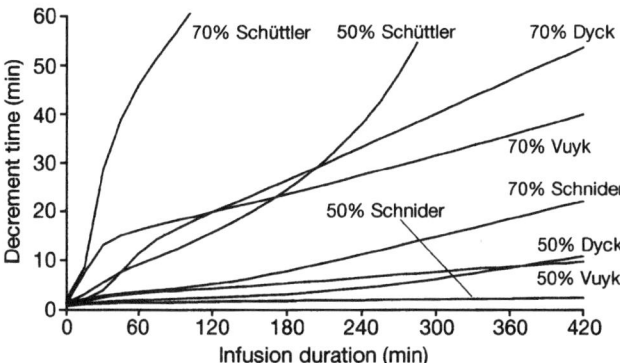

FIGURE 4.—Fifty percent and 70% decrement times (*DT*) versus infusion duration, based on the pharmacokinetic parameter sets determined by Dyck and Shafer, Schnider and colleagues, Schüttler and Ihmsen and in this study. Fifty percent and 70% decrement times are defined as the times required for the propofol concentration to drop by 50% or 70% after termination of a target controlled infusion that had been given with a constant target concentration for a given infusion duration. (Courtesy of Vuyk J, Oostwouder CJ, Vletter AA, et al: Gender differences in the pharmacokinetics of propofol in elderly patients during and after continuous infusion. *Br J Anaesth* 86:183-188, 2001. Copyright, The Board of Management and Trustees of the *British Journal of Anaesthesia*. Reproduced by permission of Oxford University Press/*British Journal of Anaesthesia*.)

Methods.—Thirty-one ASA class 1 and 2 patients who ranged in age from 65 to 91 years were assessed. Propofol 1.5 mg/kg was given intravenously over 1 minute, then 7 mg/kg/h was administered until skin closure. Alfentanil was infused at a variable rate during oxygen-air ventilation. Arterial blood samples (total 932) were obtained up to 24 hours after beginning surgery, and propofol's pharmacokinetics were assessed in 2 stages.

Results.—The patient's gender significantly influenced propofol's pharmacokinetics. Significant differences were found between men and women with respect to slow peripheral volume of distribution (V_3), metabolic clearance (Cl_1), and peripheral clearance (Cl_2) (Table 2). A weight-dependent relationship was noted with Cl_1. Specifically, elderly women had a larger V_3, a higher Cl_2, and a reduced Cl_3 than did elderly men. The 50% and 70% decrement times for elderly patients calculated from the findings of Schüttler and Ihmsen differ significantly from those of other studies (Fig 4). The predicted propofol concentrations based on these data were significantly higher than those noted in this evaluation.

Conclusions.—Gender affects the pharmacokinetics of propofol among elderly patients. The concentrations in elderly women are lower than those in elderly men who are on the same infusion regimen. Therefore elderly women require infusion rates that are about 10% higher than those for elderly men to achieve the same blood concentration of propofol.

▶ This study describes gender differences for the pharmacokinetics of propofol in an elderly patient group. These studies are important if target controlled infusion methodology is used to provide intravenous anesthesia.

As the authors point out, all studies have not shown this gender difference, and it is important to recognize that there is a small but real intraindividual variability in kinetics. If the kinetics of lidocaine were repeated for a volunteer 3 times, 1 week apart, the data would not be identical.

M. Wood, MD, FRCA

Efficacy of Propofol to Prevent Bronchoconstriction: Effects of Preservative

Brown RH, Greenberg RS, Wagner EM (Johns Hopkins School of Public Health, Baltimore, Md)
Anesthesiology 94:851-855, 2001   3–8

Background.—Patients who have asthma are given premedications and inhalation anesthetics to reduce the risk of severe bronchospasm during tracheal intubation. Propofol has been useful as a rapid induction agent in these patients. A new formulation of propofol includes the preservative metabisulfite, a substance that has caused airway narrowing in asthmatic persons. The combination was assessed for its ability to attenuate bronchoconstriction, using a sheep model.

Methods.—After anesthetizing 7 sheep using 20 mg/kg/h of pentobarbital and paralyzing them with 2 mg of pancuronium, the lungs were ventilated. Left thoracotomy was performed, the bronchial artery cannulated and perfused, and the animals were randomly assigned to receive either propofol with metabisulfite, propofol without metabisulfite, lidocaine, or metabisulfite alone. Before and after vagal nerve stimulation and methacholine challenge, airway resistance was determined, with data expressed as percent of maximal response and analyzed with variance analysis.

Results.—A significant dose effect on airway response to stimulation was noted for lidocaine, which caused a dose-dependent attenuation of the vagal nerve–stimulated bronchoconstriction. Metabisulfite increased the airway's responses to stimulation, but the increase did not reach significance over baseline values. Proprofol without metabisulfite also acted in a dose-dependent fashion, with increased vagal nerve stimulation and attenuation of the methacholine-induced bronchoconstriction at the highest dose given. Propofol with metabisulfite did not attenuate airway resistance either during vagal nerve stimulation or during methacholine infusion. Compared with propofol without metabisulfite, propofol with metabisulfite differed significantly in the ability to attenuate both vagal nerve stimulated- and methacholine-induced bronchoconstriction.

Conclusions.—At clinically relevant concentrations, propofol with metabisulfite did not attenuate vagally or methacholine-induced bronchoconstriction, whereas propofol without metabisulfite did attenuate induced bronchoconstriction.

▶ Propofol attenuates bronchoconstriction and is 1 of the intravenous anesthetics recommended for use in asthmatics. This study shows the effect of a preservative in a new propofol formulation on airway responsiveness in a sheep model. These studies underline how important it is in all clinical studies to test the vehicle for drug administration.

M. Wood, MD, FRCA

The Effect of Sevoflurane and Desflurane on Upper Airway Reactivity
Klock PA Jr, Czeslick EG, Klafta JM, et al (Univ of Halle, Germany)
Anesthesiology 94:963-967, 2001   3–9

Background.—When upper airway reactivity is increased, anesthetized patients are more likely to cough or, when the cough reflex is stimulated, the coughing intensity is increased. Upper airway reactivity has been assessed by changes in airway resistance, but a clinical maneuver was developed to assess upper airway reactivity after 2 inhaled anesthetics (sevoflurane and desflurane) were administered.

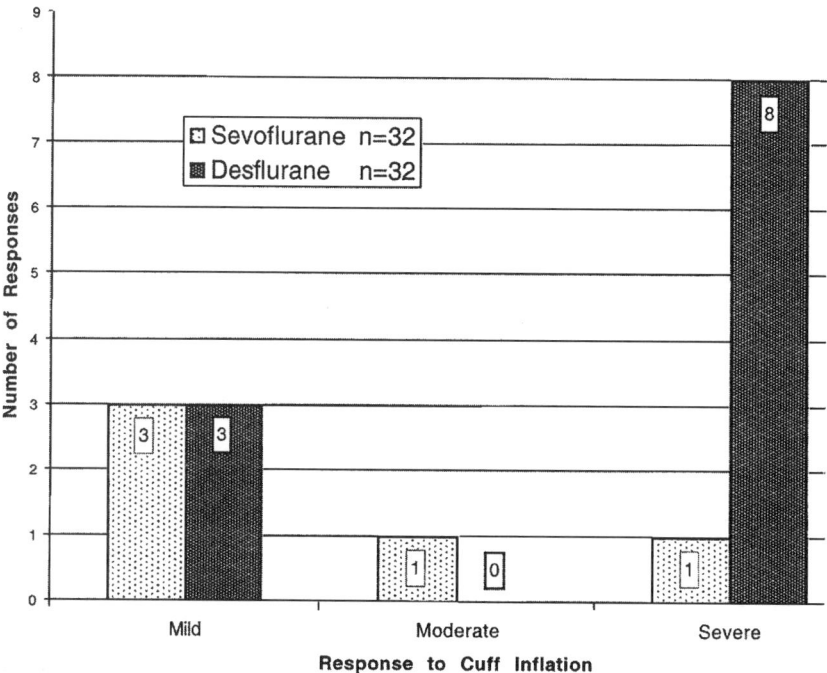

FIGURE 1.—Responses to cuff inflation during 1-MAC anesthesia with sevoflurane or desflurane. Not shown are the subjects who did not respond to cuff inflation (27 sevoflurane subjects and 21 desflurane subjects). (Courtesy of Klock PA Jr, Czeslick EG, Klafta JM, et al: The effect of sevoflurane and desflurane on upper airway reactivity. *Anesthesiology* 94:963-967, 2001. Copyright American Society of Anesthesiologists, Inc. Used with permission of Lippincott-Raven Publishers.)

Methods.—The 64 patients studied were American Society of Anesthesiologists physical status I or II. Sevoflurane or desflurane was used at 1.0 and 1.8 minimum alveolar concentration (MAC) to achieve anesthesia, then the trachea was stimulated by inflating and deflating the endotracheal tube cuff. At each of the MAC treatment conditions, the severity of patient response was assessed by a blinded observer, along with changes in hemodynamic variables.

Results.—Patients who were anesthetized with 1.0 MAC of desflurane had more severe responses to cuff inflation than did those with 1.0 MAC of sevoflurane (Fig 1). Sevoflurane prevented moderate or severe responses to cuff inflation in 94% of patients; desflurane did so in 75% of patients. Patient movement was noted in 2 of the 7 mild responses that occurred with tracheal stimulation. Including mild responses at 1.0 MAC, 5 of 32 patients anesthetized with sevoflurane and 11 of 32 with desflurane showed cuff inflation responses. With 1.8 MAC of sevoflurane, 1 patient had a mild coughing response; none responded to 1.8 MAC of desflurane. Hemodynamic changes and severity of coughing showed a significant correlation for both agents. Interestingly, cuff deflation was more likely to produce a response than cuff inflation.

Conclusions.—Inflating and deflating the endotracheal tube cuff reliably indicated upper airway reactivity. At deeper levels of anesthesia, both sevoflurane and desflurane suppressed responses to tracheal stimulation, whereas at lighter levels, sevoflurane performed better than desflurane in suppressing these responses.

▶ Desflurane and sevoflurane are 2 competing inhaled anesthetics that represent the end result of decades of research to produce the ideal inhaled anesthetic. This study attempts to use the cough response as an index of upper airway reactivity; as expected, sevoflurane was superior to desflurane in this regard.

M. Wood, MD, FRCA

Reduced Regional and Global Cerebral Blood Flow During Fenoldopam-Induced Hypotension in Volunteers
Prielipp RC, Wall MH, Groban L, et al (Wake Forest Univ, Winston-Salem, NC)
Anesth Analg 93:45-52, 2001   3–10

Background.—Cerebral blood flow is influenced by some of the receptor and pharmacologic effects of dopamine (DA). The new agent fenoldopam, a rapid-acting vasodilator indicated for in-hospital, short-term management of severe hypertension, can reduce blood pressure quickly and its effect is rapidly reversed. It has moderate α_2-receptor affinity. Its effects on the cerebral circulation were unclear, so an analysis was done with the belief that fenoldopam would decrease mean arterial blood pressure

(MAP) and cerebral blood flow (CBF) using the mechanism of vascular α_2-adrenoreceptor activation.

Methods.—Nine healthy, normotensive subjects, ranging in age from 18 to 50 years and classified as ASA physical status I or II, were assessed; only 7 completed the study (age range, 25-43 years). Positron emission tomography (PET) was used to assess CBF, with the addition of bioimpedance cardiac output and middle cerebral artery blood flow velocity monitoring.

Results.—MAP was reduced 16% from baseline when fenoldopam was infused at 1.3 µg/kg/min, decreasing from 94 mm Hg to 79 mm Hg. Cardiac output and heart rate were significantly increased during the infusion; global CBF decreased from a baseline value of 45.6 mL/100 g/min to 37.7 mL/100 g/min. When fenoldopam and phenylephrine were administered together to restore baseline MAP, global CBF remained at a lower level (37.9 mL/100 g/min). No correlation was found between the CBF changes detected on PET and changes in middle cerebral artery velocity.

Conclusions.—In addition to its unique action as a DA-agonist vasodilator, fenoldopam decreases both regional and global CBF, most likely in connection with its α_2-agonist activity. This action must be considered when choosing a vasodilator.

▶ Fenoldopam is a new rapidly acting vasodilator to manage acute perioperative hypertension. The effect on the cerebral circulation is key for any new vasodilator; this study examines the effect of fenoldopam on cerebral blood flow and on transcranial doppler velocity. Although fenoldopam increases renal plasma flow and cardiac output, it decreases both regional and global cerebral blood flow. This finding has implications for administration in the intensive care unit and for neurosurgical anesthesia.

M. Wood, MD, FRCA

Suppression of Potassium Conductance by Droperidol Has Influence on Excitability of Spinal Sensory Neurons
Olschewski A, Hempelmann G, Vogel W, et al (Justus-Liebig Univ, Giessen, Germany)
Anesthesiology 94:280-289, 2001

3–11

Background.—The dorsal horn neurons are exposed to high levels of local anesthetics or opioids during epidural and spinal anesthesia; possible side effects in this process include nausea, emesis, and pruritus. To reduce these side effects and extend the period of analgesia, droperidol is given with the opioids. It acts on dopaminergic receptors and voltage-gated Na^+ conductance. A rat model was chosen to study droperidol's action on voltage-gated K^+ channels and on membrane excitability.

Methods.—The entire soma isolation method was combined with the patch-clamp technique to evaluate the action of droperidol on fast-inactivating A-type and delayed-rectifier K^+ channels. The effect of K^+ channel block on neuronal excitability was assessed using current-clamp recordings from intact sensory neurons of spinal cord slices from 8- to 17-day-old rats.

Results.—The delayed-rectifier current was reduced in isolated somata with droperidol concentrations of 10 to 100 μm, but inactivating A-type currents were unaffected at the 100 μm level. Thus the K^+ channels appeared to have the same sensitivity to droperidol as noted with voltage-gated Na^+ channels. The half-maximum inhibiting concentration was 20.6 μm. When concentrations insufficient to suppress the action potential were evaluated, blocking the K^+ channels increased the duration of the action potential and, in response, lowered the neuron's discharge frequency.

Conclusions.—Droperidol blocked the delayed-rectifier K^+ current in spinal dorsal horn neurons, which produced alterations in the firing behavior of neurons when Na^+ conductance block was incomplete. Thus droperidol may exert an antinociceptive effect, which may be clinically relevant.

▶ The butyrophenone, droperidol, is frequently used by anesthesiologists to treat postoperative nausea and vomiting. Droperidol is known to exert many pharmacologic effects; droperidol acts not only on dopaminergic receptors but also on voltage-gated Na^+ conductance. This study shows that droperidol blocks delayed-rectifier K^+ channels as well. So, it is not surprising to note that droperidol produces many side effects. We know, for example, that droperidol has weak α-adrenoreceptor blocking activity and may cause hypotension; other adverse effects include sedation, dysphoria, and extrapyramidal side effects. In 2001, reports of death, QT prolongation, and torsade de pointes caused the manufacturers to institute a labeling change for droperidol—namely a box warning. An ECG must be performed before each administration of droperidol making droperidol more expensive than a 5HT3 receptor antagonist. This will profoundly change the way droperidol is used to treat postoperative nausea and vomiting in the perioperative period.

M. Wood, MD, FRCA

4 Anesthesia Techniques and Monitors

Noninvasive Monitoring of Carbon Dioxide During Mechanical Ventilation in Older Children: End-Tidal Versus Transcutaneous Techniques
Berkenbosch JW, Lam J, Burd RS, et al (Univ of Missouri, Columbia)
Anesth Analg 92:1427-1431, 2001   4–1

Background.—The gold standard for assessing ventilation in critically ill patients remains arterial blood gas analysis. However, an accurate, noninvasive method for monitoring arterial CO_2 levels ($PaCO_2$) would be a benefit. Such noninvasive monitoring might limit the need for repetitive, costly, and painful arterial blood gas analyses. In addition, the continuity of monitoring would stimulate proactive rather than reactive ventilator manipulations and would be valuable in weaning patients from mechanical ventilation. Currently, there are 2 types of noninvasive CO_2 monitors available for clinical use. End-tidal CO_2 ($ETCO_2$) monitoring provides an accurate estimate of ventilation in patients with normal pulmonary function but is of limited usefulness in patients with alterations in ventilation/perfusion matching caused by increased dead space or shunt fraction. Transcutaneous CO_2 ($TCCO_2$) monitoring may avoid some of the problems inherent in $CTCO_2$ monitoring. The accuracy of these 2 methods was compared.

Methods.—A total of 82 sample sets were obtained from 25 patients ranging in age from 4 to 16 years who were receiving mechanical ventilation for respiratory failure. Simultaneous monitoring of $ETCO_2$ and $TCco_2$ was performed, and values were compared with $PaCO_2$ values when arterial blood gas analysis was performed.

Results.—The difference between $ETCO_2$ and $PaCO_2$ values was 6.4 ± 6.3 mm Hg, whereas the difference in $TCCO_2$ and $PaCO_2$ values was 2.6 ± 2.0 mm Hg. In 47 of 82 measurements the absolute difference of $ETCO_2$ and $PaCO_2$ was 5 or less; the absolute difference of $TCCO_2$ to $PaCO_2$ was 5 or less in 67 of 82 measurements.

Conclusions.—The findings showed that $TCCO_2$ monitoring was superior to $ETCO_2$ monitoring in older pediatric patients with respiratory failure. $TCCO_2$ monitoring provided an accurate estimate of $PaCO_2$ over a wide range of CO_2 values.

▶ This study addresses a question from the late '70s and early '80s. Although transcutaneous techniques ended up superior, as they do here, in correlating with arterial CO_2, the side effects, potential burns, and difficulty of applying the sensors in those days limited $TCCO_2$'s usefulness compared to $ETCO_2$ monitoring. The authors do discuss the difficulty of transcutaneous monitoring; they do not appear to find tremendous difficulty or an unacceptable risk. Maybe the machinery has improved since the early '80s when I used it, or maybe these authors are better at applying it, or maybe they are just ignoring this obvious potential problem.

M. F. Roizen, MD

The Combitube in Elective Surgery: A Report of 200 Cases
Gaitini LA, Vaida SJ, Mostafa S, et al (B'nai Zion Med Ctr, Haifa, Israel; Allegheny Gen Hosp, Pittsburgh, Pa; Univ of California, San Diego)
Anesthesiology 94:79-82, 2001   4–2

Background.—The Combitube has recently been introduced for use in patients in whom airway management is difficult. The American Society of Anesthesiologists' Task Force on Management of the Difficult Airway has suggested consideration of the use of the Combitube when intubation problems occur in patients with a previously unrecognized difficult airway, particularly in "cannot ventilate, cannot intubate" situations. The Combitube has the advantages of rapid airway control without the need for neck or head movement, minimized risk for aspiration, firm fixation after inflation of the oropharyngeal balloon, and equally good performance in either the tracheal or esophageal position. In addition, the Combitube can be placed by anesthesiologists with relatively little formal training. The usefulness of the Combitube has been established in the emergency management of the difficult airway and for mechanical ventilation in intensive care, but its use in continued airway management in surgical patients has not been established. The safety and effectiveness of the Combitube in primary airway management for routine surgery with both mechanical and spontaneous ventilation of patients were investigated.

Methods.—Two hundred patients scheduled for elective surgery who met the American Society of Anesthesiologists criteria for physical status I and II, with normal airways, were randomly assigned to 1 of 2 groups. One group comprised nonparalyzed, spontaneously breathing patients, and the other group comprised paralyzed, mechanically ventilated patients. General anesthesia was induced, and the Combitube was inserted. Oxygen saturation, end-tidal carbon dioxide and isoflurane concentration, systolic and diastolic blood pressure and heart rate, and breath-by-breath spirometric data were obtained every 5 minutes.

Results.—With the Combitube, oxygenation, ventilation, respiratory mechanics, and hemodynamic stability were maintained in 97% of patients in both groups for the entire duration of surgery (15-155 minutes).

Conclusions.—The Combitube appears to be safe and effective for the continued management of the airway in nearly all patients undergoing elective surgery.

▶ Two caveats needed by the authors in the success of intubation with the Combitube are important. First, they used a laryngoscope to insert the Combitube in all the patients; and second, these are patients with normal anatomy. That obviously skews the data.

M. F. Roizen, MD

Radiofrequency Transmission to Monitoring Devices in the Operating Room: A Simulation Study
McNulty SE, Kline B, Welsh J, et al (Thomas Jefferson Univ, Philadelphia)
Anesth Analg 92:384-388, 2001   4–3

Background.—Many studies have documented the hazards of misdirection of electrosurgical unit (ESU) output through various medical devices, and the precautions necessary to avoid ESU dispersive electrode faults are well established. Although ESU generators now monitor for faulty connections of the dispersive electrode to the ESU generator and the contact between the dispersive electrode and the patient's skin, there is still the potential for dangerous current paths to occur when the ESU blade electrode is activated but is not yet directly contacting the patient's skin. Under these conditions, it is possible for the dispersive electrode to become a primary output source. The characteristics of radiofrequency current paths between the dispersive electrode and a variety of medical monitoring devices commonly found in the operating room were assessed.

Methods.—A number of medical devices, including right heart ejection fraction (REF) pulmonary artery catheters, transesophageal atrial pacing stethoscopes, and temperature-sensing esophageal stethoscopes, were subjected to radiofrequency transmission from an ESU unit with the use of circuits that simulated potentially hazardous conditions in the operating room. Peak voltage and spark intensity were measured in circuits between the electrocautery dispersive pad and the conductive elements of the devices being tested.

Results.—All the monitoring equipment that had an exposed conductive surface demonstrated induced voltages and, in some cases, spark generation. Peak voltage was lowest in the disrupted esophageal stethoscope (620 V), followed in ascending order by the transesophageal pacemaker (640 V), and the REF pulmonary artery catheter (680 V). There was a significant decrease in peak voltage measurements of the REF pulmonary artery catheter, from 388 ± 23 V to 142 ± 22 V, in a fluid medium compared with air. When the REF pulmonary artery catheter was connected to the cardiopulmonary monitor in a fluid medium, the peak voltage decreased significantly from 142 ± 22 V to 85 ± 15 V.

Conclusions.—It is possible for radiofrequency energy to be transmitted directly between the ESU dispersive electrode and the conductive elements of monitoring devices. Monitoring devices that contain conductive elements that come in contact with the patient should be observed very closely for any possible contacts with conductive surfaces outside the patient.

▶ This interesting study shows that even when usual cautions are taken with ECG and other electrode placement and with "Bovie" ground pad placement, burns can still happen. This is a fascinating article and one well worth the read.

M. F. Roizen, MD

Intraoperative Decrease in Pulse Oximeter Readings Following Injection of Isosulfan Blue
Hoskin RW, Granger R (St Mary's Hosp, New Westminster, BC, Canada)
Can J Anesth 48:38–40, 2001   4–4

Background.—Sentinel lymph node mapping is beginning to be used in patients with breast carcinoma. In this procedure, isosulfan blue dye is injected around a tumor. However, absorption of the dye into the circulation may interfere with pulse oximetry, resulting in falsely low readings. A case of a patient with carcinoma of the breast in whom changes in pulse oximeter readings occurred after injection of isosulfan blue for sentinel lymph node mapping was reported.

> *Case Report.*—Woman, 83, with biopsy-verified adenoma of the left breast was scheduled for sentinel node biopsy of the left axilla to be followed by a partial left mastectomy. After induction of anesthesia, 5 mL of 1% isosulfan blue was injected around the tumor mass, with careful aspiration to avoid intravascular injection. Pulse oximetry readings began to decrease 15 minutes after dye injection to a minimum of 89% to 90% at 30 minutes after the injection. Heart rate and blood pressure remained stable, and arterial blood gas analysis showed normal arterial partial pressure of oxygen. A grayish discoloration of the skin was evident on the patient's face. Surgery was completed 90 minutes after dye injection, and oxygen saturation at that time was 93%. By 7 hours after dye injection, pulse oximetry indicated that the patient's oxygen saturation had returned to 99%. By this time the grayish discoloration had begun to fade.

Conclusions.—A review of the literature identified a small number of case reports of low pulse oximetry readings after injection of isosulfan blue or patent blue dye for lymphatic node mapping. These reports and the report of this case suggest that there is high variability to the latency, magnitude, and duration of the effects of these dyes on pulse oximetry. It is important that other causes of low pulse oximeter readings be ruled out in these situations. Arterial blood gas analysis will verify normal oxygenation. Co-oximetry can be used to eliminate methemoglobinemia as a cause of decreased oxygen saturation in these cases.

▶ Isosulfan blue has been implicated in a number of case reports in causing a decrease in pulse oximeter saturation readings.

M. Wood, MD, FRCA

5 Cardiothoracic and Vascular Anesthesia

Ruptured Abdominal Aortic Aneurysms: The Excessive Mortality Rate of Conventional Repair
Noel AA, Gloviczki P, Cherry KJ Jr, et al (Mayo Clinic and Mayo Found, Rochester, Minn)
J Vasc Surg 34:41-46, 2001   5–1

Objective.—Rupture of abdominal aortic aneurysms (AAAs) remains lethal. In a report of patients treated in the 1980s, we recommended aggressive management. Our continued experience prompted us to re-evaluate this policy.

Methods.—We reviewed clinical variables affecting outcome, morbidity, mortality, and trends in mortality of all patients managed at our institution with ruptured AAAs between January 2, 1980, and November 30, 1998.

Results.—The study group included 413 consecutive patients, 339 men and 74 women. The mean age was 74.3 years (range, 49-96); 116 (28%) patients were older than 80 years. AAA was diagnosed before rupture in 119 (29%) patients. Eighty (19%) patients had preoperative cardiac arrest. Twenty-nine (7%) patients died before operation; 65 (17%) died during the operation. The surgical mortality rate (30-day) was 37%; the overall mortality rate was 45% and was higher in women (68%) than in men (40%) ($P < .001$). Advanced age, APACHE (*Acute Physiology and Chronic Health Evaluation*) II score, initial hematocrit, and preoperative cardiac arrest were associated multivariately with 30-day mortality rates by means of stepwise logistic regression ($P < .05$). Twelve (23%) of 53 patients with cardiac arrest survived the operation. Logistic regression, adjusted for age, sex, and APACHE II score, demonstrated a decrease in overall and 30-day mortality rates ($P < .001$) over 18 years. The mean overall mortality rate was 51% from 1980 to 1984 and 42% from 1994 to 1998.

Conclusions.—The mortality rate of ruptured AAAs remains excessive, despite improvement over 18 years. Patients older than 80 years with shock or cardiac arrest have the highest mortality rate and should be evaluated for possible endovascular treatment. Because the diagnosis of

AAA was unknown in more than 70% of patients, screening of the high-risk population and elective repair are recommended.

Stroke From Carotid Endarterectomy: When and How to Reduce Perioperative Stroke Rate?

de Borst GJ, Moll FL, van de Pavoordt HDWM, et al (St Antonius Hosp, Nieuwegein, The Netherlands)
Eur J Vasc Endovasc Surg 21:484-489, 2001   5–2

Objectives.—To analyse 4 years of CEA with respect to the underlying mechanisms of perioperative stroke and the role of intraoperative monitoring in the prevention of stroke.

Patients and Methods.—From January 1996 through December 1999, 599 CEAs were performed in 404 men and 195 women (mean age, 65 years, range, 39-88). All operations were performed under general anaesthesia using computerised electroencephalography (EEG) and transcranial Doppler (TCD). Any new or any extension of an existing focal cerebral deficit, as well as stroke-related death were registered. Perioperative strokes were classified by time of onset (intraoperative or postoperative), outcome (minor or major stroke), and side (ipsilateral or contralateral). Stroke aetiology was assessed intraoperatively by means of EEG, TCD, completion arteriography or immediate re-exploration, and postoperatively by duplex sonography, CT or MRI of the head.

Results.—Perioperative stroke or death occurred in 20 (3.3%) patients. In 4 operations stroke was apparent immediately after surgery. Mechanisms of these strokes were ipsilateral carotid artery occlusion (1) and embolisation (3). In 16 patients stroke developed after a symptom-free interval (2-72 hours, mean 18 hours) due to occlusion of the internal carotid artery on the side of surgery (9). Other mechanisms were: contralateral occlusion of the internal carotid artery (1), postoperative hyperperfusion syndrome (1), intracerebral haemorrhage (1), and contralateral ischaemia due to prolonged clamping (1). In 3 procedures the cause was unknown.

Conclusions.—In our experience, most strokes from CEA developed after a symptom-free interval and mainly due to thromboembolism of the operated artery. We suggest the introduction of additional TCD monitoring during the immediate postoperative phase.

▶ Although the suggestion of TCD monitoring during the immediate postoperative phase is made, it's not clear that TCD monitoring would show premonitory emboli. I think that a study—that is, can you intervene with such patients that prevents strokes in a study that tests such hypotheses in a randomized controlled fashion—needs to be done before routine TCD monitoring is done in the postoperative period.

M. F. Roizen, MD

Timing of Postcarotid Complications: A Guide to Safe Discharge Planning

Sheehan MK, Baker WH, Littooy FN, et al (Loyola Univ, Maywood, Ill)
J Vasc Surg 34:13-16, 2001   5–3

Objectives.—Currently, our standard of practice is that patients undergoing carotid endarterectomy (CEA) may be safely discharged on the first postoperative day. Because many patients do not appear to require overnight observation, we wanted to determine the safety and feasibility of same-evening discharge by establishing the timing of postoperative complications, which may potentially require operative intervention.

Methods.—A total of 835 consecutive patients undergoing CEA were retrospectively reviewed. Sixty-two patients had a postoperative wound hematoma or neurologic deficit (ND) (transient ischemic attack or stroke) within 24 hours of their operation, complications potentially requiring a second operation. Excluded were 64 patients not eligible for same-day discharge because of other reasons (eg, heparinization, CEA with coronary artery bypass grafting).

Results.—Sixty-two patients (8.0%) had ND (26 [3.4%]) or neck hematoma (NH) (36 [4.7%]) within 24 hours of their CEA. Nineteen (73%) of the NDs were diagnosed in the operating room or recovery room, 5 (19%) within 8 hours of the operation, and 2 (7.7%) after 8 hours but in less than 24 hours. Of the NHs, 23 (66%) were diagnosed in the recovery room, 11 (31%) within 8 hours, and 1 (2.7%) after 8 hours. Of the outliers, 1 patient experienced a blowout of the vein graft occurring on postoperative day 1, one patient had a delayed ipsilateral stroke, and 1 had a vertebrobasilar stroke. Overall, only three of 773 (0.4%) patients undergoing CEA had a complication occurring more than 8 hours after operation.

Conclusion.—NDs and NHs in post-CEA patients occurred within 8 hours of operation in 95% of those patients experiencing these complications or 99.6% of all CEA patients. These data indicate that same-evening discharge may be safely performed without increasing the adverse effects of stroke or hematoma. This plan has cautiously been initiated at this institution.

▶ This is an important study because it shows that most complications after CEA occur within 8 hours of surgery. Is this an appropriate time to discharge patients? The only problems that do occur if you do that are delayed stroke and delayed blowout of a vein graft. This is a rather large study; do you think ignoring that 2/10 of 0.2% of complications is OK?

M. F. Roizen, MD

Patient and Hospital Benefits of Local Anaesthesia for Carotid Endarterectomy

McCarthy RJ, Walker R, McAteer P, et al (Royal United Hosp, Bath, England)
Eur J Vasc Endovasc Surg 22:13-18, 2001   5–4

Objectives.—This study reviews and compares carotid endarterectomy (CEA) performed under local anaesthesia (LA) with CEA performed under general anaesthesia (GA) in a single institution.

Methods.—Data were collected prospectively from 240 CEA procedures. One hundred forty GA CEA procedures are compared to 100 LA CEA procedures in terms of outcome, operative techniques, complications, and length of stay.

Results.—The groups were similar for age, gender distribution and preoperative risk factors. There were more asymptomatic patients in the LA group. There were no significant differences in death, stroke or death/stroke rate between the two techniques. LA CEA was associated with lower shunt rate (LA 13%, GA 50%, p <0.001), lower incidence of intraoperative hypotension (LA 8%, GA 40%, p <0.001), decreased hospital stay (median [IQ], LA 2 [1-2], GA 3 [1-4]), and a cost saving of £235 per CEA procedure.

Conclusions.—Carotid endarterectomy can be performed safely under local anaesthesia with the advantage that LA CEA enables the surgeon to monitor and selectively shunt patients more accurately. In addition, LA CEA is associated with a shorter hospital stay and important cost savings.

▶ Although there were no significant differences in morbidity between local and general anesthesia, the hospital stay for patients who had local anesthesia was shorter by 1 day. Since outpatients at most institutions, for this procedure, are routinely discharged 8 hours after surgery (see Abstract 5–3), I don't think that the advantage the authors found is very substantial.

M. F. Roizen, MD

The Use of Lepirudin for Anticoagulation in Patients With Heparin-Induced Thrombocytopenia During Major Vascular Surgery

Sun Y, Greilich PE, Wilson SIO, et al (Univ of Texas, Dallas)
Anesth Analg 92:344-346, 2001   5–5

Introduction.—Individuals with previous heparin exposures are generally considered to be at increased risk for heparin-induced thrombocytopenia (HIT), an immune-mediated reaction caused by IgG antibodies. Lepirudin, a recombinant hirudin, is a direct inhibitor of thrombin and acts independently of antithrombin III. Lepirudin was administered intraoperatively to 2 patients with HIT undergoing major vascular surgery.

Case Report.—Man, 71, required revision of a femoral to posterior tibial artery bypass performed 4 months previously. Heparin was administered when graft occlusion occurred on postoperative day 1. Gangrene of the toes developed 5 days later, and the patient's platelet count fell from 208,000 µL to 103,000 µL. Acute HIT was confirmed, and lepirudin (0.4 mg/kg bolus with continuous infusion at 0.15 mg/kg/h) was administered for 2 days. When the patient was readmitted 3 months later for a second revision of the bypass graft, no heparin-containing solutions were given. Lepirudin therapy, initiated before vascular clamping, was continued for 4 days while the patient was in the surgical ICU, followed by transition to warfarin. No postoperative complications occurred.

Discussion.—Bolus-only dosing of lepirudin can be used successfully during major vascular surgery for anticoagulation in patients with a history of HIT. The lepirudin regimen described here was sufficient to maintain an activated partial thromboplastin time more than 2.5 times control values.

▶ HIT can occur in 1% to 30% of patients after heparin therapy, depending on the situation and criteria for diagnosis. Two types are known: type 1 is mild, asymptomatic, and accompanied by thrombocytopenia that is easily resolved if heparin is discontinued. Type 2 is exemplified in the case presented. Patients with this type of HIT have profound thrombocytopenia, usually associated with arteriolar thrombosis. Failure to recognize this type of HIT can result in further thrombotic complications, and mortality can reach 20% to 30%. Lepirudin is currently the only drug approved by the Food and Drug Administration for anticoagulation in HIT. The first step is to discontinue heparin; then if the patient needs further treatment lepirudin can be used. Lepirudin is a direct inhibitor of thrombin and acts independently of antithrombin III. The optimal method for administering this drug has yet to be determined; the common technique is to give an IV bolus followed by an infusion, except in patients with renal failure, in whom the half-life of lepirudin is greatly prolonged. Usually the half-life is 30 to 60 minutes, which means that normal coagulation is restored within 30 minutes after bolus administration. The use of lepirudin is still experimental, but there is increasing evidence that it can be used even during cardiopulmonary bypass surgery. For physicians with patients with HIT, and that probably includes all who do any cardiovascular anesthesia, this article is commended as an early way to learn about its use.

M. F. Roizen, MD

The Effect of Continuous Positive Airway Pressure on Cerebral Blood Flow Velocity in Awake Volunteers

Bowie RA, O'Connor PJ, Hardman JG, et al (City Hosp, Nottingham, England)

Anesth Analg 92:415-417, 2001   5–6

Introduction.—Transcranial Doppler monitoring (TCD), when used to continuously measure blood flow velocity (FV) in basal cerebral arteries, can reflect changes in cerebral blood flow (CBF). In a previous study of 9 spontaneously breathing volunteers, 12 cm H_2O continuous positive airway pressure (CPAP) caused a significant increase in middle cerebral artery (MCA) FV and a significant decrease in pulsatility index (PI). Thus the application of CPAP may confound interpretation of MCA FV data. These findings and other conflicting results led to a reexamination of the effects of CPAP on MCA FV in spontaneously breathing human volunteers.

Methods.—Inclusion criteria were age 18 to 40, body mass index 22 to 28 kg/m^2, no history of headaches or vascular problems, no previous head injury, and no vasoactive medication. Studies were performed with participants supine. A 2 MHz pulsed TCD probe with specific software was used to record data. Mean arterial pressure (MAP), heart rate, and peripheral oxygen saturation were recorded noninvasively. CPAP was administered via a tightly fitting mouthpiece attached to a high-flow air circuit. Recordings of mean FV (FVm), systolic FV (FVs), diastolic FV (FVd) and PI were obtained at baseline (before CPAP) and at 5 and 10 cm H_2O CPAP, a selection based on common practice at the study institution. Power of the reflected Doppler signal was measured continuously.

Results.—Study participants were 11 men and 4 women. At neither 5 nor 10 cm H_2O CPAP were there any statistically significant changes from baseline in the variables MAP, FVm, FVs, FVd, or PI. Throughout the study, reflected TCD power values changed by less than 5%.

Discussion.—Findings contrast with those of a previous study in which mean FV increased significantly and PI decreased during the application of 12 cm H_2O CPAP. But in this report, no significant changes in MCA FV as measured by Doppler US occurred. These results have implications for the use of TCD to evaluate changes in cerebral hemodynamic in patients receiving CPAP.

▶ This study is interesting because patients who commonly receive CPAP have obstructive sleep apnea. The study found no change in any measured variables, but it is not clear why this study differed from previous studies. Since we will see CPAP used increasingly during procedures requiring regional anesthetia as well as situations requiring no anesthesia, it probably would benefit us to ensure that this technique is safe. I think the jury is still out, although there is no doubt that CPAP has important benefits for patients with sleep apnea.

M. F. Roizen, MD

In-Hospital Mortality From Abdominal Aortic Surgery in Great Britain and Ireland: Vascular Anaesthesia Society Audit

Bayly PJM, Matthews JNS, Dobson PM, et al (Newcastle Univ, Newcastle upon Tyne, England; Northern Gen Hosp, Sheffield, England; St Mary's Hosp, London; et al)
Br J Surg 88:687-692, 2001   5–7

Introduction.—Patients requiring abdominal aortic surgery are considered a high-risk group. Factors previously reported to be associated with an increased mortality rate include older age, chronic renal impairment, hypertension, and having the surgery at centers that perform few aortic operations. A multicenter study sought to obtain current information on in-hospital mortality from abdominal aortic surgery in Great Britain and Ireland.

Methods.—Anesthesiologists involved in vascular surgery at a total of 177 hospitals expressed willingness to participate in the survey. Elective and urgent operations were included, but emergency operations excluded. Data were sought on all open infrarenal abdominal aortic aneurysm (AAA) repairs and on infrarenal aortoiliac or aortofemoral grafts for occlusive disease (AOD). The period of the audit extended from February through May of 1999. Items in the questionnaire included hospital type, size, and facilities; patient age, sex, and comorbidities; type of anesthetic and surgery; and outcome.

Results.—A total of 933 satisfactorily completed individual questionnaires were returned; 777 reported on patients who had AAA repair and 156 on patients who had aortic replacement for AOD. The majority of procedures in both groups were elective. Sixty-eight patients died for an overall mortality rate of 7.3%. The most frequently reported causes of death were "cardiac" (23 patients) and "multiorgan failure" (27 patients). Women accounted for 20.3% of patients overall and were twice as likely to have undergone surgery for AOD than for AAA (35.3% of the AOD group versus 17.2% of the AAA group). Factors increasing the risk of death were age over 74, urgent surgery, operation for occlusive disease, limited exercise capacity, a history of severe angina or cardiac failure, and the presence of ventricular ectopic beats and abnormalities suggesting ischemic heart disease on electrocardiography. Low-volume and high-volume centers yielded similar outcomes.

Conclusion.—Older studies suggested that the mortality rate for elective infrarenal aortic surgery ranges from 4% to 7%. The current overall in-hospital mortality rate in similar, but certain risk factors significantly increase mortality.

▶ This article is extremely valuable because the mandatory reporting status and audit process looks at all 177 hospitals throughout the UK and Ireland. The overall hospital death rate was 7.3%, considerably greater than that in the United States, and went up considerably as the patients aged past age 74. In the United States, we need to duplicate such a study, but the National

Hospital Discharge Data show that the increase medical cost in this country compared to Great Britain and Ireland may well be worth it because of the increasing age of our patients. The age for patients for aortic vascular surgery for example increased over 6 years in the decade between 1984 and 1994 without an increase in mortality rate in the United States. This substantial increase in age was obviously accompanied by increases in costs for intensive care unit and for preoperative preparation, which may well be worth it when one looks at the outcome of results shown in this study from the less expensive British experience. This study also shows that the more urgent cases carried much higher risk, but it does not appear that the volume of surgery done at any one center was important in outcome. That is so intuitively different from my thought processes that I have trouble with understanding how that can be. Perhaps it is because the higher volume centers accepted patients with greater risk, but this hypothesis is not borne by the data. Why did volume of surgery not affect outcome? We have no answer. One item of further interest deserves comment: there was an association of fatality rate with limited exercise capacity.

M. F. Roizen, MD

PentaLyte® Does Not Decrease Heparinoid Release but Does Decrease Circulating Thrombotic Mediator Activity Associated With Aortic Occlusion-Reperfusion in Rabbits
Nielsen VG, Armstead VE, Geary BT, et al (Univ of Alabama, Birmingham; Thomas Jefferson Univ, Philadelphia)
Anesth Analg 92:314-319, 2001   5–8

Introduction.—Hemorrhage and thrombosis are important sources of morbidity and mortality after major vascular and trauma surgery. These complications may result in part from the release of heparinoids and thrombotic mediators, findings described in rabbits after aortic occlusion-reperfusion. The hypothesis that PentaLyte administration could reduce the heparinoid and thrombotic mediator release associated with thoracic aorta occlusion-reperfusion was examined in an animal model.

Methods.—Sixteen New Zealand White rabbits were randomized to either lactated Ringer's solution or PentaLyte, a 6% pentastarch solution containing balanced electrolytes and lactate buffer. The anesthetized animals received the solutions at reperfusion after 30 minutes of ischemia. Blood samples were obtained before ischemia and after 30 minutes of reperfusion for thromboelastography assessment under 4 conditions: 1) unmodified sample, 2) platelet inhibition, 3) heparinase, and 4) platelet inhibition and heparinase. Thromboelastographic variables examined were reaction time (R), angle (α), and G, a measure of clot strength.

Results.—During reperfusion, the unmodified samples exhibited a significant increase in R and decrease in α and G that was not affected by administration of PentaLyte. No significant fluid-specific thromboelastographic differences were observed in the presence of heparinase. Thrombotic mediator release during reperfusion, as indicated by a release in *R* and an increase in α, was significantly attenuated by PentaLyte in samples with platelet inhibition and heparinase.

Conclusion.—Compared with lactated Ringer's solution, resuscitation with PentaLyte did not significantly decrease heparinoid release after aortic occlusion-reperfusion in rabbits. But in the presence of heparinase and platelet inactivation, PentaLyte decreases the release of the thrombotic mediators associated with hepatoenteric ischemia-reperfusion.

▶ This study is excellent in that it demonstrates convincingly that there is an increased thrombotic risk in the immediate perioperative period after vascular surgery. Is this true after all surgery to the same degree? We don't know the answer to that nor is it known what we should do to shut this down or if anything needs to be done. This study, like most great studies, raises more questions than it does answers.

M. F. Roizen, MD

Monitoring of End-Tidal Carbon Dioxide Partial Pressure Changes During Infrarenal Aortic Cross-Clamping: A Non-Invasive Method to Predict Unclamping Hypotension
Boccara G, Jaber S, Eliet J, et al (Med Univ of Montpellier, France)
Acta Anaesthesiol Scand 45:188-193, 2001   5–9

Introduction.—Monitoring of end-tidal partial pressure of carbon dioxide (end-tidal CO_2) can provide information about hemodynamics as well as about ventilation. A group of patients scheduled for infrarenal aortic abdominal aneurysm repair by laparotomy and insertion of conventional aorto-aortic prosthetic bypass were studied prospectively for variations in end-tidal CO_2 in response to aortic cross-clamping and the relationship with systolic arterial pressure (SAP) changes induced by unclamping.

Methods.—The 33 patients included in the study had a negative dobutamine stress echocardiography and were in New York Heart Association class I or II. All patients were anesthetized with IV midazolam, thiopentone, fentanyl, and pancuronium; anesthesia was maintained with 1% to 1.5% end-tidal isoflurane and IV fentanyl. Perioperative management was also standardized. End-tidal CO_2, central venous pressure, and SAP were measured 5 minutes before (Pre-XAA), 15 minutes after infrarenal aortic cross-clamping (XAA), 5 minutes before (Pre-UXAA), and immediately after unclamping (UXAA).

Results.—Sixteen patients (48.5%) experienced a marked decrease in SAP after aortic unclamping (>20% from pre-UXAA SAP value). Thirteen of these patients had arterial hypotension, defined as SAP <90 mm Hg. Volume loading was successful in treating hypotension, but 3 patients required vasopressors. The 2 significant postoperative complications occurred in patients with unclamping hypotension. A correlation was observed between end-tidal CO_2 variation (PreXAA-PreUXAA) induced by aortic clamping and SAP variation (PreUXAA-UXAA) induced by unclamping. An end-tidal CO_2 reduction >15% after aortic cross-clamping had a 100% sensitivity to detect a SAP decrease >20% after unclamping. Patients with and without unclamping hypotension were similar in demographic characteristics, preoperative diseases, and medications.

Conclusion.—Monitoring of end-tidal CO_2 variations during aortic cross-clamping may have potential as a reliable and noninvasive method for predicting unclamping hypotension. Upon release of the aortic clamp, systolic hypotension occurred in patients who had a >15% decrease in end-tidal CO_2 during aortic cross-clamping.

▶ This is one of my favorite studies of 2001. Why? Because it shows what a prepared mind can discover. These authors saw in several cases that end-tidal CO_2 decreases on unclamping correlated with unclamping hypotension. They then started to study the issue, and found that is in fact true. This is thus in my mind a great study because of their approach to evaluation. If the end-tidal CO_2 decreases by more that 15% on unclamping, you're bound to have unclamping hypotension.

M. F. Roizen, MD

Experience in the United States With Intact Abdominal Aortic Aneurysm Repair
Huber TS, Wang JG, Derrow AE, et al (Univ of Florida, Gainesville; Shands HealthCare Incorporated, Royal Oak, Mich)
J Vasc Surg 33:304-311, 2001   5–10

Objectives.—The purpose of this study was to determine the current outcome in the United States and to identify predictors of mortality and "bad outcome" after open, intact abdominal aortic aneurysm (AAA) repair.

Methods.—In a retrospective analysis, data were obtained from the Nationwide Inpatient Sample during 1994 to 1996. The Nationwide Inpatient Sample is a 20% all-payer stratified sample of nonfederal United States hospitals. Patients older than 49 years were identified by the presence of primary diagnostic (441.4-intact AAA) and procedure (38.44-resection of abdominal aorta with replacement) codes of the *International Classification of Diseases, Ninth Revision (ICD-9)*. In-hospital mortality rate, discharge disposition, bad outcome (death or discharge to an institution), complications (*ICD-9* postoperative codes), length of stay, and charges were determined. The mortality rate and bad outcome were analyzed by the use of patient demographics (age, sex, race), patient comorbidities (*ICD-9* diagnostic codes), calendar year, and hospital characteristics (size, location, teaching status) with univariate and multivariate analyses.

Results.—We identified 16,450 intact AAA repairs during the study years. The mean patient age was 72 ± 7 (± SD) years, and most patients were male (79.7%) and white (94.6%). Most repairs were performed at large (67.3%), urban (92.5%), and nonteaching (66.7%) institutions. The in-hospital mortality rate was 4.2%, the overall complication rate was 32.4%, and 91.2% of patients were discharged home, whereas the bad outcome rate was 12.6%. The median length of stay was 8 days (mean, 10.0 ± 8.1), and median hospital charges were $28,052 (mean, $35,681 ± $33,006) in 1996 dollars. Multivariate analysis showed that the mortality rate ($P < .05$) increased with age (70-79 years, 1.8 odds ratio [OR] [95% CI, 1.4-2.3], >79 years, 3.8 OR [95% CI, 2.9-4.9]), sex (female, 1.6 OR [95% CI, 1.3-1.9]), cerebral vascular occlusive disease (1.8 OR [95% CI, 1.3-2.5]), preoperative renal insufficiency (9.5 OR [95% CI, 7.7-11.7]), and more than three comorbidities (11.2 OR [95% CI, 3.6-35.4]). Multivariate analysis also showed that bad outcome was associated with the same variables in addition to hospital size (small/medium), year of procedure (1996), chronic obstructive pulmonary disease, and 2 to 3 comorbidities.

Conclusions.—Outcome after open repair of intact AAA across the United States is quite good. Older, sicker patients may benefit from nonoperative treatment or the potentially lower risk endovascular approaches.

▶ This article is important because of recent data showing that when inpatient mortality increased to 10%, there would be no benefit to open aortic aneurysm repair in the elective case. This article shows that the overall mortality rate in the United States, even when one considers that the average age of patients between 1994 and 1996 was 72 years, was only 4.2%, with 91.2% of patients being discharged home. The mortality rate went down as the size of the hospital increased and the health of the patient increased, with patients without other preexisting conditions having essentially no mortality. Thus, mortality rate increased to approximately 9-fold greater than the average mortality if a creatinine above 2.3 was present.

M. F. Roizen, MD

Age Versus Comorbidities as Risk Factors for Complications After Elective Abdominal Aortic Reconstructive Surgery
Berry AJ, Smith RB III, Weintraub WS, et al (Emory Univ, Atlanta, Ga)
J Vasc Surg 33:345-352, 2001   5–11

Introduction.—Because older individuals are now being considered for major operations, it is important to understand the effect increasing age has on surgical morbidity and mortality. The relationship between age and in-hospital postoperative complications was examined in a series of patients undergoing elective abdominal aortic reconstructive (AAR) surgery. The risks associated with age were compared with other comorbidities in a retrospective cohort investigation at a tertiary care, university-affiliated hospital.

Methods.—A total of 856 consecutive patients undergoing elective AAR surgery between January 1, 1986 to August 1, 1996 were included. Significant risk factors were controlled for, and an estimate was made of the odds ratio (OR) and 95% CI for the relationship between patient age and in-hospital major mortality.

Results.—One hundred seventy patients had nonfatal complications (136 major and 34 minor). Eleven patients died. The final logistic model showed a mild correlation between increasing age and the rate of major postoperative complications, including death (for each increase in age of 10 years: OR, 1.23; 95% CI, 1.00-1.52; $P = .052$). Other significant covariates in the final model were cardiac disease (OR, 2.84; 95% CI, 1.18-6.86; $P = .020$), pulmonary disease (OR, 1.96; 95% CI, 1.35-2.84; $P = .0004$), and renal disease (OR, 2.57; 95% CI, 1.66-3.99; $P = .0001$). Increasing age was correlated with a moderate increase in the rate of death (for each increase in age of 10 years: OR, 2.74; 95% CI, 1.22-6.16; $P = .015$) in a model with cardiac disease as the only significant covariate (OR, 14.67; 95% CI, 3.46-62.16; $P = .0003$).

Conclusion.—In patients undergoing elective AAR surgery, increasing age was correlated with a small increase in the risk of in-hospital morbidity or mortality. Significant cardiac, pulmonary, or renal disease was correlated with a much greater risk of postoperative complications. Thus, advanced age should not be the only factor excluding otherwise suitable candidates for elective AAR surgery.

▶ I should say that, as someone who developed RealAge, I love this study; however, I clearly have a conflict of interest, as I believe that it is physiologic age, not calendar age, that matters most, which is why I did the work on RealAge. That's also what Berry et al at Emory University found: although increasing patient age is associated with a small increase in risk, it is mainly physiologic age (that which is related to significant cardiac, pulmonary, and arterial disease) that is associated with a much greater risk of mortality. The authors should be congratulated for such a clear study and results.

M. F. Roizen, MD

Relative Cost of Autologous Red Cell Salvage Versus Allogeneic Red Cell Transfusion During Abdominal Aortic Aneurysm Repair
Gardner A, Gibbs N, Evans C, et al (Sir Charles Gairdner Hosp, Perth, Western Australia)
Anaesth Intensive Care 28:646-649, 2000   5–12

Background.—Autologous red cell concentrate obtained by intraoperative red blood cell salvage provides many advantages of allogeneic packed red cell concentrate, but the additional costs of autologous blood may be difficult to justify given the low risks associated with the use of allogeneic blood transfusion. The high costs associated with intraoperative red cell salvage are related to the costs of the disposable equipment needed for collection and processing of the scavenged blood and the labor needed to run the cell salvage equipment. However, the use of allogeneic blood also has associated costs, which are incurred in the collection of blood from donors, typing of the blood, and screening for antibodies and infectious agents. Little current data are available regarding the relative costs of these alternative sources of blood. These costs in Australia during infrarenal abdominal aortic aneurysm (AAA) repair were compared.

Methods.—In a prospective review, the costs of washed autologous red cell concentrate obtained by intraoperative red cell salvage were compared with the costs associated with use of allogeneic paced red cell transfusion in 110 consecutive elective and emergency AAA repairs.

Results.—The mean volume of scavenged blood during elective AAA repairs was 1350 mL, whereas the mean volume scavenged in emergency AAA repairs was 2750 mL. The mean volume of washed blood returned in elective repairs was 759 mL, and the mean volume of washed blood returned in emergency repairs was 1117 mL. At $151 per 285 mL unit, the cost of routine autologous red cell salvage was only slightly higher than the estimated costs of cross-matched, leukocyte-reduced, allogeneic blood ($143 per 285 mL unit).

Conclusions.—These findings indicate that the use of autologous red cell concentrate by intraoperative red blood cell salvage in emergency AAA repair can be justified on an economic basis alone. Routine salvage of red cells during elective repair can provide the benefits of autologous blood at little additional cost.

▶ This is an excellent study and one that which many of us will be forced to read as spending is cut tremendously in the inpatient environment and as costs come under pressure again. Clearly red cell salvage can be beneficial in emergency situations and is also cost effective. As we get better surgical techniques, red cell salvage will be less useful on an elective basis but still extremely beneficial for emergencies. But how can one be prepared for emergencies if not using a technique routinely? Will the service cost more in that case? That is a major question.

M. F. Roizen, MD

Anterior Spinal Artery Syndrome After Aortic Surgery in a Child
Servais LJ, Rivelli SK, Dachy BA, et al (Free Univ, Brussels, Belgium)
Pediatr Neurol 24:310-312, 2001   5–13

Background.—Anterior spinal artery syndrome (ASAS) was first described almost 100 years ago. ASAS is characterized by flaccid paralysis of sudden onset evolving toward spasticity, dissociated sensory impairment, and sphincter paralysis after acute ischemia in the territory of the anterior spinal artery. ASAS is rare in children and is observed most frequently in adults after resection of thoracoabdominal aortic aneurysms. Spinal MRI is considered the first-line investigation for confirmation of the clinical diagnosis. This study reports a case of ASAS in a child after surgery for aortic coarctation.

> *Case Report.*—Boy, 3 years, was admitted for palliative cardiac surgery for a complex cardiac malformation associated with aortic coarctation. The patient's history included an uncomplicated pregnancy by his mother and full-term delivery, and his development was normal with the exception of a failure to thrive. The cardiac malformation included a single ventricle, mitral valve dysplasia, atrial communication, and coarctation of the aorta. Surgery was indicated because of significant pulmonary hypertension, low peripheral blood flow, and congestive heart failure despite treatment with furosemide, aldactone, and digoxin. The patient subsequently presented with ASAS, and a clinical diagnosis of anterior horn cell impairment below the L2 level was confirmed by electromyography and F-wave studies. Sparing of dorsal sensory tracts was documented by normal somatosensory-evoked potentials, which confirmed the anterior localization of the lesion. Findings on spinal MRI performed on postoperative days 15 and 105 were normal. The neurologic deficits, including flaccid paraplegia, remained stable with the exception of the reappearance of patellar reflexes on day 83. Neurophysiologic conduction studies were consistent were lower motoneuron loss.

Conclusions.—In this patient, somatosensory-evoked potentials did not detect the insult, demonstrating that MRI was less sensitive than clinical neurophysiology. The prevention of ASAS may necessitate the use of other neurophysiologic monitoring techniques.

▶ This case report is important for those involved in spinal surgery in children. It shows an unusual complication and has an even more unusual finding in the difficulty of detection with usual monitoring systems.

M. F. Roizen, MD

Ischaemia/Reperfusion Contributes to Colonic Injury Following Experimental Aortic Surgery

Reber PU, Peter M, Patel AG, et al (Univ of Bern, Switzerland)
Eur J Vasc Endovasc Surg 21:35-39, 2001   5–14

Objectives.—Ischemia of the colon is an important complication of abdominal aortic aneurysm (AAA) repair. The aim of this animal study was to investigate the effect of sequential ischemia and reperfusion on sigmoid mucosal pO_2 and its association with local endothelin-1 (ET-1) release.

Material and Methods.—Twelve pigs underwent colonic ischemia followed by complete reperfusion. Six other animals were sham controls. A Clark-type microcatheter was used for continuous mucosal pO_2 measurements. Serial systemic and inferior mesenteric vein blood samples were obtained for determination of ET-1 concentration. Neutrophil extravasation was assessed by tissue myeloperoxidase (MPO) activity.

Results.—Arterial occlusion was associated with a gradual decrease of mucosal pO_2 and local release of ET-1. After restoration of blood flow, mucosal pO_2 returned to near baseline values, whereas ET-1 reached its maximum concentration during the reperfusion period. MPO activity was significantly increased.

Conclusions.—Colonic ischemia and reperfusion causes neutrophil extravasation and local ET-1.

▶ This article is one that attributes reperfusion injury during aortic surgery to release of ET-1. An excellent study that may lead us to therapeutic options when bypass times have to be long, or your surgeons are not as good technically as the ones I've been lucky enough to work with.

M. F. Roizen, MD

Operation for Acute Type A Aortic Dissection in Octogenarians: Is it Justified?
Neri E, Toscano T, Massetti M, et al (Université de Caen, France)
J Thorac Cardiovasc Surg 121:259-267, 2001   5–15

Background.—With the progressive aging of Western populations, cardiac surgeons are faced with treating an increasing number of elderly patients. Controversy exists as to whether the expenditure of health care resources on the growing elderly populations represents a cost-effective approach to resource management. The potential to avoid surgery in patients with little chance of survival and poor quality of life would spare unnecessary suffering, reduce operative mortality, and enhance the use of scarce resources.

Methods.—We reviewed the records of 24 consecutive patients aged 80 years or older (mean age, 83 years; range, 80-93 years) who underwent operations for acute type A dissection from 1985 through 1999. No patient with acute type A dissection was refused surgery because of age or concomitant disease. Seventeen patients were men. Preoperatively, none of the patients was moribund, although 66% had hemodynamic instability and 41% experienced cerebral ischemia. All patients had 1 or more associated pathologic conditions. Hospital mortality and morbidity models, based on our overall experience with 197 patients operated on for acute type A aortic dissection during the period of the study, were developed by means of multivariate logistic regression with preoperative and intraoperative variables used as independent predictors of outcome.

Results.—Overall hospital mortality was 83%. Intraoperative mortality was 33%. All patients who survived the operation had 1 or more postoperative complications. Mean hospital stay was 37 days with a total of 314 days in the intensive care unit (average, 19 days; median, 17 days). None of the survivors (4 patients) discharged from the hospital was able to function independently and their survival at 6 months was 0%. Statistical analysis of the overall experience with operations for type A acute aortic dissection confirmed that age in excess of 80 years is the most important independent patient risk factor associated with 30-day mortality and morbidity.

Conclusions.—Operations for acute type A dissection performed on octogenarians involve increased hospital mortality and morbidity. Short-term survival is unfavorable and is associated with a poor quality of life. Without additional corroborative studies to endorse the present findings, the use of age as a parameter to limit access of patients to expensive medical resources remains an unsubstantiated concept. In the context of acute type A aortic dissection, however, the hypothesis that older patients should be denied such a complicated surgical intervention to conserve resources is supported by the presented data.

▶ This is an experienced group of surgeons, and the mortality rate for patients under age 80 is 16% but their mortality rate once you hit 80 years is 83%. Perhaps mortality relates more to physiologic and not calendar age, but these patients are really quite old based on other factors: 100% had chronic hypertension, 66% of them smoked, 30% of them had bad diabetes, and 40% had angina. This is a very old group of people physiologically and the mortality rate is high because of that.

M. F. Roizen, MD

Sudden Respiratory Arrest Resulting From Brainstem Embolism in a Patient Undergoing Endovascular Abdominal Aortic Aneurysm Repair
Zaugg M, Lachat ML, Pfammatter T, et al (Univ Hosp Zurich, Switzerland)
Anesth Analg 92:335-337, 2001   5–16

Background.—Stent-graft procedures are increasingly being used to repair abdominal aortic aneurysms (AAAs) because of the reduced perioperative stress response, the improved intraoperative hemodynamic stability, and the decreased incidence of embolic complications associated with this approach. A case of an extremely rare fatal intraoperative cerebral insult in a patient undergoing endovascular AAA repair was reported.

Case Report.—Man, 72, was admitted for coronary revascularization and repair of a 2 × 5 cm infrarenal AAA. The patient's medical history included previous myocardial infarction, mild renal insufficiency, and pulmonary embolism as a result of a deep venous thrombosis of his right leg about 1 year earlier. The patient underwent uneventful coronary artery bypass surgery with revascularization of the left descending and left circumflex coronary arteries. Significant atheromatous plaques were observed by intraoperative transesophageal echocardiography (TEE) in the aortic arch and the descending thoracic aorta. Postoperative TEE demonstrated decreased anterolateral hypokinesia and a slightly improved ejection fraction of 70%. The increasing and partially thrombosed infrarenal AAA was repaired during the same hospital stay by means of endovascular technique. The procedure was performed in the patient under monitored anesthesia care by using IV analgesia with remifentanil and local anesthetic infiltration with lidocaine 0.5% in the right and left groins. During preparation of the operative field, the patient was completely free of pain, responsive, and breathing adequately, with an oxygen saturation of more than 95%. After 90 minutes, the endovascular prosthesis was deployed via the right common femoral artery and positioned by means of balloon inflation, with the proximal end below the lower renal artery. The patient began to gasp for breath and within seconds stopped breathing. There were no signs of seizures. The mean arterial blood pressure was unchanged, but the heart rate was slightly decreased to 55 beats/min, and the oxygen saturation decreased to 83%. The patient was immediately ventilated by mask with 100% oxygen, and the trachea was intubated. Duplex sonography did not reveal any occlusion or uncommon flow patterns, and TEE demonstrated well-preserved cardiac function and no change in the pattern of atheromatous plaques in the aorta. The endograft procedure was completed. Postoperative CT demonstrated a massive ischemic brain stem insult with multiple foci, including the pons, cerebellum, and thalamus. A diagnosis of massive ischemic brain stem insult, likely the result of a thromboembolic event, was made. The patient died 3 days after the endovascular procedure.

Conclusions.—Cerebral embolization is a possibility during the critical episodes of endovascular repair of AAA and can be detected easily in a patient who is sedated but conscious. The potential mechanisms underlying this complication are both antegrade and retrograde migration of emboli released by surgical manipulations of the aorta. It is important to avoid the forceful large-volume flushing of aortic cannulas, particularly in patients with extensive luminal pathology of the aorta.

▶ Brain stem embolism is an extremely unusual cause of respiratory arrest, perhaps resulting from dislodgment of a plaque in the aorta and retrograde transmission caused by vigorous flushing. It's an interesting case report and one that any of us involved in anesthesia for endovascular surgery should read.

M. F. Roizen, MD

Carotid Endarterectomy in Diabetic Patients

Raimondo Pistolese G, Appolloni A, Ronchey S, et al (Univ of Rome)
J Vasc Surg 33:148-154, 2001   5–17

Objective.—The purpose of the current study was to identify the possible short- and long-term effects of diabetes on the outcome of carotid endarterectomy.

Methods.—Medical records were reviewed for 781 carotid endarterectomies (in 734 patients) performed by the same vascular surgeon in a university medical center between January 1994 and December 1998. Patients were divided into 2 groups: those with diabetes (n = 181 patients; 193 operations) and those without diabetes (n = 553; 588 operations). The 2 groups were similar with respect to mean age, male-female ratio, and contralateral lesions. The only significant differences were a higher prevalence of peripheral vascular disease and dyslipidemia in the diabetic group and a higher prevalence of hemispheric transient ischemic attacks among the nondiabetic patients. Carotid color duplex ultrasound scan had been performed in all patients, and in 56 patients from the diabetic group and 56 patients from the nondiabetic group (matched for age, sex, and contralateral lesions), the distal extension of the lesion from the carotid bifurcation had also been defined. Both of these subgroups were fully representative of their respective groups of origin. Carotid endarterectomy was performed after the induction of general anesthesia; electroencephalographic monitoring was continuous.

Results.—Except for the significantly higher prevalence of calcified plaques in the diabetic patients (P <.0001), the characteristics of the carotid disease in the 2 groups were similar. In the 56-member subgroups, 73.2% of the diabetic and 35.7% of the nondiabetic patients (P <.0001) had lesions extending more than 2 cm beyond the carotid bifurcation. Mean length of plaque beyond the bifurcation was 2.3 ± 0.09 cm for the diabetic and 1.7 ± 0.08 cm for the nondiabetic patients (P <.0001). Diabetes was the only factor significantly correlated with plaque length. In the diabetic subgroup, surgery was characterized by significantly longer carotid arteriotomies (P = .03) and clamp times (P < .003). Operative mortality was 1.5% in the diabetic group (2 myocardial infarctions + 1 stroke) and 0.5% in the nondiabetic group (1 myocardial infarction + 2 strokes; P value not significant); stroke rates were 1.5% (3 major strokes) and 0.5% (2 major strokes + 1 minor stroke), respectively (P = not significant). Long-term survival (5 years) was not significantly lower among the diabetic patients.

Conclusions.—Diabetes mellitus does not seem to significantly increase the surgical risk for carotid endarterectomy. The presence of more extensive plaques has no significant effect on the results of surgery.

▶ The authors state that survival is not any different for the diabetic patients, but that's based on inadequate statistics. If I was diabetic and had a 66% chance of having a heart attack versus a 50.8% in the rest of the group or had 3 times the mortality rate and 4 times the mobility, I would say that was an increased risk in diabetes. But the numbers don't allow them to find it. If you study too few patients, even if it is large in number—but too few with the disease, you're unlikely to find statistical differences. But this study, like every other in diabetics, has shown that diabetic patients have 3 to 10 times the morbidity and mortality for the same operation as non-diabetic patients. But it's all in the patients who have associated end-organ effects of diabetes, such as hypertension or renal dysfunction.

M. F. Roizen, MD

Impact of Increasing Comorbidity on Infrainguinal Reconstruction: A 20-Year Perspective
Conte MS, Belkin M, Upchurch GR, et al (Harvard Med School, Boston)
Ann Surg 233:445-452, 2001   5–18

Background.—During the past 20 years, these authors have noted that more patients are requiring treatment for infrainguinal arterial occlusive disease. These patients seem to have more comorbidities, and demographics appear to have shifted as well (eg, more women are being treated). Changes in demographics and risk factors and their impact on surgical outcomes of patients undergoing lower extremity vascular reconstruction (LER) were reviewed over a 20-year period at Brigham and Women's Hospital in Boston.

Methods.—Medical records were used to identify all patients who had undergone LER by means of an autogenous vein conduit between 1978 and 1997. For analysis, patient data were examined in 4 time frames: 1978 to 1982 (group 1), 1983 to 1987 (group 2), 1988 to 1992 (group 3), and 1993 to 1997 (group 4). Patient demographics, risk factors, and outcomes were compared among these 4 intervals.

Results.—Between 1978 and 1997, 1274 patients underwent 1642 autogenous vein LER procedures at the authors' institution. Follow-up was complete for 70% of patients overall (mean follow-up, 968 days), including 56%, 68%, 63%, and 82% of patients in groups 1, 2, 3, and 4, respectively. Compared with groups 1 and 2, patients in group 4 were significantly older (median age, 65 and 67 vs 70 years, respectively); more likely to be female (26% and 40% vs 47%); and more likely to have diabetes mellitus (37% and 36% vs 52%), prior coronary artery bypass grafting (6% and 5% vs 21%), and renal insufficiency (6% and 7% vs 21%).

These changes in patient demographics and risk factors were reflected by changes in indications and procedural variables. When groups 1 and 2 were compared with group 4, the proportion of patients undergoing LER for claudication decreased significantly (30% and 31% vs 20%), whereas the proportions of patients undergoing LER for ulceration (18% and 20% vs 37%) or tissue necrosis (31% and 35% vs 53%) increased significantly. As time passed, the use of nonreversed greater saphenous vein (0% and

5% vs 38%) and ectopic (4% and 3% vs 7%) or composite (0.4% and 2% vs 12%) vein grafts increased significantly. In addition, the level of outflow used during LER became more distal, and significantly more tibial/pedal outflow sites were used in the most recent interval (23% and 45% vs 68%).

Despite these trends, the surgical mortality rate remained unchanged throughout this period, at 2%. The incidence of complications decreased as well, and a significant decrease was seen in early graft occlusion between groups 1 and 4 (9% vs 5%). The patient survival rate did not differ significantly according to interval (overall 5-year survival, 70%) nor did primary graft patency (overall at 5 years, 63%), secondary graft patency (overall at 5 years, 73%), or limb salvage rates (overall at 5 years, 85%).

However, among LER procedures performed exclusively for limb salvage indications, 5-year limb salvage rates improved significantly between the earliest and latest intervals (75% vs 86%). Finally, the length of the hospital stay decreased significantly between groups 3 and 4 (from 15.7-11.7 days, which is a 25% decrease).

Conclusion.—The demographics and risk factors of patients undergoing LER procedures have changed substantially over the past 20 years. The management of these patients is increasingly complex, yet the safety, durability, and effectiveness of LER with autogenous vein grafts has remained consistently excellent.

▶ This is a fascinating study because it shows that infrainguinal vascular reconstruction over a 20-year period was progressively done in older patients (the average age of patients got older by 4.5 years). This is a change that you would expect to more than double morbidity and mortality rates, but it didn't. This shows the incredible benefits of excellent anesthesia and ICU care, as well as, perhaps, surgical techniques.

M. F. Roizen, MD

Cardiac Response and Complications During Endovascular Repair of Abdominal Aortic Aneurysms: A Concurrent Comparison With Open Surgery

Cuypers PWM, Gardien M, Buth J, et al (Catharina Hosp, Eindhoven, The Netherlands; St Joseph Hosp, Veldhoven, The Netherlands; Erasmus Univ, Rotterdam, The Netherlands)
J Vasc Surg 33:353-360, 2001   5–19

Purpose.—The purpose of this study was to assess and to compare perioperative changes in left ventricular function and the incidence of adverse cardiac events in 2 groups of patients with abdominal aortic aneurysms, 1 during endovascular aneurysm repair (EAR) and the other during open aneurysm repair (OAR).

Methods.—One hundred twenty consecutive patients who underwent EAR (49 patients) or OAR (71 patients) were prospectively studied. During the operation, the left ventricular function was assessed by the recording of the left ventricle stroke work index (SWI) and the cardiac index (CI) with a pulmonary artery catheter. Measurements were performed before, during, and after stent-graft deployment or aortic cross-clamping. Both maneuvers were defined as aortic occlusion (AO). Transesophageal echocardiography was performed to identify signs of wall motion abnormalities of the left ventricular wall, which indicated myocardial ischemia. Six-lead electrocardiograph monitoring was maintained until discharge from the intensive care unit. Postoperative cardiac complications were diagnosed by clinical observation, 12-lead ECG analysis at 1, 3, and 7 days after the operation, transthoracic echocardiography at 1 month, and measurement of cardiac enzymes.

Results.—The 2 study groups were comparable with regard to most clinical aspects. Baseline myocardial performance was worse in patients who underwent EAR compared with patients who underwent OAR, as indicated by a reduced SWI (33.1 and 37.4, respectively; $P = .03$). During AO there was a comparable increase of the CI in both groups. However, after AO the rise in CI was higher in patients who underwent OAR compared with patients who underwent EAR (0.7 and 0.2, respectively; $P <.01$), representing a more pronounced hyperdynamic state. In addition, the SWI demonstrated a decrease in patients who underwent OAR compared with an increase in patients who underwent EAR during AO (-1.4 and $+1.9$, respectively; $P = .04$) and after AO (-0.9 and $+2.6$, respectively; $P = .01$). These findings represent more severe myocardial stress in patients who underwent OAR. The incidence of postoperative clinical cardiac adverse events was comparable in the 2 study groups. However, myocardial ischemia, as indicated by electrocardiography and transesophageal echocardiography, had a higher incidence in patients who underwent open surgery as compared with patients whose condition was managed endovascularly (57% and 33%, respectively; $P = .01$).

Conclusion.—Hemodynamic alterations during endovascular repair were not as severe as those in patients with open surgery and indicated less myocardial stress in the former category. These findings may explain a lower incidence of myocardial ischemia that was observed during endovascular repair. A lower frequency of clinical perioperative cardiac events in patients undergoing endovascular treatment may ultimately be expected.

▶ Although the hemodynamic changes weren't that severe in the endovascular group, the perioperative events, the ICU stay, and other factors, except for total hospital stay, were the same between groups. While the hospital stay in the endovascular group was 5 days, it was 11 days in the open group. Because this is extremely long compared with that I'm used to, I'd say that both can be shortened dramatically.

M. F. Roizen, MD

Perioperative Activation of Hemostasis in Vascular Surgery Patients

Samama CM, Thiry D, Elalamy I, et al (La Pitié-Salpêtrière Hosp, Paris; Hôtel-Dieu Hosp, Paris)
Anesthesiology 94:74-78, 2001   5–20

Background.—It is possible that the perioperative activation of hemostasis could have an important role in the occurrence of postoperative cardiac events. Some studies have observed extensive changes in the plasma levels of coagulation factors and in thromboelastographic parameters leading to a hypercoagulable state, and impaired postoperative fibrinolysis has been reported in patients undergoing vascular surgery. Many studies have documented an increase in platelet response in patients with ischemic heart disease or peripheral vascular disease. However, few studies have addressed perioperative platelet function. Platelet function, coagulation, and fibrinolysis status were assessed during and after infrarenal aortic surgery.

Methods.—Blood samples were obtained from 17 patients before induction of anesthesia (T1), 1 hour after incision (T2), 1 hour after extubation (T3), 24 hours postoperatively (T4), 48 hours postoperatively (T5), and at day 7 (T6). Tests that were performed included platelet count, platelet aggregation, platelet flow cytometry for CD62 and CD63, usual coagulation tests, thrombin-antithrombin complexes, and plasminogen activator inhibitor 1.

Results.—A significant increase in adenosine diphosphate–induced platelet aggregation occurred postoperatively at T4 and T5 that was not associated with an alteration in flow cytometry profile. No increase in levels of thrombin-antithrombin complexes was observed. A higher fibrinogen rate was noted at T5 and T6, and greater amounts of plasminogen activator inhibitor 1 were detected at T3 and T4. Thrombin generation was limited and fibrinolysis was impaired in the postoperative period. Flow cytometry demonstrated that platelets were not activated postoperatively, but aggregation studies indicated that they were prone to activation.

Conclusions.—An association was observed between more easily activated platelets with a higher fibrinogen rate and temporary shutdown of fibrinolysis in the early postoperative period. This association may be indicative of an increased risk of thrombosis in patients undergoing major vascular surgery.

▶ This is an excellent study which confirms that platelet aggregation is increased postoperatively accompanied by a decrease in fibrinolysis. One wonders whether this occurs in patients undergoing more minor surgery-that is, less stressful surgery—as well as in patients undergoing vascular surgery. I wish there were a control group to look at to determine whether this phenomenon relates to the degree of stress the patient has, and whether it could be affected by stress-free anesthetic.

M. F. Roizen, MD

Long-term Use of a Left Ventricular Assist Device for End-Stage Heart Failure

Rose EA, for the Randomized Evaluation of Mechanical Assistance for the Treatment of Congestive Heart Failure (REMATCH) Study Group (Columbia Univ, New York; Brigham and Women's Hosp, Boston; Sharp Mem Hosp, San Diego, Calif; et al)
N Engl J Med 345:1435-1443, 2001   5–21

Background.—Many patients with end-stage heart failure receive a left ventricular assist device (LVAD) while awaiting cardiac transplantation.

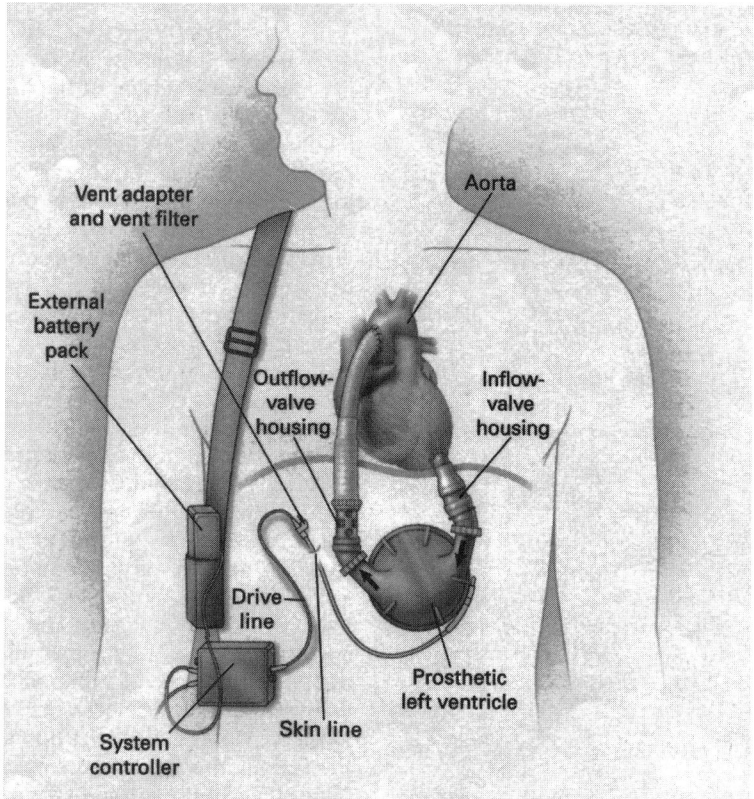

FIGURE 1.—Components of the left ventricular assist device. The inflow cannula is inserted into the apex of the left ventricle, and the outflow cannula is anastomosed to the ascending aorta. Blood returns from the lungs to the left side of the heart and exits through the left ventricular apex and across an inflow valve into the prosthetic pumping chamber. Blood is then actively pumped through an outflow valve into the ascending aorta. The pumping chamber is placed within the abdominal wall or peritoneal cavity. A percutaneous drive line carries the electric cable and air vent to the battery packs (only the pack on the right side is shown) and electronic controls, which are worn on a shoulder holster and belt, respectively. (Reprinted by permission of *The New England Journal of Medicine*, from Rose EA, for the Randomized Evaluation of Mechanical Assistance for the Treatment of Congestive Heart Failure (REMATCH) Study Group. *N Engl J Med* 345:1435-1443. Copyright 2001, Massachusetts Medical Society. All rights reserved.)

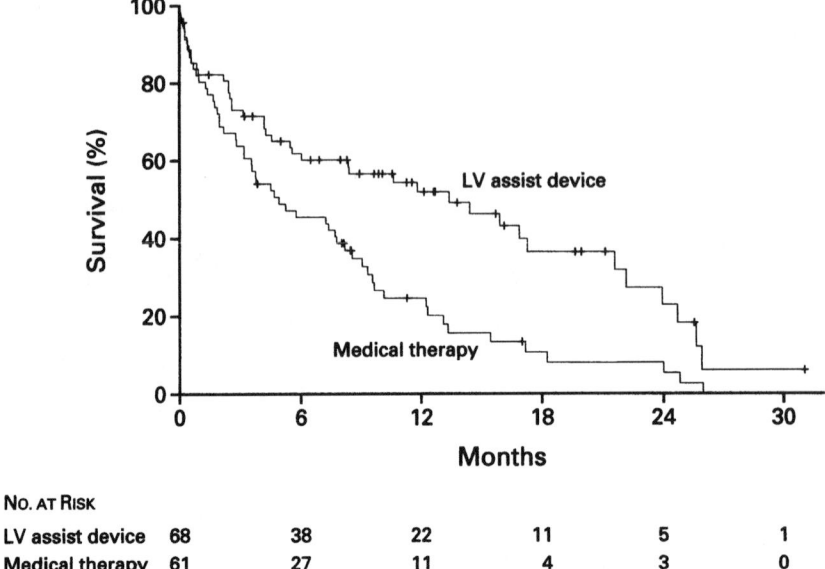

FIGURE 2.—Kaplan-Meier analysis of survival in the group that received left ventricular (LV) assist devices and the group that received optimal medical therapy. *Crosses* depict censored patients. Enrollment in the trial was terminated after 92 patients had died; 95 deaths had occurred by the time of the final analysis. (Reprinted by permission of *The New England Journal of Medicine*, from Rose EA, for the Randomized Evaluation of Mechanical Assistance for the Treatment of Congestive Heart Failure (RE-MATCH) Study Group. *N Engl J Med* 345:1435-1443, Copyright 2001, Massachusetts Medical Society. All rights reserved.)

Over the short term, LVADs normalize hemodynamics and provide a reasonable quality of life for these patients. Whether these devices have similar effects over a longer period and, thus, may be useful as myocardial replacement therapy for patients with end-stage heart failure who are ineligible for cardiac transplantation was examined in a multicenter, randomized trial.

Methods.—The research subjects were 129 adults with chronic end-stage heart failure (New York Heart Association class IV, left ventricular ejection fraction <25%) and contraindications for heart transplantation. Patients were randomly assigned to receive either optimal medical therapy (n = 61; 82% men; mean age, 68 years) or an LVAD (n = 68; 78% men; mean age, 66 years). The LVAD was a vented electric device that was implanted into a preperitoneal pocket or the peritoneal cavity (Fig 1). It was predetermined statistically that enrollment in the trial would end once 92 deaths had occurred. Patients were followed up to determine all-cause mortality, serious adverse events, quality of life, and functional status.

Results.—Kaplan-Meier estimates of survival were significantly higher in the LVAD group than in the medical therapy group both at 1 year (52% vs 25%) and at 2 years (23% vs 8%). The risk of all-cause mortality in the LVAD group was reduced by 48% compared with that in the medical therapy group (relative risk, 0.52) (Fig 2). Adverse events were significantly more common in the LVAD group (6.45 vs 2.75 events per patient-year; rate ratio, 2.35) and were primarily caused by infection, bleeding, and device malfunction. At 1 year, patients in the LVAD group reported significantly better quality of life and functional status compared with baseline than did patients in the medical therapy group.

Conclusions.—Long-term use of an LVAD significantly improved the survival rate, quality of life, and functional status in these patients with end-stage heart failure. Statistically, for every 1000 patients with end-stage heart failure, an LVAD could prevent 270 deaths annually compared with a treatment effect for β-blocker or angiotensin-converting enzyme therapy of 70 deaths per 1000 patients. However, use of an LVAD greatly complicates therapy and was associated with high rates of drive-line tract or pocket infection (0.41 events per patient-year), pump infection (0.23 events per patient-year), perioperative bleeding (0.46 events per patient-year), and LVAD dysfunction (0.75 events per patient-year). Nonetheless, an LVAD should be considered for select patients with end-stage heart failure who are ineligible for cardiac transplantation. In addition, given the shortfall in donor hearts, trials should be undertaken to compare the efficacy and safety of this approach with that of heart transplantation.

▶ LVADs have been used by many cardiac surgeons as a bridge to cardiac transplantation. This study suggests that they have benefit for patients with advanced heart failure who are not candidates for cardiac transplantation. At the present time, anesthesiologists in academic health centers see these patients relatively frequently. If this study can be extrapolated to all centers, then I predict that this operation will become more frequent.

M. Wood, MD, FRCA

Predictors of Atrial Fibrillation After Conventional and Beating Heart Coronary Surgery: A Prospective, Randomized Study
Ascione R, Caputo M, Calori G, et al (Bristol Royal Infirmary, England; San Raffaele Hosp, Milan, Italy)
Circulation 102:1530-1535, 2000   5–22

Introduction.—Atrial fibrillation (AF) is a common complication of coronary artery bypass grafting and increases the mortality rate in patients undergoing this procedure. Myocardial ischemia and inadequate cardioplegic protection of the atrium may increase the incidence of postoperative AF. The roles of cardiopulmonary bypass (CPB) and cardioplegic arrest in the pathogenesis of AF were examined.

Methods.—Between March 1997 and August 1998, 200 of 538 patients undergoing first-time bypass grafting were randomly assigned to receive myocardial revascularization with either (1) on-pump conventional surgery (normothermic CPB and cardioplegic arrest of the heart) or (2) off-pump surgery on the beating heart. Mean patient age for both groups was 63 years. Heart rate and rhythm were continuously monitored with an

TABLE 3.—Postoperative Arrhythmias

Variable	On Pump (n = 100 Patients)	Off Pump (n = 100 Patients)	P*
Arrhythmia incidence, n	49	14	0.001
Total AF, n	45	11	0.001
Sustained AF, n	39	8	0.001
Unsustained AF, n	6	3	0.3
Duration of sustained AF, h	14 (6-67)	13 (8-71)	0.3
Atrial flutter, n	2	1	0.8
Transient second-degree AV block, n	1	1	1.0
Third-degree AV block, n	1	1	1.0
Permanent pacemaker, n	1	1	1.0
Temporary pacing over first 24 h	7	1	0.03

Data are presented as median with minimum-maximal values or number of patients (in parentheses).
*χ^2 test.
(Courtesy of Ascione R, Caputo M, Calori G, et al: Predictors of atrial fibrillation after conventional and beating heart coronary surgery: A prospective, randomized study. *Circulation* 102:1530-1535, 2000.)

automated arrhythmia detector during the first 72 postoperative hours. Patients underwent routine clinical evaluation. Continuous monitoring was performed in the presence of arrhythmias. The relation between perioperative factors and AF was examined by univariate analysis. Significant variables were included in a stepwise logistic regression model to determine their independent effect on the occurrence of AF.

Results.—There were no significant between-group differences at baseline in age, sex, severity of coronary disease, diabetes mellitus, angina class, or surgical data, including number of distant anastomoses. Thirty-nine and 8 patients, respectively, in the on-pump and off-pump groups had sustained postoperative AF (P = .001) of similar duration (Table 3). Compared with the on-pump group, the off-pump group had decreased inotropic use, chest infection, blood loss and transfusion requirement, intubation time, and length of ICU and hospital stay (Table 4). Univariate

TABLE 4.—Postoperative Data

Variable	On Pump (n = 100)	Off Pump (n = 100)	P*
Deaths	2	0	0.7
MI	4	1	0.2
Chest infection	22	8	0.006
Transient stroke	2	2	1.0
Inotropic requirement	23	6	0.001
Total blood loss, mL	900 (90-4220)	690 (110-2300)	0.0001
Intubation time, h	8 (3-192)	6 (3-21)	0.0001
ICU length of stay, d	1 (1-8)	1 (0-6)	0.0001
Hospital length of stay, d	7 (5-17)	5 (4-23)	0.0001

Data are presented as median with minimum-maximal values or number of patients (in parentheses).
*Mann-Whitney or χ^2 test.
(Courtesy of Ascione R, Caputo M, Calori G, et al: Predictors of atrial fibrillation after conventional and beating heart coronary surgery: A prospective, randomized study. *Circulation* 102:1530-1535, 2000.)

analysis revealed that CPB inclusive of cardioplegic arrest, postoperative inotropic support, intubation time, chest infection, and hospital length of stay were predictors of AF (all $P < .05$). Stepwise multivariate analysis showed that CPB inclusive of cardioplegic arrest was the primary independent predictor of postoperative AF (OR, 7.4; CI, 3.4-17.9).

Conclusion.—CPB inclusive of cardioplegic arrest is the primary independent predictor of postoperative AF in patients undergoing coronary revascularization.

Influence of Diabetes on Mortality and Morbidity: Off-Pump Coronary Artery Bypass Grafting Versus Coronary Artery Bypass Grafting With Cardiopulmonary Bypass
Magee MJ, Dewey TM, Acuff T, et al (Cardiopulmonary Research and Technology Inst, Dallas)
Ann Thorac Surg 72:776-781, 2001   5–23

Introduction.—Myocardial revascularization in patients with diabetes is challenging. No established optimum treatment approach exists. Eliminating cardiopulmonary bypass (CPB) in coronary artery bypass grafting (CABG) usually has favorable outcomes on morbidity and mortality rates, but some findings conflict or are confusing. Experience with CABG was reviewed to ascertain the influence of eliminating CPB on outcomes in diabetic versus nondiabetic patients.

Methods.—Between January 1995 through December 1999, 9965 patients underwent isolated CABG; 2891 (29%) patients had diabetes. Diabetic and nondiabetic patients were further classified according to CPB use. Twelve percent (346 of 2891) of diabetic and 12% (829 of 7074) of nondiabetic patients underwent CABG without CPB; the remaining patients underwent CABG with CPB. Nineteen preoperative variables were compared among treatment groups by univariate analysis.

TABLE 4.—Significant Postoperative Complications and Outcomes

Variable	Diabetic OPCABG	Diabetic CABG-CPB	*p* Value	Nondiabetic OPCABG	Nondiabetic CABG-CPB	*p* Value
LOS*	6.6 ± 5.96	7.8 ± 6.27	0.1100	5.9 ± 4.83	7.2 ± 6.40	0.0001
ARDS	0.58%	1.14%	0.3411	0.36%	1.78%	0.0024
MI	1.16%	1.61%	0.5208	0.97%	1.97%	0.0437
Atrial fibrillation	15.90%	23.26%	0.002	19.66%	22.59%	0.0584
RF-Dialysis	0.87%	2.75%	0.0361	0.97%	1.28%	0.4403
Prolonged ventilation	6.94%	12.10%	0.0047	4.83%	9.45%	0.0001
Blood use	34.39%	58.47%	0.0001	29.31%	54.27%	0.0001

*Days in hospital from operation to discharge. Data are mean ± SD.
Abbreviations: ARDS, adult respiratory distress syndrome; *LOS,* length of stay; *MI,* myocardial infarction; *OPCABG,* CABG without CPB; *RF-dialysis,* renal failure requiring dialysis.
(Courtesy of Magee MJ, Dewey TM, Acuff T, et al: Influence of diabetes on mortality and morbidity: Off-pump coronary artery bypass grafting versus coronary artery bypass grafting with cardiopulmonary bypass. *Ann Thorac Surg* 72:776-781, 2001. Reprinted with permission of the Society of Thoracic Surgeons.)

Results.—Patients who underwent CABG without CPB had nonsignificantly higher mean predicted mortality rates versus those who underwent CABG with CPB (diabetic, 3.96% vs 3.72%, $P = .83$; nondiabetic, 3.03% vs 2.86%, $P = .79$). In nondiabetic patients, CABG without CPB offers an actual and risk-adjusted survival advantage over CABG with CPB (1.81% vs 3.44%, $P = .0127$; risk-adjusted mortality rate, 1.79% vs 3.61%, $P = .007$). The survival benefit of CABG without CPB was not observed in patients with diabetes (2.89% vs 3.69%, $P = .452$; risk-adjusted mortality rate, 2.19% vs 2.98%, $P = .42$). Diabetic patients who underwent CABG without CPB had fewer complications, including reduced blood product use (34.39% vs 58.4%; $P = .001$) and decreased incidence of prolonged ventilation (6.94% vs 12.10%; $P = .005$), and renal failure necessitating dialysis (0.87% vs 2.75%; $P = .036$) (Table 4).

Conclusion.—The survival advantage in nondiabetic patients who undergo CABG without CPB is not observed in patients with diabetes. Why this occurs is not understood. By contrast, CABG without CPB in diabetic patients is correlated with a significant decrease in morbidity rate.

Perfusion-Assisted Direct Coronary Artery Bypass: Selective Graft Perfusion in Off-Pump Cases

Guyton RA, Thourani VH, Puskas JD, et al (Emory Univ, Atlanta)

Ann Thorac Surg 69:171-175, 2000   5–24

Introduction.—Hemodynamic instability during multivessel off-pump coronary artery bypass grafting can produce hypotension, progressive myocardial ischemia, further hypotension, and requirement for cardiopulmonary bypass. An adjunctive technology in multivessel off-pump coronary artery bypass has been used that promotes early perfusion and rapid recovery of grafted segments that may reduce ischemia during subsequent anastomoses. Reported are the initial 10 patients in whom this selective graft perfusion technology was used.

Methods.—The perfusion-assisted direct coronary artery bypass system (Fig 1) uses a servo-controlled pump to allow delivery of blood at systemic or suprasystemic pressures and allows the option for infusion of supplemental additives for myocardial resuscitation, myocardial vasodilation, and enhancement of myocardial performance.

Results.—Myocardial perfusion was successfully enhanced with 1 or 2 grafts in all 10 patients. The average graft flow was 98 mL/min. A 27% increase in perfusion pressure produced a 59% increase in perfusate flow in 3 patients. All patients were hemodynamically stable after selective graft perfusion was started.

Conclusion.—The selective perfusion of grafted vessels appears to facilitate multivessel off-pump coronary artery bypass grafting. The advantages to this approach are (1) immediate perfusion of grafted myocardial regions to meet oxygen demands and prevent cumulative ischemic dysfunction; (2) enhanced hemodynamic stability during multivessel grafting;

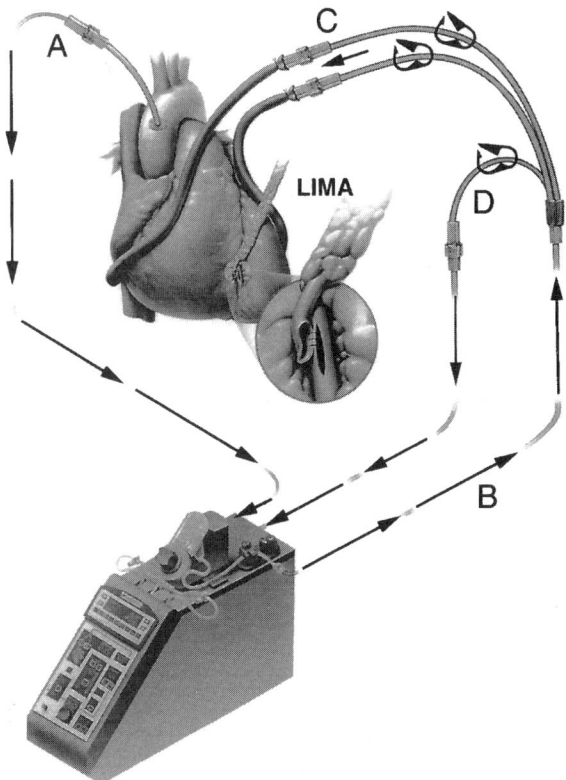

FIGURE 1.—Perfusion-assisted direct coronary artery bypass system. Aortic blood is directed from aortic cannula (**A**) through the Quest MPS to the multiple perfusion set (**B**) and finally the proximal vein or arterial grafts (**C**). Vein infusion pressure is monitored by the MPS system from a feedback line (**D**) located at the proximal portion of the multiple perfusion set. (Courtesy of Guyton RA, Thourani VH, Puskas JD, et al: Perfusion-assisted direct coronary artery bypass: Selective graft perfusion in off-pump cases. *Ann Thorac Surg* 69:171-175, 2000. Reprinted by permission of the Society of Thoracic Surgeons.)

(3) potential for administration of drugs in the perfusate that can facilitate recovery and function; and (4) a logistic advantage to the surgeon regarding the appropriate sequence of grafting.

Off-Pump Coronary Artery Bypass Grafting Decreases Risk-Adjusting Mortality and Morbidity

Cleveland JC Jr, Shroyer ALW, Chen AY, et al (Univ of Colorado, Denver; Duke Univ, Durham, NC)
Ann Thorac Surg 72:1282-1289, 2001   5–25

Introduction.—Cardiopulmonary bypass (CPB) can induce a proinflammatory state with various adverse consequences. CPB-associated death includes neurologic dysfunction, pulmonary dysfunction, renal dysfunction, and possibly infectious-related complications. Off-pump coronary

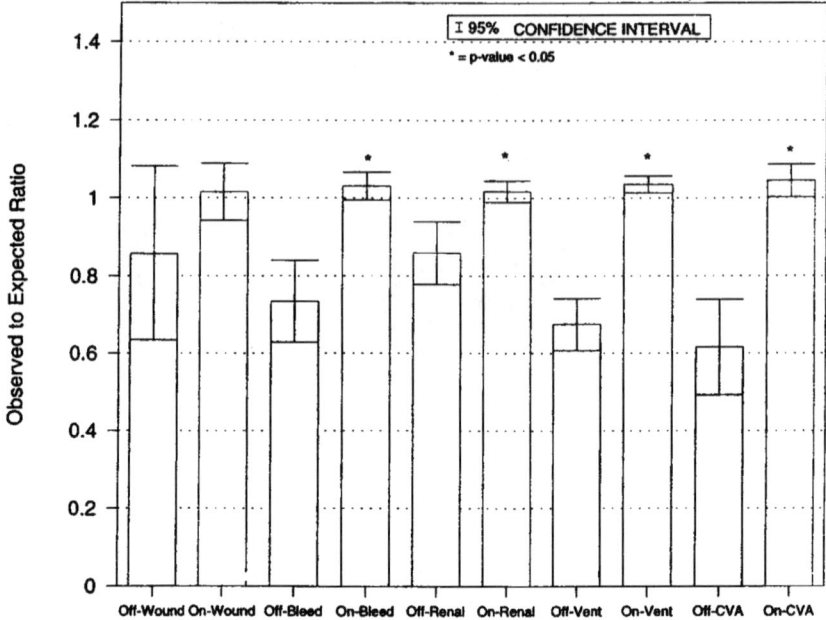

FIGURE 2.—Observed-to-expected ratio of the 5 major complications. Graph shows effect of off-pump CABG in decreasing observed-to-expected occurrences of acute postoperative renal failure; bleeding complications; cerebral vascular accidents (*CVA*), such as stroke or coma; and prolonged ventilator dependence. There was no observed decrease in deep sternal infections between the 2 groups. *, $P < .05$ between on and off-pump groups. (Courtesy of Cleveland JC Jr, Shroyer ALW, Chen AY, et al: Off-pump coronary artery bypass grafting decreases risk-adjusting mortality and morbidity. *Ann Thorac Surg* 72:1282-1289, 2001. Reprinted with permission of the Society of Thoracic Surgeons.)

artery bypass grafting (CABG) was examined to ascertain if it reduces risk-adjusted operative death and major complications in selected patients.

Methods.—Data from January 1, 1998, through December 31, 1999, were obtained from the Society of Thoracic Surgeons National Adult Cardiac Surgery Database. Outcomes were compared for conventional

TABLE 4.—Comparison of Key Morbidity Types

Major Morbidity Type (%)	Off-Pump Patients	On-Pump Patients	*p* Value
Neurologic (CVA/stroke)	1.25	1.99	< 0.001
Renal (postoperative ARF)	3.85	4.26	0.036
Infection (mediastinitis)	0.55	0.68	0.121
Cardiac (postoperative arrest)	1.42	1.74	0.010
Respiratory (prolonged mechanical ventilation)	4.13	6.51	< 0.001
Bleeding (reexploration)	2.07	2.80	< 0.001

Abbreviations: ARF, acute renal failure; *CVA,* cerebrovascular accident.
(Courtesy of Cleveland JC Jr, Shroyer ALW, Chen AY, et al: Off-pump coronary artery bypass grafting decreases risk-adjusting mortality and morbidity. *Ann Thorac Surg* 72:1282-1289, 2001. Reprinted with permission of the Society of Thoracic Surgeons.)

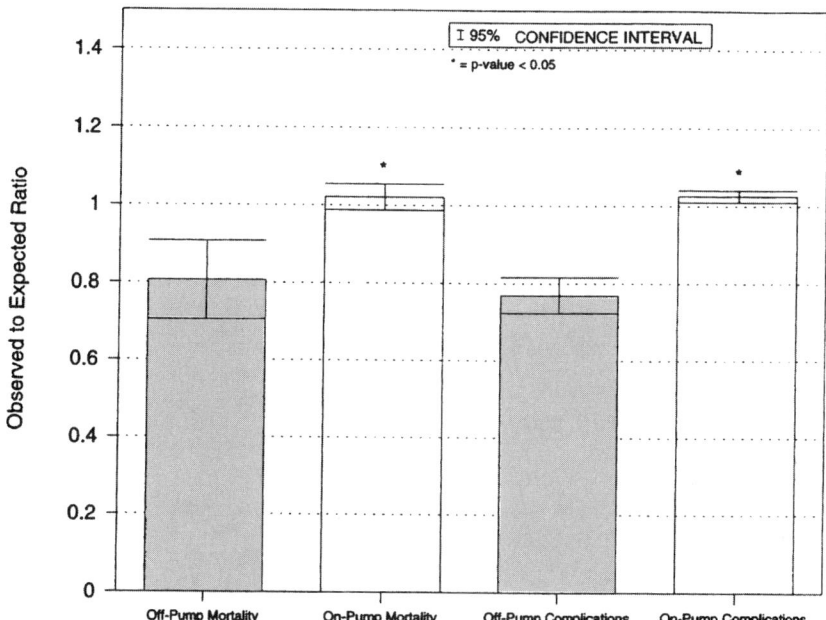

FIGURE 1.—Observed-to-expected ratio of death and any major complications. Shown is effect of off-pump CABG in decreasing observed-to-expected death and occurrence of any of the 5 major complications analyzed. *, *P* < .05 between on-pump and off-pump groups. (Courtesy of Cleveland JC Jr, Shroyer ALW, Chen AY, et al: Off-pump coronary artery bypass grafting decreases risk-adjusting mortality and morbidity. *Ann Thorac Surg* 72:1282-1289, 2001. Reprinted with permission of the Society of Thoracic Surgeons.)

versus off-pump CABG procedures. Death and major complications were assessed, both as unadjusted rates and after adjusting for known baseline patient risk factors.

Results.—Data were available from 126 experienced centers that performed a total of 118,140 CABG procedures. Of these, 9.9% (11,717)

TABLE 6.—Subgroup Analysis for Risk of Renal, Neurologic, and Pulmonary Complications in Patients With Preoperative Risk Factors

Percent Morbidity in Subgroup at Risk	Off-Pump	On-Pump	*p* Value
Percent with postop renal failure with baseline creatinine > 1.5	16.2	18.9	0.14
Percent with postop CVA with CVD	2.5	4.6	> 0.001
Percent with postop ventilator dependence with COPD	8.9	11.3	< 0.001

Abbreviations: COPD, chronic obstructive pulmonary disease; *CVA,* cerebrovascular accident; *CVD,* cerebrovascular disease; *postop,* postoperative.

(Courtesy of Cleveland JC Jr, Shroyer ALW, Chen AY, et al: Off-pump coronary artery bypass grafting decreases risk-adjusting mortality and morbidity. *Ann Thorac Surg* 72:1282-1289, 2001. Reprinted with permission of the Society of Thoracic Surgeons.)

were off-pump CABG procedures. The use of an off-pump procedure was correlated with a reduction in risk-adjusted operative death (2.9% with conventional CABG vs 2.3% in the off-pump group; $P < .001$). Use of an off-pump procedure reduced the risk-adjusted major complication rate from 14.15% with conventional CABG to 10.62% for the off-pump group ($P < .0001$) (Fig 2) (Table 4). Patients who underwent off-pump procedures were less likely to die (adjusted OR, 0.81; 95% CI, 0.70-0.91) and less likely to have major complications (adjusted OR, 0.77; 95% CI, 0.72-0.82) (Fig 1) (Table 6).

Conclusion.—Off-pump CABG is correlated with reduced mortality and morbidity rates after CABG. This approach may be superior to conventional CABG in selected patients.

Off-Pump Coronary Artery Bypass Is Associated With Improved Risk-Adjusted Outcomes

Plomondon ME, Cleveland JC Jr, Ludwig ST, et al (Univ of Colorado, Denver; Dept of Veterans Affairs Med Ctr, Denver; Univ of Alabama, Birmingham)
Ann Thorac Surg 72:114-119, 2001   5–26

Introduction.—Since April 1987, the Continuous Improvement in Cardiac Surgery Program (CICSP) has collected data concerning risk, descriptive procedural classification, and outcome data on all cardiac surgical procedures performed within the Department of Veterans Affairs (VA) medical centers. These data were used to examine the impact of off-pump median sternotomy coronary artery bypass grafting (CABG) procedures on rates of risk-adjusted mortality and morbidity compared with conventional on-pump procedures. The impact of off-pump procedures on resource consumption was evaluated.

Methods.—CICSP data from October 1997 through March 1999 were used to evaluate 9 VA centers that performed at least 8% CABG procedures off-pump. By using all other 34 VA cardiac surgery programs, baseline logistic regression models were created to predict the risk of 30-day operative mortality and morbidity. These models were used to predict patient outcomes at the 9 centers being evaluated. A final model assessed the impact of the off-pump approach within the 9 centers, adjusting for preoperative risk. A total of 680 patients were treated off-pump and 1733 were treated on-pump.

Results.—Patients in the off-pump group had lower 30-day complication (8.8% vs 14.0%; $P = .001$) and mortality (2.7% vs 4.0%; $P .101$) rates compared with the on-pump group. Risk-adjusted morbidity and mortality rates were better in the off-pump versus on-pump group (0.52 and 0.56 multivariable odds; $P = .05$), respectively. Patients in the off-pump group were more likely to be emergent and had a higher frequency of chronic obstructive pulmonary disease, a higher rate of diuretic use,

TABLE 1.—Comparison of Off-Pump and On-Pump Patients in the Study Population

Preoperative Clinical Risk Variable	Off-Pump (n = 680)	On-Pump (n = 1733)	p Value
Priority of surgery			0.016
Elective	78.1	82.8	
Urgent	15.2	12.6	
Emergent	6.8	4.6	
Angina functional class			0.001
I	5.2	11.4	
II	13.5	18.5	
III	34.0	32.5	
IV	47.4	37.6	
COPD	36.2	22.8	0.001
Diabetes	31.3	36.7	0.048
Congestive heart failure (NYHA FC)			0.001
I	44.1	60.7	
II	29.1	22.9	
III	19.0	12.4	
IV	7.8	4.1	
Creatinine			0.046
< 1.5	84.0	86.5	
1.5-3.0	14.0	12.6	
> 3.0	2.1	0.9	
Current digoxin use	9.4	7.0	0.049
Current diuretic use	26.8	21.4	0.004
Three or more major arteries with stenosis > 50%	66.5	74.1	0.001
CICSP CABG-only mortality risk estimate	4.4	3.9	0.0022
CICSP CABG-only morbidity risk estimate	13.2	11.9	0.0008

Note: Values expressed as percentages unless otherwise indicated.
Abbreviations: COPD, chronic obstructive pulmonary disease; NYHA FC, New York Heart Association functional class.
(Courtesy of Plomondon ME, Cleveland JC Jr, Ludwig ST, et al: Off-pump coronary artery bypass is associated with improved risk-adjusted outcomes. *Ann Thorac Surg* 72:114-119, 2001. Reprinted by permission of the Society of Thoracic Surgeons.)

worse ratings for angina function and congestive heart failure, and generally fewer major arteries with stenosis greater than 50% (Table 1). The preoperative length of stay for patients without a catheterization procedure performed during the same admission was significantly longer for off-pump versus on-pump procedures ($P < .0001$). There were no between-group differences in preoperative length of stay for patients with catheterization during the same admission ($P = .11$). The postoperative length of stay was significantly shorter for the off-pump group versus the on-pump group ($P = .0005$). The percent of same-day surgeries was significantly lower for the off-pump versus on-pump group (20.6% vs 27.6%; $P = .001$). The operating room time was significantly less for the off-pump vs on-pump group ($P = .0001$) (Table 4). Generally, the observed-to-expected ratio was less than 1 for off-pump patients and more than 1 for on-pump

TABLE 4.—Resource Consumption Use: Nine Study Hospitals

Variable	Off-Pump			On-Pump			p Value
	Mean	SD	Median	Mean	SD	Median	
% Same-day surgery*	20.6%			27.6%			0.001
Postoperative length of stay (days)†	9.2	11.0	6	10.8	15.2	7	0.0005
Operating room time (hours)‡	4.0	1.1	4.0	2.8	54.9	4.5	0.0001

*χ^2 test.
†Survival analysis.
‡Wilcoxon rank sum test.
(Courtesy of Plomondon ME, Cleveland JC Jr, Ludwig ST, et al: Off-pump coronary artery bypass is associated with improved risk-adjusted outcomes. *Ann Thorac Surg* 72:114-119, 2001. Reprinted by permission of the Society of Thoracic Surgeons.)

patients for both 30-day operative death and perioperative morbidity outcomes (Fig 1).

Conclusion.—An off-pump approach for CABG procedures is correlated with lower risk-adjusted morbidity and mortality rates. Improvements in several resource consumption measures may be realized when using an off-pump procedural approach.

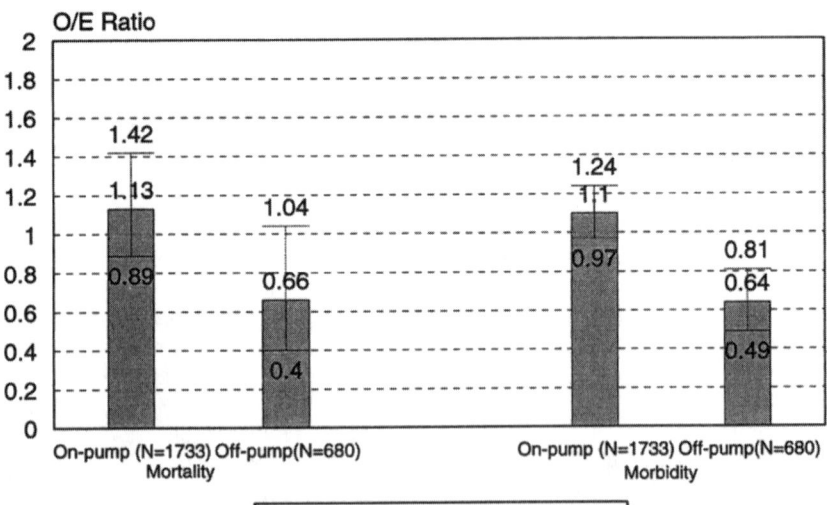

FIGURE 1.—Observed-to-expected (O/E) ratios for on-pump versus off-pump patients. *Bars*, mean values; *lines*, 95% confidence intervals (CI). (Courtesy of Plomondon ME, Cleveland JC Jr, Ludwig ST, et al: Off-pump coronary artery bypass is associated with improved risk-adjusted outcomes. *Ann Thorac Surg* 72:114-119, 2001. Reprinted by permission of the Society of Thoracic Surgeons.)

Clinical Outcomes, Angiographic Patency, and Resource Utilization in 200 Consecutive Off-Pump Coronary Bypass Patients
Puskas JD, Thourani VH, Marshall JJ, et al (Emory Univ, Atlanta)
Ann Thorac Surg 71:1477-1484, 2001   5–27

Introduction.—Although several reports on off-pump coronary artery bypass grafting (OPCAB) have noted excellent mortality rates, there is concern over a reduction in graft patency rates. Clinical outcome and resource utilization were retrospectively compared in patients undergoing OPCAB versus conventional coronary artery bypass grafting (CABG). Angiographic patency was documented in patients who underwent OPCAB.

Methods.—Data were collected concerning 200 consecutive patients who underwent OPCAB between April 1997 and November 1999. These findings were compared with those from a matched control group of 1000 patients undergoing CABG. Patients were matched for age, sex, pre-existing disease (renal failure, diabetes, pulmonary disease, stroke, hypertension, peripheral vascular disease, and previous myocardial infarction), and primary or repeat status. Follow-up was 93% and an average of 13.4 months in the OPCAB group.

Results.—Hospital death, postoperative stroke, myocardial infarction, and re-entry for bleeding were rare in the OPCAB group (1.0%, 1.5%, 1.0%, and 1.5%, respectively). Compared with the conventional CABG group, the OPCAB group had reduced rates of transfusion (70.0% vs 33.0%; P = .001) (Table 3) and deep sternal wound infection (2.2% vs 0%; P = .067). Angiography was performed before hospital discharge for 421 grafted arteries in 167 patients (83.5%) in the OPCAB group. All except 5 arteries were patent (98.8%) (93.3% FitzGibbon A, 5.5% FitzGibbon B, 1.2% FitzGibbon O). All 163 internal mammary artery grafts were patent. The OPCAB group had a lower rate of hospital stay compared with the CABG group (5.7 vs 3.9 days; P < .001). Hospital cost was 15% less in the OPCAB versus CABG group ($14,898 vs $17,501; P < .001).

Conclusion.—Hospital cost, postoperative length of stay, and morbidity rate are lower with OPCAB than with CABG. A large, prospective, ran-

---

TABLE 3.—Transfusion Requirements

Variable	OPCAB (%)	CABG (%)	*p* Value
Any transfusion	33.0	70.0	< 0.001
Packed RBCs	33.0	69.0	< 0.001
Platelets	3.5	16.19	< 0.001
FFP	1.5	5.3	0.032
Cryoprecipitate	0.5	6.7	< 0.001

Abbreviations: FFP, fresh frozen plasma; *RBC*, red blood cells.
(Courtesy of Puskas JD, Thourani VH, Marshall JJ, et al: Clinical outcomes, angiographic patency, and resource utilization in 200 consecutive off-pump coronary bypass patients. *Ann Thorac Surg* 71:1477-1484, 2001. Reprinted with permission of the Society of Thoracic Surgeons.)

domized, longitudinal comparison of graft patency and clinical outcomes after coronary bypass surgery performed with and without the use of cardiopulmonary bypass is needed to validate the safety, efficacy, and superiority of the off-pump approach.

Further Reduction in Stroke After Off-Pump Coronary Artery Bypass Grafting: A 10-Year Experience
Trehan N, Mishra M, Sharma OP, et al (Escorts Heart Inst and Research Centre, New Delhi, India)
Ann Thorac Surg 72:S1026-S1032, 2001   5–28

Introduction.—The rate of neurologic complications after conventional coronary artery bypass grafting (CABG) is between 3% and 7%. The aorta has been shown to be a risk of atheroemboli and a risk factor for perioperative stroke (25% in patients with mobile plaques of aortic arch). Carotid artery stenosis is often linked to severe aortic atherosclerosis, yet has a positive predictive value of only between 16% to 57%. The incidence of neurologic sequelae were examined in patients who underwent off-pump coronary artery bypass (OPCAB).

Methods.—Between January 1990 and September 2000, 2800 patients underwent OPCAB among 18,037 who underwent CABG during that 10-year period. Initially, OPCAB was performed selectively in patients at high risk (including having atheromatous aorta, renal impairment, and chronic obstructive pulmonary disease as well as being octogenarians). Multivessel OPCABs were performed electively in approximately 60% to 65% of patients who underwent CABG during the latter part of the evaluation period (Fig 1).

Results.—Neurologic complications, including stroke and transient ischemic attack, occurred in 0.14% of patients (Table 6). The overall hospital mortality rate was 2.14% (Table 8) for the OPCAB group; the neurologic complications rate was 0.07%. By using the National Society of Thoracic Surgeons Cardiac Surgery Database Risk Model for CABG, the predicted mortality rate for the entire patient cohort was 3.86% ($P <$ .001).

Conclusion.—These data strongly support the use of OPCAB to further decrease the rate of stroke after CABG, particularly in high-risk patients.

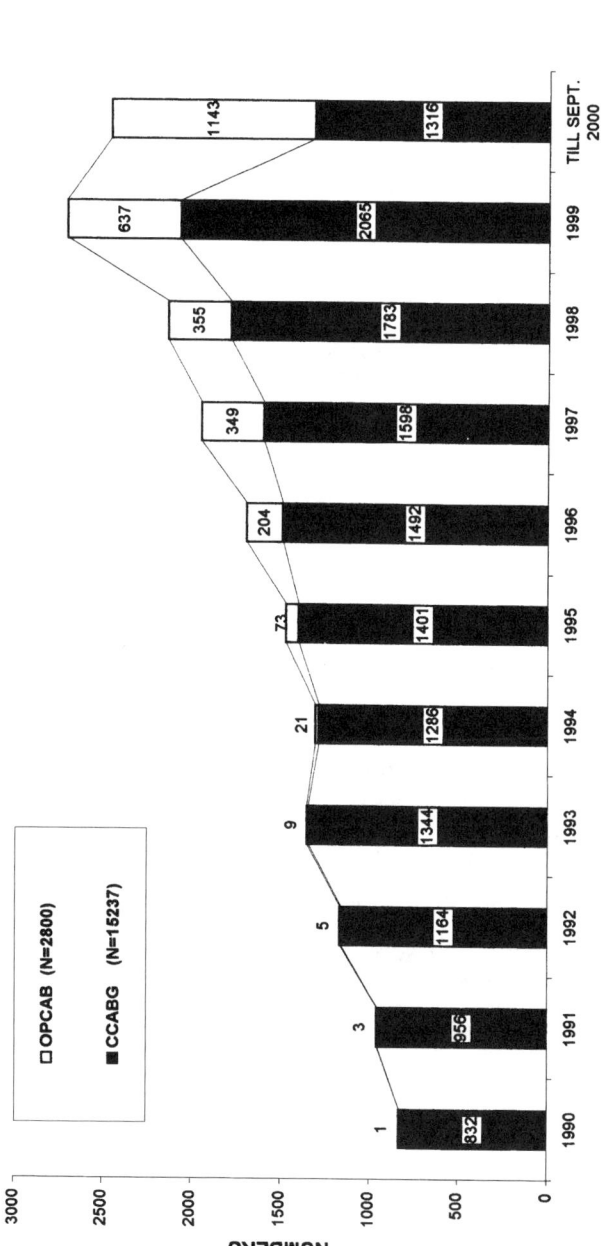

FIGURE 1.—Comparative growth of off-pump CABG over a 10-year period (1990 to 2000). N = 18,037. *Abbreviation: CCABG,* conventional CABG. (Courtesy of Trehan N, Mishra M, Sharma OP, et al: Further reduction in stroke after off-pump coronary artery bypass grafting: A 10-year experience. *Ann Thorac Surg* 72:S1026-S1032, 2001. Reprinted with permission of the Society of Thoracic Surgeons.)

TABLE 6.—Postoperative Complications and 30-Day Mortality
Rate (n = 2800)

Complication	n	Percent (%)
Blood transfusion requirement	540	19.28
Reexplorations	31	1.10
Wound infection	27	0.96
Superficial	13	0.46
Deep	14	0.50
Renal dysfunction	148	5.28
Perioperative myocardial infarction	30	1.07
Ventricular arrhythmias	31	1.10
Prolonged ventilation	30	1.07
Tracheostomy	18	0.64
Average ICU stay (hours)	41 ± 11.4	
Average hospital stay (days)	6.8 ± 1.3	
Mortality	60	2.14

(Courtesy of Trehan N, Mishra M, Sharma OP, et al: Further reduction in stroke after off-pump coronary artery bypass grafting: A 10-year experience. *Ann Thorac Surg* 72:S1026-S1032, 2001. Reprinted by permission of the Society of Thoracic Surgeons.)

TABLE 8.—Causes of Death After CABG (n = 60)

Causes	n
Cardiac	19
Neurological	2
Pulmonary	7
Renal	9
Multiorgan failure	23

(Courtesy of Trehan N, Mishra M, Sharma OP, et al: Further reduction in stroke after off-pump coronary artery bypass grafting: A 10-year experience. *Ann Thorac Surg* 72:S1026-S1032, 2001. Reprinted by permission of the Society of Thoracic Surgeons.)

Coronary Artery Bypass Performed Without the Use of Cardiopulmonary Bypass Is Associated With Reduced Cerebral Microemboli and Improved Clinical Results

Bowles BJ, Lee JD, Dang CR, et al (Univ of Hawaii, Honolulu)
Chest 119:25-30, 2001

5–29

Introduction.—Microembolic phenomena have been recognized as unwanted complications of cardiopulmonary bypass (CPB) and may even be a source of neurologic complications in patients who undergo CPB. The results of off-pump coronary artery bypass (OPCAB) were compared with those of traditional coronary artery bypass grafting (CABG) to ascertain whether, and to what degree, OPCAB diminishes the cerebral microembolic burden.

Methods.—Data from 137 patients who underwent CABG were retrospectively reviewed. Of these, 70 underwent elective CABG and 67 underwent OPCAB. Forty patients underwent transcranial Doppler ultrasonography (20 CABG, 20 OPCAB). They were continuously monitored intraoperatively for the occurrence and pattern of cerebral microemboli. The quantity and distribution of microemboli were compared. Factors related to increasing numbers of microemboli were examined.

Results.—Patients did not differ significantly in age, sex, or underlying comorbidities. The CABG group had a slightly lower preoperative ejection fraction (50.9% vs 55.5%; $P = .03$). Compared with the CABG group, the OPCAB group had significant reductions in cerebral microemboli (27 vs 1766; $P = .003$) (Table 3), transfusion requirement (29.9% vs 47.1%; $P = .04$), intubation time (3.3 vs 9.5 hours; $P < .001$), ICU length of stay (1.5 vs 2.8 days; $P = .02$), and overall hospitalization (4.9 vs 6.6 days; $P = .01$) without an increase in mortality rate (Table 2). The OPCAB group had nonsignificantly fewer strokes and deaths than the CABG group.

Conclusion.—A significant reduction in the number of microemboli and a trend toward a decrease in the stroke rate was observed in patients undergoing OPCAB compared with CABG. The clinical significance of the dramatic decrease in cerebral microemboli has yet to be determined.

TABLE 3.—Comparison of Microemboli OPCAB vs CABG

Microemboli	OPCAB (n = 20)	CABG (n = 20)	p Value
Mean No. of emboli/patient	27 ± 35	1766 ± 2455	0.003
Median No. of emboli/patient	12	1041	
Range	0 to 133	131 to 10703	
Distribution of microemboli (mean)			
	Left MCA	Right MCA	p Value
OPCAB	12 ± 13 (42%)	17 ± 26 (58%)	NS
CABG	1237 ± 1608 (56%)	975 ± 1238 (44%)	NS

(Courtesy of Bowles BJ, Lee JD, Dang CR, et al: Coronary artery bypass performed without the use of cardiopulmonary bypass is associated with reduced cerebral microemboli and improved clinical results. *Chest* 119:25-30, 2001.)

TABLE 2.—Comparison of Operative Results and Complications

Variable	OPCAB (n = 67)	CABG (n = 70)	p Value
No. of grafts	2.5 ± 0.9	3.0 ± 0.8	0.004
Required transfusion, %	29.9	47.1	0.04
Intubation postoperatively, h	3.3 ± 7.4	9.5 ± 8.1	<0.001
ICU stay, d	1.5 ± 1.0	2.8 ± 4.2	0.02
Total length of stay, d	4.9 ± 2.2	6.6 ± 4.2	0.01
Atrial fibrillation, %	32.8	34.3	NS
CVA, %	0	2.9	NS
Death, %	0	2.9	NS

Abbreviations: CVA, cerebrovascular accident.
(Courtesy of Bowles BJ, Lee JD, Dang CR, et al: Coronary artery bypass performed without the use of cardiopulmonary bypass is associated with reduced cerebral microemboli and improved clinical results. *Chest* 119:25-30, 2001.)

Analysis of Hemodynamic Changes During Beating Heart Surgical Procedures

Mathison M, Edgerton JR, Horswell JL, et al (Cardiopulmonary Research Science and Technology Inst, Dallas)
Ann Thorac Surg 70:1355-1361, 2000   5–30

Introduction.—Coronary artery bypass grafting on the beating heart produces significant hemodynamic compromises during displacement of the heart. The exact mechanisms that cause altered hemodynamics are not

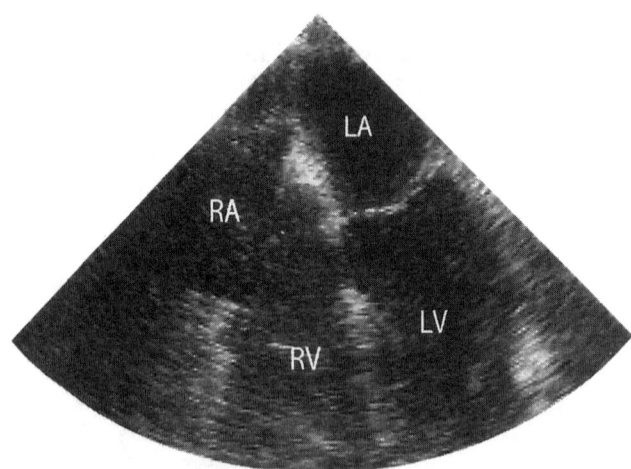

FIGURE 2.—Preoperative transesophageal midesophageal 4-chamber echocardiogram. *Abbreviations: RA,* right atrium; *RV,* right ventricle; *LA,* left atrium; *LV,* left ventricle. (Courtesy of Mathison M, Edgerton JR, Horswell JL, et al: Analysis of hemodynamic changes during beating heart surgical procedures. *Ann Thorac Surg* 70:1355-1361, 2000. Reprinted by permission of the Society of Thoracic Surgeons.)

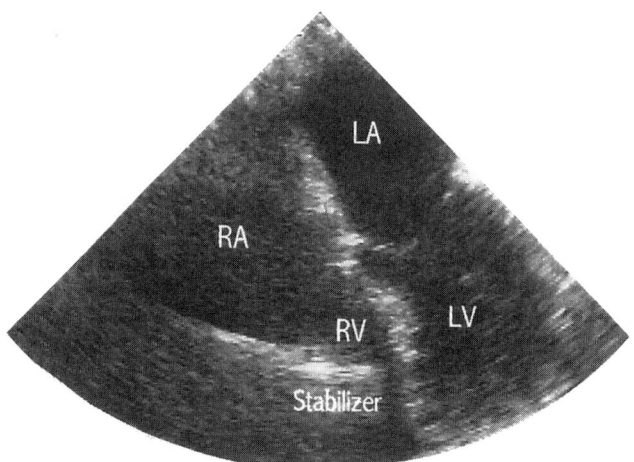

FIGURE 4.—Transesophageal midesophageal 4-chamber echocardiogram for a very proximal posterior descending artery positioning. *Abbreviations: RA*, right atrium; *RV*, right ventricle; *LA*, left atrium; *LV*, left ventricle. (Courtesy of Mathison M, Edgerton JR, Horswell JL, et al: Analysis of hemodynamic changes during beating heart surgical procedures. *Ann Thorac Surg* 70:1355-1361, 2000. Reprinted by permission of the Society of Thoracic Surgeons.)

well understood. The hemodynamic changes caused by displacing the heart were assessed in 44 patients undergoing beating-heart surgeries.

Methods.—The patients were 35 men and 9 women with a mean age of 64.5 years. Intraoperative transesophageal echocardiography was performed in 31 patients (Fig 2). Hemodynamic variables were measured before and after positioning the heart for anastomosis of the left anterior, descending, circumflex, and posterior descending coronary arteries.

Results.—During positioning for all vessels, right ventricular end-diastolic pressure rose significantly (Fig 4) (Table 3); left ventricular end-diastolic pressure rose significantly during positioning for the left anterior descending and circumflex coronary arteries (Fig 1). Positioning for the circumflex artery demonstrated the highest rise in left and right ventricular end-diastolic pressure, resulting in the greatest hemodynamic compromise (Fig 3).

TABLE 3.—Comparison of Hemodynamic Changes on the Basis of Ejection Fraction

Group	ΔMAP (mm Hg)			ΔCO (L/min)		
	CX	PDA	LAD	CX	PDA	LAD
EF ≤ 40	−12.1 ± 22.0	−1.2 ± 10.8	−9.1 ± 15.8	−1.98 ± 1.52	−0.10 ± 1.15	−0.73 ± 1.19
EF > 40	−18.8 ± 18.1	−12.2 ± 14.8	−2.7 ± 18.0	−1.16 ± 1.08	−1.46 ± 1.27	−0.42 ± 1.27

Abbreviations: CO, cardiac output; ΔCO, (CO during positioning) - (CO of baseline); CX, circumflex artery; EF, ejection fraction; LAD, left anterior descending artery; MAP, mean arterial pressure; ΔMAP, (MAP during positioning) - (MAP of baseline); PDA, posterior descending artery.

(Courtesy of Mathison M, Edgerton JR, Horswell JL, et al: Analysis of hemodynamic changes during beating heart surgical procedures. *Ann Thorac Surg* 70:1355-1361, 2000. Reprinted by permission of the Society of Thoracic Surgeons.)

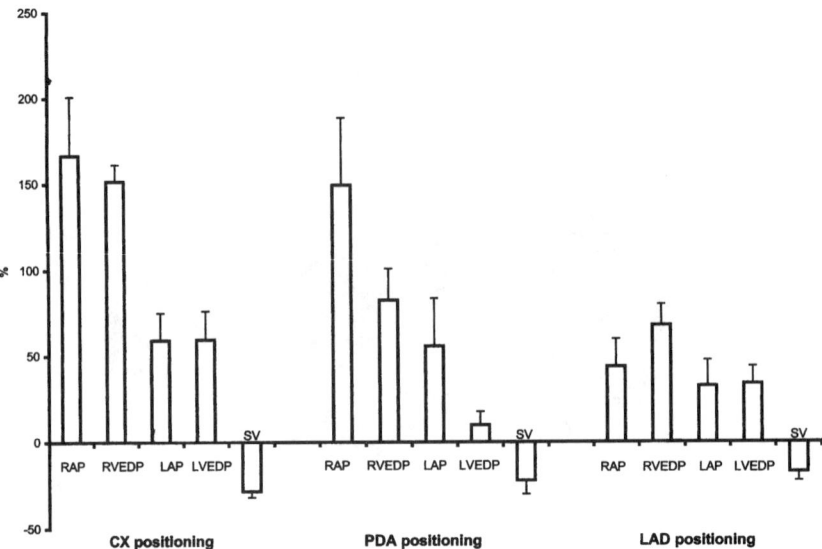

FIGURE 1.—Hemodynamic changes during positioning of heart. Graphs are mean + SE for a percentage of baseline values. *Abbreviations: RAP*, right arterial pressure; *RVEDP*, right ventricular end-diastolic pressure; *LAP*, left arterial pressure; *LVEDP*, left ventricular end-diastolic pressure; *SV*, stroke volume; *CX*, circumflex artery; *PDA*, posterior descending artery; *LAD*, left anterior descending artery. (Courtesy of Mathison M, Edgerton JR, Horswell JL, et al: Analysis of hemodynamic changes during beating heart surgical procedures. *Ann Thorac Surg* 70:1355-1361, 2000. Reprinted by permission of the Society of Thoracic Surgeons.)

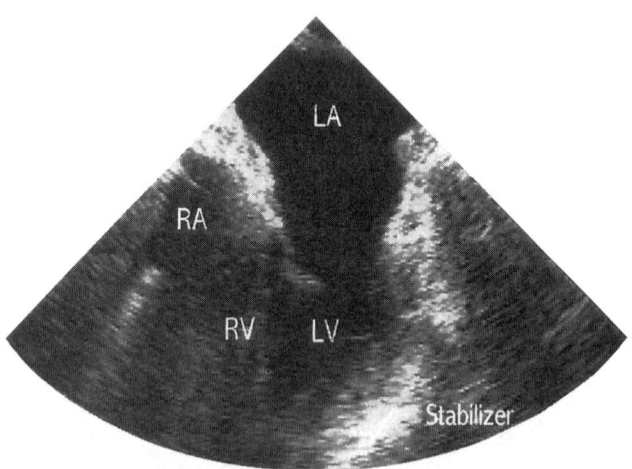

FIGURE 3.—Transesophageal midesophageal 4-chamber echocardiogram for circumflex positioning. *Abbreviations: RA*, right atrium; *RV*, right ventricle; *LA*, left atrium; *LV*, left ventricle. (Courtesy of Mathison M, Edgerton JR, Horswell JL, et al: Analysis of hemodynamic changes during beating heart surgical procedures. *Ann Thorac Surg* 70:1355-1361, 2000. Reprinted by permission of the Society of Thoracic Surgeons.)

Conclusion.—There is a biventricular contribution to altered hemodynamics when displacing the heart during off-pump coronary artery bypass grafting. The increase in right ventricular end-diastolic pressure in all positions indicates that the most important cause of hemodynamic change is disturbed diastolic filling of the right ventricle, particularly by direct ventricular compression.

Heart Displacement During Off-Pump CABG: How Well Is It Tolerated?
Nierich AP, Diephuis J, Jansen EWL, et al (Utrecht Univ, The Netherlands)
Ann Thorac Surg 70:466-472, 2000   5–31

Introduction.—Heart displacement during off-pump coronary artery bypass grafting (CABG) is required to expose the sites of anastomosis. The hemodynamic consequences of cardiac dislocation and stabilization in relation to the location of the anastomoses were examined, along with the mechanisms of cardiovascular changes.

Methods.—The association between surgical exposure and hemodynamic management was examined in 150 consecutive patients undergoing off-pump CABG with the Octopus Tissue Stabilization System. Surgical access was achieved by either anterolateral thoracotomy (ALT group) or medial sternotomy (STERN group).

Results.—Surgical exposure by ALT demonstrated no significant hemodynamic changes. With the STERN approach, stroke volume was significantly decreased by dislocation at all target sites: 6% at the left anterior descending artery (LAD), 25% at the diagonal branch artery (D), 14% at the right coronary artery (RCA), and 21% at the obtuse marginal artery (OM). The most challenging site to graft on the beating heart was the posterior wall. The first phase of rotating and elevating the heart to inspect the OM vessels compressed the heart and produced hemodynamic deterioration (Fig 3). Head-down positioning (LAD, 56%; D, 74%; RCA, 90%; OM, 96%) increased surgical exposure and preload, creating correction of ventricular filling pressures and output. Some patients required dopamine 3 to 5 µg/kg per minute to maintain baseline hemodynamic values (LAD, 5%; D, 15%; RCA, 7%; OM, 28%).

Conclusion.—Revascularization during ALT was not eventful. STERN caused right heart compression. Fluid redistribution was adequate to correct cardiac output. Once stabilized, systemic circulation was unchanged during revascularization.

▶ Atrial fibrillation (AF) is the most common complication occurring after cardiac surgery.[1,2] Despite advances in CPB, cardioplegia, and surgical techniques, the incidence has paradoxically increased in recent years as the result of CABG patients being older.[3] The first selection, from Ascione et al (Abstract 5–22), is one of the best thus far regarding off-pump coronary artery bypass (OPCAB). The literature is replete with either retrospective or nonrandomized "series" describing outcomes. By contrast, this manuscript

FIGURE 3

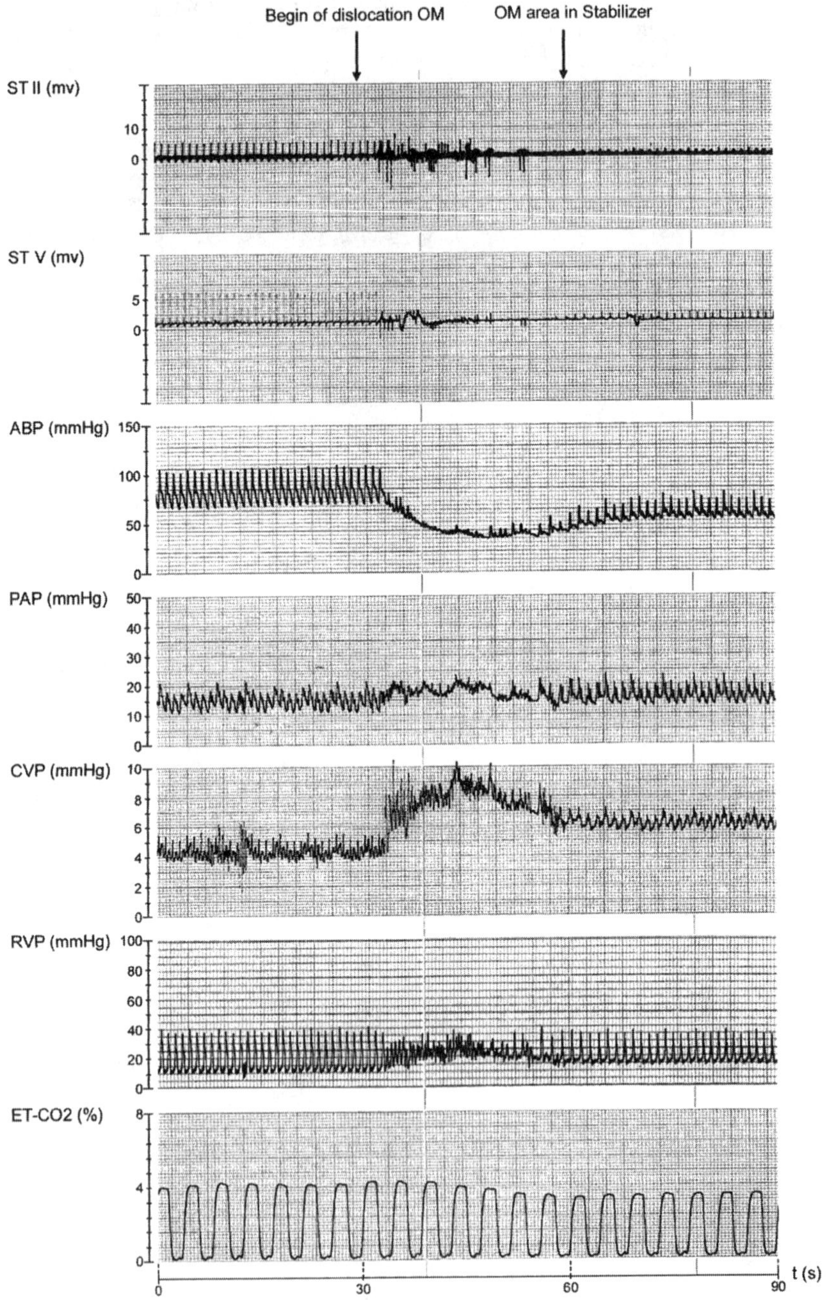

(Continued)

tackles a significant question—that of AF after CABG. The study is well designed and carefully carried out. The conclusions are well supported by the research. Several subsequent papers have concluded the opposite, but are of inferior study design.[4,5] An excellent review of the subject was recently published that should be read by those interested in this costly event.[6] Further articles are reviewed below.

Coronary artery disease (CAD) is a significant problem for diabetics that tends to be extensive and involves multiple vessels. The Bypass Angioplasty Revascularization trial data suggest a decreased mortality rate in diabetics when CABG is used to treat CAD compared with angioplasty.[7,8,9] The question then becomes: What type of surgical procedure should be performed in diabetics with CAD? Magee et al (Abstract 5–23) attempt to answer this question by using a nonrandomized retrospective analysis of 9965 patients undergoing CABG over a 5-year period by 22 different surgeons. The study suffers from surgical bias with surgeons using different selection criteria and having different outcomes. Despite these shortcomings, the study demonstrates a survival advantage in nondiabetics treated with OPCAB, fewer blood transfusions, decreased duration of postoperative ventilation, decreased length of stay, and—as in the last article—a decreased incidence of AF. All these findings are consistent with other studies. In contrast, OPCAB in diabetics did not show a survival advantage, but the group did have a lower mortality rate. Of interest, there was no difference in outcomes between diabetics treated with insulin versus oral agents. Despite the flaws, this manuscript suggests that OPCAB may offer some advantage in diabetics, so the anesthesiologist can expect to care for these patients more often during OPCAB. Management of serum glucose during these procedures has not yet been studied.

Renal dysfunction after CABG is a costly complication associated with an increased postoperative mortality rate. The mechanism of this insult is unclear, but increased CPB time is associated with postoperative renal dysfunction.[10,11] Data were collected prospectively but reviewed retrospectively and used the institutions' first OPCAB cases. Earlier small series have suggested less renal insult with OPCAB.[12] This study compared preoperative and highest postoperative calculated creatinine clearances. This approach is reasonable and should detect renal function changes. The study conclusion that OPCAB does not offer renal protection is reasonable despite the shortcomings of the study design. The study did, however, confirm the findings of Mangano et al[11] that preoperative renal insufficiency, diabetes mellitus, and increasing age are risk factors for post-CABG renal dysfunction. Similar findings were noted in a recent series from Emory of 200 OPCAB patients in

---

FIGURE 3.—Acute hemodynamic alterations during tilting of heart to reach posterior wall. Note decrease of ECG voltage, mean arterial pressure (MAP), wedging of the pulmonary artery catheter, and the decrease of end-tidal carbon dioxide (ET-CO2) but increase of central venous pressure (CVP) during the phase of placement of the stabilizer by the surgeon. After placement, these values normalized. *Abbreviations: ABP*, arterial blood pressure; *PAP*, pulmonary artery pressure; *RVP*, right ventricular pressure. (Courtesy of Nierich AP, Diephuis J, Jansen EWL, et al: Heart displacement during off-pump CABG: How well is it tolerated? *Ann Thorac Surg* 70:466-472, 2000. Reprinted by permission of the Society of Thoracic Surgeons.)

which no difference in renal outcome was noted compared with patients undergoing CPB.[13]

Temporary occlusion of a coronary vessel in addition to nonanatomic positioning of the heart during grafting with OPCAB is of major concern. Various strategies have been developed to minimize risk during these periods, including coronary shunting, creative positioning/stabilization, and "proximals first." Emory is developing a new device, described by Guyton et al (Abstract 5–24), that allows selective perfusion of distal grafts through a computerized delivery system. This series, although small, suggests some additional use compared with other techniques. The authors mention (1) immediate perfusion of the grafted area, (2) enhanced hemodynamic stability, (3) a system to add medications directly to the myocardium at risk, and (4) increased flexibility for surgical sequence of grafting. I would add a fifth: only 1 aortic cross-clamping (partial occlusion) is necessary. I have witnessed several surgeons place the clamp on the aorta for every proximal vessel. I suspect that is not optimal from a central nervous system or embolic point of view. One could envision that future anesthesiologists might be called on to add medications directly into a similar system, and our understanding of drug delivery, therefore, would be very much altered by this technology. In addition, this system could potentially prevent the "crash on CPB" that occurs occasionally during OPCAB when a patient becomes unstable.

The media, as well as patients, is driving the increase in OPCAB procedures. Many manuscripts have reported improved clinical outcomes after OPCAB.[14-19] Most are retrospective or underpowered and include significant surgical selection bias. The report by Cleveland et al (Abstract 5–25), which uses the Society of Thoracic Surgeons voluntary database in 118,140 CABG procedures, is the largest to date and therefore probably is the best available. Many limitations are inherent: retrospective observational data, patient selection bias, differences in surgical technique, no evaluation of graft patency, and surgical experience. Despite the problems, the analysis suggests that OPCAB may reduce postoperative morbidity rates, mortality rates, and length of stay. OPCAB appears to have special value in patients with preexisting cerebrovascular and pulmonary disease. The authors speak of a mandate that a prospective, randomized trial be undertaken. I am aware of 2 large multicenter groups applying for funding to undertake such a study— spear-headed by an anesthesiologist!

In a similar study, Plomondon et al (Abstract 5–26) used the Veterans Affairs database to come to conclusions similar to those of Cleveland et al. Despite the OPCAB patients having higher estimated preoperative risk, both mortality and morbidity rates were lower in the OPCAB group. In addition, length of stay and operating room time were reduced in the OPCAB group. Taken together, the last 2 manuscripts present a strong argument that OPCAB improves outcomes and reduces costs. It is hoped that a true randomized trial, to decrease selection bias, will be funded in the near future. Long-term graft patency must also be addressed.

Puskas et al (Abstract 5–27), in a nonrandomized trial, again sees trends toward improved outcomes and decreased costs but in a single-surgeon series with a large level of experience. The outcomes were particularly striking for decreased wound infections, blood transfusion, and length of stay in the OPCAB group. I included this article because 83.5% of the OPCAB patients had postoperative angiography with results superior to traditional CABG.[20] Follow-up was more than 1 year, with excellent early outcomes. To date, the relatively limited amount of studies available suggests that OPCAB has the potential to achieve consistent good graft function. Again, a randomized trial of graft patency would be superior to this study, but I suspect the chance of that occurring is low because of costs and the increased risk to patients.

Neurologic injury after CABG continues to be a great source of frustration to all those involved. The mechanisms of neuropsychologic impairment after CABG are multifactorial, and the exact role of CPB in this is still controversial. OPCAB has been suggested as a possible way of improving neurologic outcome,[21] especially if aortic manipulation is reduced.[22] The reported incidence of neurologic complications after traditional CABG is 3% to 7%.[23-28] Trehan et al (Abstract 5–28), in a 10-year observational study of 2800 patients, had only a neurologic complication rate of 0.14%. Overall mortality rate was significantly lower than predicted by the Society of Thoracic Surgeons risk model. They attribute their success to the use of individualized surgical techniques with OPCAB and careful manipulation of the aorta. This manuscript highlights the potential for improved neurologic outcomes with OPCAB but by no means proves its superiority.

Murkin et al, in 1997, suggested that OPCAB could decrease the cerebral embolic load and improve outcomes.[29] Bowles et al (Abstract 5–29) sought to detect if patients revascularized with OPCAB would indeed have a reduced embolic load. The results that can be noted in their Table 3 were striking. Unfortunately, their study was retrospective and did not achieve significance for improved outcomes.

My residents often are skeptical when I tell them that the decrease in blood pressure, cardiac output, and SVO_2 are caused by right heart compression. Grundeman et al first described this in an animal model.[30] Mathison et al (Abstract 5–30), in a well-done study, is the first to investigate the phenomenon in human beings. Not only is the left ventricle involved, but also unlike in animals, Trendelenburg positioning did not restore cardiac output and SVO_2.

In contrast, the study by Nierich et al (Abstract 5–31) did see restoration of hemodynamics by the use of the Trendelenburg position. This article was included because it is a good review of surgical positioning and manipulations. Clearly, positioning of the heart, especially for the posterior circulation, is a surgical art that continues to evolve in both technique and technology (eg, the Starfish stabilizer).

In summary, observational studies have suggested a reduced incidence of pulmonary, renal, and neurologic damage after OPCAB. The few prospective randomized trials, including the recent van Dijk manuscript,[31] have shown no detectable differences in end-organ damage. Neurologic outcome was identical, as were neuropsychological and quality-of-life measures. This might be a result of the relatively small number of patients or, alternatively, the fact that there is no difference between the 2 groups in that regard. Cardiopulmonary bypass is also known to interfere with blood coagulation and therefore can cause excessive blood loss. Several studies have documented reduced blood loss or need for blood products in OPCAB. OPCAB is clearly establishing its position in the practice at many institutions, but we anesthesiologists should be aware of the controversies involved with its evolution.

M. F. Trankina, MD

References

1. Aranki SF, Shaw DP, Adams DH, et al: Predictors of atrial fibrillation after coronary artery surgery: Current trends and impact on hospital resources. *Circulation* 94:390-397, 1996.
2. Kalman JM, Munawar M, Howes LG, et al: Atrial fibrillation after coronary artery bypass grafting is associated with sympathetic activation. *Ann Thorac Surg* 60:1709-1715, 1995.
3. Creswell LL, Damiano RJ Jr: Postoperative atrial fibrillation: An old problem crying for new solutions. *J Thorac Cardiovasc Surg* 121:638-641, 2001.
4. Hravnak M, Hoffman LA, Saul MI, et al: Atrial fibrillation: Prevalence after minimally invasive direct and standard coronary artery bypass. *Ann Thorac Surg* 71:1491-1495, 2001.
5. Siebert J, Anisimowicz L, Lango R, et al: Atrial fibrillation after coronary artery bypass grafting: Does the type of procedure influence the early postoperative incidence? *Eur J Cardiothorac Surg* 19:455-459, 2001.
6. Maisel WH, Rawn JD, Stevenson WG: Atrial fibrillation after cardiac surgery. *Ann Intern Med* 135:1061-1073, 2001.
7. Brooks MM, Jones RI-I, Bach RG, et al: Predictors of morbidity and mortality from cardiac causes in the bypass angioplasty revascularization investigation (BARI) randomized trial and registry. *Circulation* 101:2682-2689, 2000.
8. Detre KM, Lombardero MS, Brooks MM, et al: The effect of previous coronary-artery bypass surgery on the prognosis of patients with diabetes who have acute myocardial infarction. Bypass Angioplasty Revascularization Investigation Investigators. *N Engl J Med* 342:989-997, 2000.
9. Gum PA, O'Keefe JH Jr, Borkon AM, et al: Bypass surgery versus coronary angioplasty for revascularization of treated diabetic patients. *Circulation* 96:II-10, 1997.
10. Conlon PJ, Stafford-Smith M, White WD, et al: Acute renal failure following cardiac surgery. *Nephrol Dial Transplant* 14:1158-1162, 1999.
11. Mangano CM, Diamondstone LS, Ramsay JG, et al: Renal dysfunction after myocardial revascularization: Risk factors, adverse outcomes, and hospital resource utilization. The Multicenter Study of Perioperative Ischemia Research Group. *Ann Intern Med* 128:194-203, 1998.
12. Ascione R, Lloyd CT, Underwood MJ, et al: On-pump versus off-pump coronary revascularization: Evaluation of renal function. *Ann Thorac Surg* 68:493-498, 1999.
13. Puskas JD, Thourani VII, Marshall JJ, et al: Clinical outcomes, angiographic patency, and resource utilization in 200 consecutive off-pump coronary bypass patients. *Ann Thorac Surg* 71:1477-1483, 2001.
14. Yokoyama T, Baumgarmer FJ, Gheissafi A, et al: Off-pump versus on-pump coronary bypass in high-risk subgroups. *Ann Thorac Surg* 70:1546-1550, 2000.
15. Arom KV, Flavin TF, Emery RW, et al: Is low ejection fraction safe for off-pump coronary bypass operation? *Ann Thorac Surg* 70:1021-1025, 2000.
16. Lee IH, Abdelhady K, Capdeville M: Clinical outcomes and resource usage in 100 consecutive patients after off-pump coronary bypass procedures. *Surgery* 128:548-555, 2000.

17. Arom KV, Flavin TF, Emery RW, et al: Safety and efficacy of off-pump coronary artery bypass grafting. *Ann Thorac Surg* 69:704-710, 2000.
18. Puskas JD, Wright CE, Ronson RS, et al: Clinical outcomes and angiographic patency in 125 consecutive off-pump coronary bypass patients. *Heart Surg Forum* 2:216-221, 1999.
19. Ascione R, Williams S, Lloyd CT, et al: Reduced postoperative blood loss and transfusion requirement after beating-heart coronary operations: A prospective randomized study. *J Thorac Cardiovasc Surg* 121:689-696, 2001.
20. The thrombolysis in Myocardial Infarction (TIMI) trial: Phase I findings. TIMI Study Group. *N Engl J Med* 312:932-936, 1985.
21. Gaudino M, Glieca F, Alessandrini F, et al: The unclampable ascending aorta in coronary artery bypass patients: A surgical challenge of increasing frequency. *Circulation* 102:1497-1502, 2000.
22. Hartman GS, Yao FS, Bruefach M, et al: Severity of aortic atheromatous disease diagnosed by transesophageal echocardiography predicts stroke and other outcomes associated with coronary artery surgery: A prospective study. *Anesth Analg* 83:701-708, 1996.
23. Breuer AC, Furlan AJ, Hanson MR, et al: Central nervous system complications of coronary artery bypass graft surgery: Prospective analysis of 421 patients. *Stroke* 14:682-687, 1983.
24. Gardner TJ, Horneffer PJ, Manolio TA, et al: Stroke following coronary artery bypass grafting: A ten-year study. *Ann Thorac Surg* 40:574-581, 1985.
25. Newman MF, Wolman P, Kanchuger M, et al: Multicenter preoperative stroke risk index for patients undergoing coronary artery bypass graft surgery. Multicenter Study of Perioperative Ischemia (McSPI) Research Group. *Circulation* 94:II74-II80, 1996.
26. Nussmeier NA: Adverse neurologic events: Risks of intracardiac versus extracardiac surgery. *J Cardiothorac Vasc Anesth* 10:31-37, 1996.
27. Roach GW, Kanchuger M, Mangano CM, et al: Adverse cerebral outcomes after coronary bypass surgery. Multicenter Study of Perioperative Ischemia Research Group and the Ischemia Research and Education Foundation Investigators. *N Engl J Med* 335:1857-1863, 1996.
28. Shaw PJ, Bates D, Cartlidge NE, et al: Early neurological complications of coronary artery bypass surgery. *Br Med J Clin Res Ed* 291:1384-1387, 1985.
29. Murkin JM: Attenuation of neurologic injury during cardiac surgery. *Ann Thorac Surg* 72:S1838-S1844, 2001.
30. Grundeman PF, Borst C, van Herwaarden JA, et al: Hemodynamic changes during displacement of the beating heart by the Utrecht Octopus method. *Ann Thorac Surg* 63:S88-S92, 1997.
31. van Dijk D, Nierich AP, Jansen EW, et al: Early outcome after off-pump versus on-pump coronary bypass surgery: Results from a randomized study. *Circulation* 104:1761-1766, 2001.

Safety and Efficacy of O-Raffinose Cross-Linked Human Hemoglobin (Hemolink™) in Cardiac Surgery

Cheng DCH (Univ of Toronto)

Can J Anesth 48:S41-S48, 2001

5–32

Introduction.—The search for a safe and effective oxygen therapeutic is spurred primarily by concerns regarding the risks associated with blood transfusion. There are presently 2 main classes of oxygen therapeutics: hemoglobin-based oxygen carriers (HBOCs) and synthetic perfluorocarbons (PFCs). Described is the use of o-raffinose cross-linked human hemoglobin (Hb raffimer) in cardiac surgery.

Methods.—The literature on HBOCs was reviewed and the development and clinical trials on Hb raffimer were examined.

Major Findings.—The benefits of HBOCs include bypassing of known viruses, pathogens, and cross-matching; increased stability and product storage times; and effective oxygen delivery to tissues. Limitations of HBOCs include binding the exogenous vasodilator nitric oxide, thus inducing transient hypertension, esophageal dysfunction, and abdominal discomfort. The short half-life of HBOCs makes them best suited for acute anemia.

The Hb raffimer is prepared from outdated red blood cells, cross-linked with o-raffinose, a polyaldehyde acquired from the oxidation of the trisaccharide raffinose. The Hb is a covalently cross-linked (β-β) within the 2,3 DPG binding pocket, which forms a stable 64 kDa tetramer.

More than 500 patients have been enrolled and more than 300 have received Hb raffimer. Preliminary evaluation of data from recent phase II and III clinical trials of Hb raffimer in routine coronary artery bypass grafting surgery indicate that HBOCs are well tolerated and may facilitate avoidance of allogeneic blood product transfusions in the surgical setting.

Conclusion.—The HBOCs have the potential to provide hemoglobin and oxygen carrying capacity to tissues to treat acute anemia during surgery. It may be that Hb raffimer will be used to facilitate intraoperative autologous donation and become an important alternative to allogeneic blood transfusions during cardiac surgery.

Intraoperative Plateletpheresis and Autologous Platelet Gel Do Not Reduce Chest Tube Drainage or Allogeneic Blood Transfusion After Reoperative Coronary Artery Bypass Graft
Wajon P, Gibson J, Calcroft R, et al (Royal Prince Alfred Hosp, Camperdown, NSW, Australia)
Anesth Analg 93:536-542, 2001   5–33

Background.—Platelet-rich plasma (PRP) is thought to reduce mediastinal chest tube drainage (MCTD) and allogeneic blood transfusions (ABT) after cardiopulmonary bypass surgery. However, a recent meta-analysis of available studies found few good-quality trials demonstrating this benefit. The effects of plateletpheresis on MCTD, ABT, and hemodynamic stability in patients undergoing reoperative coronary artery bypass grafting were documented.

Methods.—By random assignment, 90 patients received pheresis or no pheresis. All patients received ϵ-aminocaproic acid. Part of the sequestered platelet volume was used to make autologous platelet gel for use as a wound sealant.

Findings.—The mean pheresis yield was 30% of the circulating platelet mass, or 6.4 allogeneic platelet unit equivalents. The pheresis and control groups did not differ in total MCTD or mean packed red blood cell, platelet, or plasma transfusion rates. Fifty-two percent of the pheresis group and 55% of the control group received ABT. Fifty-three percent of the pheresis recipients and 27% of the control group had significant hemodynamic instability.

Conclusions.—Although plateletpheresis may offset platelet dysfunction from aspirin or increased blood exposure to nonbiologic surfaces, it did not reduce MCTD or ABT in the current series. The significantly increased incidence of hemodynamic instability in patients receiving pheresis in this trial underscores the need to determine risk-benefit ratios for cardiac surgical units.

Failure of Autologous Fresh Frozen Plasma to Reduce Blood Loss and Transfusion Requirements in Coronary Artery Bypass Surgery

Kasper S-M, Giesecke T, Limpers P, et al (Univ of Cologne, Germany)
Anesthesiology 95:81-86, 2001   5–34

Background.—Previous research has not shown that fresh frozen plasma (FFP) prophylaxis is beneficial in patients undergoing cardiopulmonay bypass (CPB) procedures. However, earlier studies have been retrospective or have used subtherapeutic doses of FFP. Whether a therapeutic dose of FFP decreases blood loss and transfusion requirements in patients undergoing elective coronary artery bypass surgery was investigated.

Methods.—Sixty adults were randomly assigned to receive an IV infusion of 15 mL/kg of autologous FFP or 6% hydroxyethyl starch 450/0.7 (HES) after CPB. Data on 56 patients who completed the study according to protocol were used in the final analysis.

Findings.—Median postoperative blood loss was 630 mL in the FFP group and 830 mL in the HES group. The groups did not differ significantly in postoperative or total perioperative erythrocyte transfusion requirements.

Conclusions.—Prophylactic administration of a therapeutic dose of autologous FFP after CPB did not decrease blood loss or transfusion needs in these patients undergoing uncomplicated, elective, primary coronary artery bypass surgery. This use of FFP exposes patients to unnecessary risks and increases costs.

▶ Blood transfusion and conservation continue to be of concern both to anesthesiologists and our patients. Risk of infection and cost have continued to drive the search to prevent reliance on allogeneic blood transfusion.[1] Pharmacologic methods, such as the use of aprotinin and ε-aminocaproic acid, were introduced in the 1980s. During the 1990s, efforts were focused on blood substitutes. Hemolink is 1 approach that appears to have promise. Cheng (Abstract 5–32) nicely reviews the studies to date involving this compound. It has been safely used in hundreds of patients and appears to significantly reduce the transfusion of allogeneic blood during coronary artery bypass grafting (CABG). Hemolink is now undergoing FDA phase II trials here in the United States in CABG patients. I look forward to the future when we can offer our patients an alternative to RBC transfusion. This article was part of an excellent supplement on blood conservation in cardiac surgery that should be read by all who take care of cardiac patients.[2-6]

Over the last 2 decades various approaches to blood conservation have come and gone. Attempts to protect platelet number and function during cardiopulmonary bypass have been described since 1977. Newer technologies have emerged to increase yields and ease of use.[7] Wajon et al (Abstract 5–33) have described the best study of plateletpheresis to date despite several problems. The study was not blinded, no intraoperative salvage was used, and ε-aminocaproic acid was used in all patients. In addition, few patients had received recent aspirin, and none had received any of the other platelet inhibitors that are so commonly seen today.[8] I have used this technology myself under the guise of "platelet protection." It is time-consuming, distracting, and costly. This study calls the practice into question, even in reoperative CABG, and highlights the hemodynamic instability that I have noted on many occasions. We all continue to search for conservation strategies. It appears that the new plateletpheresis machines are not the answer. A recent article even calls acute normovolemic hemodilution, a technique used at numerous institutions,[9] into question.[10]

Despite practice guidelines to the contrary,[11] many institutions continue to use FFP at high frequencies.[9] Kasper et al (Abstract 5–34), in a good study design, appear to have put the question to rest. To correct earlier study design flaws, this study was randomized, included an adequate dosing scheme, and used autologous donation to decrease the risk of infection. No clinical difference was noted in chest tube drainage. The authors' conclusions that prophylactic use of FFP is inappropriate in CABG surgery and increases costs are quite reasonable. Perhaps our own guidelines should be more closely adhered to.[12]

M. F. Trankina, MD

References

1. Glyrm SA, Kleinman SH, Schreiber GB, et al: Trends in incidence and prevalence of major transfusion-transmissible viral infections in US blood donors, 1991 to 1996: Retrovirus Epidemiology Donor Study (REDS). *JAMA* 284:229-235, 2000.
2. Feindel CM: Medical legal issues in allogeneic blood transfusion. *Can J Anaesth* 48:S2-S5, 2001.
3. Thurer RL: Blood transfusion in cardiac surgery. *Can J Anaesth* 48:S6-12, 2001.
4. Ruel MA, Rubens FD: Non-pharmacological strategies for blood conservation in cardiac surgery. *Can J Anaesth* 48:S13-S23, 2001.
5. Hardy JF: Pharmacological strategies for blood conservation in cardiac surgery: Erythropoietin and antifibrinolytics. *Can J Anaesth* 48:S24-S31, 2001.
6. Hill SE: Oxygen therapeutics—Current concepts. *Can J Anaesth* 48:S32-S40, 2001.
7. Boldt J: Acute platelet-rich plasmapheresis for cardiac surgery. *J Cardiothorac Vasc Anesth* 9:79-88, 1995.
8. Lee LY, DeBois W, Krieger KH, et al: The effects of platelet inhibitors on blood use in cardiac surgery. *Perfusion* 17:33-37, 2002.

9. Stover EP, Siegel LC, Body SC, et al: Institutional variability in red blood cell conservation practices for coronary artery bypass graft surgery. Institutions of the MultiCenter Study of Perioperative Ischemia Research Group. *J Cardiothorac Vasc Anesth* 14:171-176, 2000.
10. Hohn L, Schweizer A, Licker M, et al: Absence of beneficial effect of acute normovolemic hemodilution combined with aprotinin on allogeneic blood transfusion requirements in cardiac surgery. *Anesthesiology* 96:276-282, 2002.
11. Practice parameter for the use of fresh-frozen plasma, cryoprecipitate, and platelets. Fresh-Frozen Plasma, Cryoprecipitate, and Platelets Administration Practice Guidelines Development Task Force of the College of American Pathologists. *JAMA* 271:777-781, 1994.
12. Practice Guidelines for blood component therapy: A report by the American Society of Anesthesiologists Task Force on Blood Component Therapy. *Anesthesiology* 84:732-747, 1996.

Cause-Specific Mortality Risks of Anesthesiologists

Alexander BH, Checkoway H, Nagahama SI, et al (Univ of Minnesota, Minneapolis; Univ of Washington, Seattle)
Anesthesiology 93:922-930, 2000   5–35

Background.—The operating room (OR) environment chronically exposes anesthesiologists and other OR personnel to trace concentrations of anesthetic gases, low-dose radiation, and psychological stresses. The health effects of such exposure have not been documented. The mortality risk of anesthesiologists was compared with that of internal medicine physicians between 1979 and 1995.

Methods.—A cohort of 40,211 internists was frequency-matched to a cohort of 40,242 anesthesiologists by sex, decade of birth, and US citizenship. Data from the National Death Index were used to confirm death status as well as causes of death.

Findings.—For all physicians, the standardized mortality ratios were well below 1.0 for all causes except suicide. Internists and anesthesiologists did not differ significantly in all-cause mortality ratios or risk of death from cancer and heart disease. Among anesthesiologists, the risk of death from suicide, drug-related causes, other external causes, and cerebrovascular disease was increased, the rate ratios being 1.45, 2.79, 1.53, 1.39, respectively. Male anesthesiologists had an increased risk of death from HIV, with a rate ratio of 1.82, and viral hepatitis, with a rate ratio of 7.98. The risk of drug-related death among anesthesiologists was greatest in the first 5 years after medical school but remained increased over that of internists throughout their careers.

Conclusions.—Substance abuse and suicide appear to be significant occupational hazards among anesthesiologists. These issues need to be addressed.

▶ This is an important article for all anesthesiologists. Reviewing cause of death and mortality rates for anesthesiologists and comparing those to both the general population and general internists identify health risks associated with our profession. The authors point out that anesthesiologists, like all physicians, have a lower mortality rate than the general population. This is attributed to a healthier lifestyle (or at least greater awareness of health issues), lower rates of tobacco abuse, and the fact that people who are working are generally healthier than those who are not working. It is comforting that there is no higher incidence of any type of cancer as a cause of death in anesthesiologists, in spite of higher exposures to potential carcinogens present in the OR. The authors correctly warn that, given the young mean age (50) of the study cohort, cancer death related to occupational risks may not be detected from this study and that longer follow-up would be needed. Of great concern is the increased incidence of suicide and drug-related deaths in anesthesiologists as compared with internists. These findings are no surprise, given both the nature of our profession and the relatively easy access to potent drugs of abuse. These deaths account for the significantly younger age at death and the greater number of life-years lost in anesthesiologists. Also of concern is the observation that the rate of drug-related death is unchanged by both our recognition of the risk and institution of educational programs during residency. Clearly, what we are doing is not working. Also of interest is the higher rate of death among anesthesiologists due to boating, biking, airplane accidents, drowning, etc. Is there something about the OR environment that contributes to risk-taking behavior outside the work place? In light of observations such as these, we must carefully evaluate only our training programs and try to develop ways to reduce this risk in our new colleagues. We must also evaluate our own professional environment and what can be done to address these serious health risks.

M. F. Trankina, MD

Use of the Internal Mammary Artery Graft and In-Hospital Mortality and Other Adverse Outcomes Associated With Coronary Artery Bypass Surgery
Leavitt BJ, for the Northern New England Cardiovascular Disease Study Group (Fletcher Allen Health Care, Burlington, Vt; et al)
Circulation 103:507-512, 2001   5–36

Introduction.—Although clear evidence exists that coronary artery bypass grafting (CABG) surgeries using the internal mammary artery (IMA) have better long-term survival rates, widespread differences in IMA use are found. Patients who are female, older, of smaller size, of urgent or emergent priority, and with reduced left ventricular ejection fraction receive an IMA graft less frequently. More patients could benefit from an IMA as a conduit for CABG surgery. There is concern that the likely protective effect of IMA on short-term mortality rate has been confounded by other risk factors. The independent effects of use of IMA grafts on in-hospital mortality rate was evaluated while adjusting for patient and disease factors.

Methods.—The use of the left IMA (LIMA) was examined in 21,873 consecutive, isolated, first-time CABG procedures performed between

TABLE 2.—Use of LIMA and In-Hospital Outcomes: Risk-Adjusted* Rates

| | LIMA Used? | | |
Outcome	No	Yes	*P*
n (total=21 873)	2857	19 016	
In-hospital mortality, %	4.9	2.2	<0.001
Intraoperative or postoperative cerebrovascular accident, %	1.9	1.6	0.096
Return to bypass,† %	4.3	3.7	0.319
Return to operating room for treatment of postoperative thoracic bleeding, %	3.2	2.7	0.365
Mediastinitis or sternal dehiscence requiring reoperation, %	1.3	1.1	0.810

*Event rates are adjusted for age, sex, surface area, body mass index ≥30, comorbidity (chronic obstructive pulmonary disease, diabetes, peripheral vascular disease, congestive heart failure, pre-existing renal failure), preoperative left ventricular end-diastolic pressure, preoperative ejection fraction, left main stenosis, 3-vessel disease, and priority at surgery.

†Data available for 10,048 procedures. This variable was collected only since 1996.

(Courtesy of Leavitt BJ, for the Northern New England Cardiovascular Disease Study Group: Use of the internal mammary artery graft and in-hospital mortality and other adverse outcomes associated with coronary artery bypass grafting. *Circulation* 103:507-512, 2001.)

1992 and 1999 at 6 medical centers (34 cardiothoracic surgeons). Of these, 87% received a LIMA graft. Pertinent data were collected from medical records.

Results.—Use of a LIMA graft was correlated with a significant reduction in risk of death. The overall in-hospital adjusted mortality rate was 2.2% for patients who underwent LIMA grafting and 4.9% in patients who did not receive a LIMA graft ($P < .001$) (Table 2). The overall crude OR for in-hospital death was 0.26 (95% CI, 0.22-0.31; $P < .001$). Use of the LIMA grafts was protective across all major patient and disease subgroups. ORs for the subgroups ranged from 0.13 to 0.48. The OR for death was 0.40 (95% CI, 0.33-0.48; $P < .001$) after adjustment was made for all major risk factors. The rates of cerebrovascular accident, return to cardiopulmonary bypass, reoperation for bleeding, and mediastinitis or sternal dehiscence necessitating surgery were nonsignificantly less in the LIMA group.

Conclusion.—In addition to well-documented patency and long-term beneficial effects, LIMA grafting provides a strong protective effect on perioperative death.

▶ The LIMA often is not recommended for emergent situations or in patients with numerous complications. Also, the longer harvest time of the IMA and the increased bleeding tendency of the emergent patient, especially those undergoing interventional procedures in the cardiac catheterization laboratory who may be receiving some form of anticoagulation and in the fragile elderly, are also considered contraindications to the use of the LIMA. Therefore, the LIMA is not always used in the compromised patient. This prospective study of more than 21,000 patients undergoing CABG for the first time who had their surgery performed in the "modern" era has refuted many of these long-held beliefs. In every clinical situation, including the ones mentioned, the use of this conduit for left anterior descending coronary bypass was positively correlated with improved survival rate when compared with the use of a venous conduit to the left anterior descending artery. This is an important study when one looks at the current trends in CABG surgery and the pathophysiologic characteristics of failed grafts. I am always happy when the surgeon selects the LIMA, even though it takes longer.

M. F. Trankina, MD

The Cardiac Anesthesia Risk Evaluation Score: A Clinically Useful Predictor of Mortality and Morbidity After Cardiac Surgery
Dupuis J-Y, Wang F, Nathan H, et al (Univ of Ottawa, Canada)
Anesthesiology 94:194-204, 2001   5–37

Background.—The Cardiac Anesthesia Risk Evaluation (CARE) score, which provides a simple risk classification for patients undergoing cardiac surgery, is based on clinical judgment and 3 clinical variables (comorbid conditions categorized as controlled or uncontrolled, surgical complexity, and urgency of procedure). The CARE score was compared with the Parsonnet, Tuman, and Tu multifactorial risk indices for predicting mortality and morbidity after cardiac surgery.

Methods.—A total of 3548 patients undergoing cardiac surgery were prospectively stratified by risk according to the CARE score and the 3 indices. The first 2000 patients served as a reference group for discriminating each classification with receiver operating characteristic curves, and the remainder were used to determine calibration with the Pearson χ^2 goodness-of-fit test.

Findings.—The CARE score had areas under the receiver operating characteristic curves of 0.801 and 0.721 for mortality and morbidity, respectively. The corresponding values were 0.808 and 0.726 for the Parsonnet index, 0.782 and 0.697 for the Tuman index, and 0.770 and 0.724 for the Tu index. All risk models but the Parsonnet had acceptable calibration in predicting mortality and morbidity.

Conclusions.—The performance of the CARE score in predicting outcomes in patients undergoing cardiac surgery is equal to that of multifactorial risk indices. Cardiac anesthesiologists may use this score to predict outcomes with acceptable accuracy.

▶ It is important that anesthesiologists understand and participate in the perioperative risk assessment of our patients. The American Society of Anesthesiologists (ASA) classification is of less value for patients undergoing cardiac surgery than for patients undergoing noncardiac surgery in predicting perioperative morbidity and mortality. In this study, a very simple risk assessment system, which is very similar to the ASA risk classification system, was developed and tested. The CARE score was compared with more complex multifactorial risk indices as well as with single factors (such as left ventricular function, New York Heart Association classification for heart failure, age, renal failure, ASA physical status) shown to influence risk after cardiac surgery. The outcomes evaluated included major morbidity, mortality, and prolonged length of stay. The CARE score was as accurate at predicting outcome in the individual patient as the more complex indices and was significantly better than any single factor. It has the advantage of being simple, easy to remember, and, as demonstrated in this study, capable of being used in a consistent fashion in clinical practice. It allows for some subjectivity in risk classification, such as determining "controlled" versus "uncontrolled" comorbid medical conditions and in the determination of "complex" versus "simple" operative procedures. This subjectivity did not impair predictive value of the CARE score in this large prospective series (more than 3000 patients). Preoperative assessment by anesthesiologists routinely involves definition of adequate "control" of medical conditions. I have greater concern with the lack of definition of complex versus simple surgical procedures. What is simple for 1 surgeon may be complex for another, dramatically changing the CARE score and the predictive risk. Nonetheless, I would agree with the authors' conclusion. This is a simple, reliably predictive preoperative risk assessment for cardiac surgery patients that is likely to be used clinically rather than simply as a research tool.

M. F. Trankina, MD

Outcome With High Blood Lactate Levels During Cardiopulmonary Bypass in Adult Cardiac Operation

Demers P, Elkouri S, Martineau R, et al (Montreal Heart Inst)
Ann Thorac Surg 70:2082-2086, 2000   5–38

Introduction.—High blood lactate levels during cardiopulmonary bypass (CPB) are correlated with tissue hypoperfusion and may contribute to postoperative morbidity and mortality. The relation between blood lactate

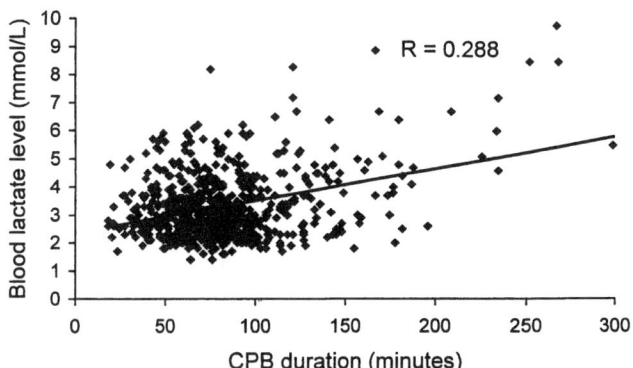

FIGURE 1.—Correlation between CPB time and peak blood lactate level (R = .288; *P* = .001). (Courtesy of Demers P, Elkouri S, Martineau R, et al: Outcome with high blood lactate levels during cardiopulmonary bypass in adult cardiac operation. *Ann Thorac Surg* 70:2082-2086, 2000. Reprinted by permission of the Society of Thoracic Surgeons.)

TABLE 2.—Operative Data of 1259 Patients Undergoing Cardiac Operation According to
Peak Blood Lactate Levels During Cardiopulmonary Bypass

| | Lactates | | |
Variable	< 4.0 mmol/L (n = 1,032)	≥ 4.0 mmol/L (n = 227)	p Value
CPB time (min)	77.9 ± 30.4	101.3 ± 52.8	< 0.001
Ischemic time (min)	49.8 ± 24.7	63.5 ± 37.8	< 0.001
Lowest hemoglobin (g/L)	72.1 ± 11.4	63.5 ± 11.3	< 0.001

(Courtesy of Demers P, Elkouri S, Martineau R, et al: Outcome with high blood lactate levels during cardiopulmonary bypass in adult cardiac operation. *Ann Thorac Surg* 70:2082-2086, 2000. Reprinted by permission of the Society of Thoracic Surgeons.)

levels during CPB and perioperative complications and death were examined in patients who underwent cardiac surgery with CPB.

Methods.—Of 1376 patients evaluated, 101 had abnormal preoperative blood lactate levels and were excluded. Retrospective data were collected regarding blood lactate concentration during CPB, clinical data, and perioperative events.

Results.—Peak blood lactate levels of 4.0 mmol/L or higher during CPB were observed in 227 (18.0%) patients. There was a significant link between CPB time and peak blood lactate levels (Fig 1) ($P = .001$) (Table 2). The postoperative mortality rate was higher in this group compared with those who had peak blood lactate levels of below 4.0 mmol/L during CPB (11.0% vs 1.4%; $P < .001$; RR, 9.0). Postoperative hemodynamic

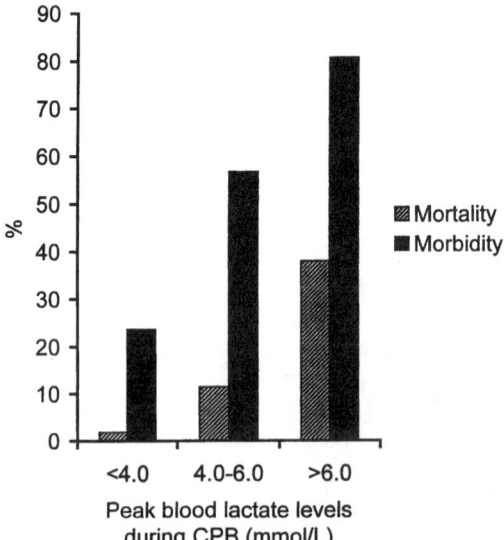

FIGURE 2.—Positive correlation between peak blood lactate levels during CPB and the rate of postoperative morbidity and mortality ($P < .001$). (Courtesy of Demers P, Elkouri S, Martineau R, et al: Outcome with high blood lactate levels during cardiopulmonary bypass in adult cardiac operation. *Ann Thorac Surg* 70:2082-2086, 2000. Reprinted by permission of the Society of Thoracic Surgeons.)

TABLE 3.—Postoperative Mortality, Morbidity, and Hospital Length of Stay of 1259 Patients Undergoing Cardiac Operation According to Peak Blood Lactate Levels During CPB

| | Lactates | | |
| | < 4.0 mmol/L | ≥ 4.0 mmol/L | |
Variable	(n = 1,032)	(n = 227)	*p* Value
Death within 30 days	1.4%	11.0%	< 0.001
Neurologic	1.7%	9.3%	< 0.001
Myocardial infarction	6.8%	17.2%	< 0.001
Hemodynamic	10.9%	29.5%	< 0.001
Pulmonary	3.6%	8.8%	< 0.001
Digestive	3.0%	7.5%	0.003
Renal	3.5%	9.3%	<0.001
Infectious	4.2%	7.1%	0.063
Length of stay (days)			
Intensive care unit	4.5 ± 3.8	5.8 ± 4.7	< 0.001
Hospital	8.4 ± 6.4	11.1 ± 8.2	< 0.001

(Courtesy of Demers P, Elkouri S, Martineau R, et al: Outcome with high blood lactate levels during cardiopulmonary bypass in adult cardiac operation. *Ann Thorac Surg* 70:2082-2086, 2000. Reprinted by permission of the Society of Thoracic Surgeons.)

instability was observed in 29.5% of patients with elevated levels of lactate during CPB compared with 10.9% of patients who had lower lactate levels ($P < .001$; RR, 3.4). Overall, the main postoperative complications occurred in 43.2% of patients in the elevated lactate level group and 21.8% of those in the lower lactate level group ($P < .001$; RR = 2.7). Logistic regression analysis showed that peak blood lactate levels of 4.0 mmol/L or higher during CPB were strongly correlated with postoperative death ($P = .0001$) and morbidity ($P = .013$) (Fig 2) (Table 3).

Conclusion.—Blood lactate concentration of 4.0 mmol/L or higher during CPB is associated with increased risk of postoperative morbidity and mortality.

▶ When this study surfaced last year, it caused quite a stir among some of the surgeons I work with. In that particular practice, it is not unusual to see lactate levels during CPB at more than 4 mmol/L. It led to changes in assays and a look at CPB practices at that hospital. Although this study is imperfect (retrospective, isolated lactate measurements, Ringer's lactate used in pump prime), I believe it has value in alerting the cardiac team to potential problem patients. Perhaps patients with elevated lactate levels should be more closely monitored, perhaps by pulmonary artery catheters, and additional therapies instituted, such as the use of inotropes, inodilators, red blood cells, and the intra-aortic balloon pump. Surprisingly, CPB time only weakly correlated with peak lactates (R = 0.288). Only with further prospective studies will we better understand this interesting finding.

M. F. Trankina, MD

Postoperative Prophylactic Administration of β-Adrenergic Blockers in Patients at Risk for Myocardial Ischemia

Urban MK, Markowitz SM, Gordon MA, et al (Cornell Univ, New York)
Anesth Analg 90:1257-1261, 2000   5–39

Background.—Cardiac morbidity can result from perioperative myocardial ischemia (MI). A study was undertaken to determine whether postoperative sympatholysis could decrease the incidence of MI in at-risk patients undergoing total knee arthroplasty.

Methods.—One hundred seven patients undergoing elective total knee arthroplasty with epidural anesthesia and postoperative epidural analgesia were randomly assigned to a control group or to a β-blocker group. Patients in the latter group received postoperative esmolol infusions on the day of surgery and metoprolol for the next 48 hours to maintain a heart rate of less than 80 bpm. A Holter monitor was used to monitor patients' ST segment depression.

Findings.—Postoperative electrocardiographic ischemia occurred significantly more in the control group than in the β-blocker recipients during esmolol blockade. In addition, ischemia tended to be more common in the control group in the following 2 days. The 2 groups also differed significantly in the number of ischemic events being (50 and 16 events in the control and treatment groups, respectively) and in total ischemic time (709 and 236 minutes, respectively). Myocardial infarction and cardiac events were more common in the control group but not significantly so.

Conclusions.—Prophylaxis with β-blockers appears to reduce the number of postoperative ischemic episodes in patients at risk of MI who are undergoing elective total knee arthroplasty with epidural anesthesia and postoperative epidural analgesia. This lower incidence may be associated with prevention of increased heart rate.

The Case for β-Adrenergic Blockade as Prophylaxis Against Perioperative Cardiovascular Morbidity and Mortality

Selzman CH, Miller SA, Zimmerman MA, et al (Univ of Colorado, Denver)
Arch Surg 136:286-290, 2001   5–40

Background.—Myocardial ischemia is still the main cause of postoperative morbidity and death in patients with known cardiovascular disease undergoing cardiac or noncardiac surgery. The physiologic and clinical basis for the use of β-adrenergic antagonists in such patients was discussed.

Discussion.—The neurohormonal stress induced by elective surgery begins as soon as the procedure is scheduled and persists until about 1 week after surgery. This period, called the adrenergic-corticosteroid phase, is characterized by neuroendocrine substance hypercatabolism and hypersecretion. The surgery itself then requires increased myocardial work, a demand that patients with coronary artery disease are not able to meet. The

4 main determinants of oxygen demand—heart rate, preload, afterload, and contractility—are increased by catecholamines. Several studies have demonstrated that β-adrenergic blockade can reduce perioperative myocardial ischemia. However, few studies have shown a positive correlation between this physiologic effect and clinical outcomes.

The use of β-adrenergic blockade in patients with cardiopulmonary disease has been shown to be well tolerated. Reactive airway disease is not an automatic contraindication to the use of β-adrenergic blocking agents. Judicious titration of cardioselective adrenergic antagonists appears to be appropriate in patients with mild to moderately severe asthma and coronary artery disease.

Recommendations.—Specific recommendations for patients undergoing major elective noncardiac surgery were provided. Patients at high risk must be identified, commonly through history and physical examination. If men older than 40 years and women older than 45 years are already taking a β-adrenergic blocking agent, therapy should be continued to lower heart rate and systolic blood pressure to 70 bpm and 110 mm Hg, respectively. Patients who are not taking a β-adrenergic blocking agent should begin an oral regimen as soon as possible before surgery. β-Adrenergic blocking agents should be continued throughout hospitalization and the outpatient period.

▶ This is yet another study evaluating the effect of perioperative prophylactic β-blockade on myocardial ischemia and cardiac complications. Although there are some issues of concern related to study design, primarily the high rate of β-blocker use in the control group and the lack of treating physician blinding during the β-blocker treatment period, there are some unique features to this study that make it noteworthy. First, all patients underwent the same procedure, total knee arthroplasty (an intermediate-risk procedure) according to AHA guidelines, and all patients were given epidural anesthesia with sedation intraoperatively. Most other studies addressing this issue include high-risk surgical procedures such as major vascular surgery,[1,2] and most examine patients who are given general anesthesia. In spite of a number of factors likely to decrease the demonstrated impact of prophylactic β-blocker use, the study demonstrates a lower incidence of myocardial ischemia during intravenous esmolol administration (early postoperative period) and a shorter total period of myocardial ischemia in the patients in the β-blocker group. The lack of significant difference in cardiac events and morbidity is not surprising, given the small study size. The particular manner of administration of β-blockade—esmolol infusion and ICU admission in the immediate postoperative period—is impractical for most practices. Nonetheless, this study is noteworthy as giving yet further evidence of the benefits of prophylactic perioperative β-blockade in patients with known or suspected coronary artery disease—even in clinical situations not routinely considered to involve high risk, such as uncomplicated orthopedic procedures under regional anesthesia.

Selzman et al (Abstract 5–40) provide a concise and clear review of prophylactic perioperative β-blockade in the surgical literature. Although this issue has been addressed numerous times in the anesthesia literature, it is important to note this review article in the surgical literature that provides specific recommendations regarding preoperative evaluation and management of the patient with likely coronary artery disease. The recommendations are clear and are derived from both the ACC/AHA guidelines (updated 1/2002, www.acc.org) and several of the larger trials of perioperative β-blockade. I am happy to note that our surgical colleagues are becoming supportive of these strategies.

M. F. Trankina, MD

References

1. Wallace A, Layug B, Tateo I, et al, for the McSPI Research Group: Prophylactic atenolol reduces postoperative myocardial ischemia. *Anesthesiology* 88:7-17, 1998.
2. Mangano DT, Layug EL, Wallace A, et al, for the Multicenter Study of Perioperative Ischemia Multicenter Study of Perioperative Ischemia Research Group: Effect of atenolol on mortality and cardiovascular morbidity after noncardiac surgery. *N Engl J Med* 335:1713-1720, 1996.

Vasopressin for Refractory Hypotension During Cardiopulmonary Bypass

Talbot MP, Tremblay I, Denault AY, et al (Univ of Montreal)
J Thorac Cardiovasc Surg 120:401-402, 2000   5–41

Background.—Vasopressin, a potent endogenous vasoconstricting agent, is effective in treating refractory hypotension. The use of this agent for refractory hypotension during cardiopulmonary bypass (CPB) was reported.

> *Case Report.*—Woman, 72, weighing 42 kg, was referred for coronary arteriography and hemodynamic assessment because of aortic stenosis. She had a history of aorta-bifemoral bypass, hypothyroidism, and non–Q-wave myocardial infarction after a carotid endarterectomy. Medications included remipril, metoprolol, aspirin, oral nitrates, furosemide, levothyroxine sodium, and pravastatin. On evaluation, coronary arteriography demonstrated severe tritruncular disease. Hemodynamic evaluation and transthoracic echocardiography showed severe aortic disease and grade 2/4 mitral regurgitation. In addition, the patient had severe diastolic dysfunction and reduced ejection fraction. Revascularization and aortic valve replacement were scheduled. General anesthesia was induced with sufentanil, 60 µg, midazolam, 5 mg, and pancuronium, 5 mg. Hemodynamics remained stable until CPB was initiated, after which the patient became hypotensive. The hypotension worsened with each bolus of cardioplegic solution. Multiple 100 and 200 µg boluses were given. A phenylephrine infusion was

begun, followed shortly thereafter by norepinephrine. However, the patient's hypotension was refractory to this therapy. Thus, 1 unit of vasopressin was given. Mean arterial pressure normalized at about 80 mm Hg, enabling tapering of the phenylephrine and norepinephrine infusions. Hypotension recurred during CPB, and a second vasopressin dose was given. After surgery, the patient was taken to the ICU. She received norepinephrine, 4 µg/min, and nitroglycerin, 17 µg/min. Vasopressors were discontinued, and the patient was extubated. On postoperative day 6, the patient was discharged with no apparent sequelae.

Conclusions.—This patient was successfully treated with vasopressin for refractory hypotension during CPB. The efficacy and safety of this promising pressor agent during CPB need to be confirmed in a randomized study.

▶ Talbot describes, in a case report, the use of arginine vasopressin for refractory hypotension during CPB. I included this article to highlight the potential of this drug when other therapies are failing. I tell my residents to have vasopressin "in their back pocket" as a backup. Vasopressin has been used with good success in heart transplantation,[1] sepsis, left ventricular assist device patients,[2] and during CPB.[3] Its potential for harm is poorly elucidated in this population, and the drug may be harmful as evidenced by its ability to cause vasoconstriction in saphenous vein grafts.[4] Until good studies are performed, the routine use of vasopressin should be reserved for cases such as the one described in this article.

M. F. Trankina, MD

References

1. Argenziano M, Chert JM, Cullinane S, et al: Arginine vasopressin in the management of vasodilatory hypotension after cardiac transplantation. *J Heart Lung Transplant* 18:814-817, 1999.
2. Morales DL, Gregg D, Helman DN, et al: Arginine vasopressin in the treatment of 50 patients with postcardiotomy vasodilatory shock. *Ann Thorac Surg* 69:102-106, 2000.
3. Argenziano M, Chen JM, Choudhri AF, et al: Management of vasodilatory shock after cardiac surgery: Identification of predisposing factors and use of a novel pressor agent. *J Thorac Cardiovasc Surg* 116:973-980, 1998.
4. Medina P, Acuna A, Martinez-Leon JB, et al: Arginine vasopressin enhances sympathetic constriction through the V1 vasopressin receptor in human saphenous vein. *Circulation* 97:865-870, 1998.

Effects of Biatrial Pacing in Prevention of Postoperative Atrial Fibrillation After Coronary Artery Bypass Surgery

Fan K, Lee KL, Chiu CSW, et al (Queen Mary Hosp, Hong Kong, China)
Circulation 102:755-760, 2000   5–42

Background.—Atrial fibrillation (AF) occurs commonly after coronary artery bypass surgery (CABG), resulting in prolonged hospitalization. The efficacy of biatrial pacing in preventing this complication was compared with that of single-site atrial pacing.

Methods.—One hundred thirty-two patients with no history of AF who were undergoing CABG were enrolled in a prospective study. By random assignment, patients received biatrial pacing (BiA), left atrial pacing (LA), right atrial pacing (RA), or no atrial pacing (control) postoperatively. Overdrive atrial pacing was continued for 5 days.

Findings.—The BiA group had a significantly lower incidence of AF than the LA, RA, and control groups, with incidences of 12.5%, 36.4%, 33.3%, and 41.9%, respectively. Mean hospitalization time was also significantly lower in the BiA group. Biatrial pacing was associated with the most significant percentage of decrease in P-wave dispersion compared with the LA and RA groups. Neither P-wave duration nor dispersion differed significantly between patients in whom AF developed and those who remained in sinus rhythm at baseline. However, only patients remaining in sinus rhythm had significantly decreased P-wave duration and dispersion after pacing therapy.

Conclusions.—Biatrial overdrive pacing appears to be more effective than single-site atrial pacing in preventing post-CABG AF. Biatrial pacing also reduced length of hospital stay. A reduction in P-wave dispersion reflected the overall decrease in atrial activation time with BiA pacing.

Magnesium Infusion Dramatically Decreases the Incidence of Atrial Fibrillation After Coronary Artery Bypass Grafting

Toraman F, Karabulut EH, Alhan HC, et al (Acibadem Hosp, Istanbul, Turkey)
Ann Thorac Surg 72:1256-1262, 2001   5–43

Introduction.—There are 2 factors consistently associated with atrial fibrillation (AF) after cardiac surgery: preoperative withdrawal of β-adrenoceptor antagonist therapy and advancing age. The latter is correlated with increasing circulating norephinephrine level that may be caused by increasing sympathetic outflow. Varying degrees of success have been observed with postoperative administration of magnesium. The dose and timing of magnesium prophylaxis have yet to be ascertained. The effect of intermittent magnesium infusion on postoperative AF was examined in 200 consecutive patients who underwent elective, isolated, first-time coronary artery bypass grafting (CABG).

Methods.—Patients were prospectively randomly assigned to treatment with either magnesium, 6 mmol $MgSO_4$ infusion in 100 mL, or 0.9% NaCl solution, 25 mL/hr the day before surgery, immediately after cardiopulmonary bypass, and once daily for 4 days postoperatively. Controls received 100 mL 0.9% NaCl solution at the same time points.

Results.—Two patients (2%) in the magnesium group and 21 controls (21%) experienced postoperative AF ($P < .001$). Atrial fibrillation began an average of 49.4 hours postoperatively. The postoperative length of hospital stay was similar in patients with AF (7.4 days), compared with those who did not have AF (5.4 days) ($P = .236$).

Conclusion.—Administration of magnesium in the preoperative and early postoperative periods is highly effective in diminishing the incidence of AF after CABG. The mechanism by which magnesium decreases myocardial irritability and tachyarrhythmias is not yet understood.

Randomized Controlled Study Investigating the Effect of Biatrial Pacing in Prevention of Atrial Fibrillation After Coronary Artery Bypass Grafting

Levy T, Fotopoulos G, Walker S, et al (Harefield Hosp, Middlesex, England)
Circulation 102:1382-1387, 2000   5–44

Introduction.—The prevention of atrial fibrillation (AF) with prophylactic drug therapy after coronary artery bypass grafting (CABG) has limited success. Biatrial pacing is a technique of simultaneous activation of the right and left atrium that can prevent the reoccurrence of AF in paced patients with marked intra-atrial conduction delay. The role of biatrial pacing was compared with no pacing on AF incidence after isolated first-time CABG.

Methods.—Temporary pacing leads were placed in the lateral wall on the right atrium and on the roof of the left atrium in Bachmann's bundle during surgery to provide bipolar pacing and sensing at each site. After surgery, all patients were connected to an external pacemaker that was also a Holter monitor. One hundred and thirty-one patients were consecutively randomly assigned to undergo either 4 days of biatrial pacing at a base rate of 80 beats/min or to no pacing (controls, base rate 30 beats/min). The major end points included an episode of AF lasting more than 1 hour on pacemaker Holter monitor, clinically detected AF, ICU and hospital stay, and postoperative complications.

Results.—Biatrial pacing significantly decreased both monitored (13.8% vs 38.5%; $P = .001$) and clinical (10.8% vs 33.8%; $P = .002$) episodes of AF. The median ICU (19 vs 24 h; $P = $ NS) and mean hospital stay (7.7 vs 9.7 d; $P = $ NS) were not significantly changed. The biatrial group had a significantly lower number of postoperative complications (13 vs 35; $P = .001$).

Conclusion.—Biatrial pacing after CABG significantly reduces the incidence of AF. This is correlated with decreased postoperative complications and a trend toward decreased ICU and hospital stay.

▶ AF is the most common complication occurring after cardiac surgery. Despite advances in cardiopulmonary bypass, cardioplegia, and surgical techniques, the incidence has paradoxically increased in recent years as the result of CABG patients being older. AF is frequently not well tolerated, and patients may have symptoms including temporary hemodynamic instability and thromboembolic events, and has been shown to increase costs, ICU times, and lengthen hospital stay. Many preoperative and postoperative factors have been suggested to increase the incidence of postoperative AF after conventional CABG, such as advanced age, hypertension, withdrawal of β-blocker therapy, right coronary artery stenosis, respiratory complications, and bleeding. Strategies directed toward reduction of postoperative AF have focused on several prophylactic drugs, such as β-blockers, calcium-channel blockers, amiodarone, and propafenone—all with conflicting results. However, little is known about intraoperative mechanisms through which the incidence of postoperative AF could be reduced.[1-9] Both pacing articles (Abstracts 5–42 and 5–44) show a significant reduction in AF when biatrial pacing is instituted. I have tried this therapy, and it is relatively easy to implement in the operating room if the surgeon is willing. Fan (Abstract 5–42) also showed a decreased length of hospital stay in patients receiving biatrial therapy. This group saw a decrease in postoperative complications. An even more recent article confirmed the use of biatrial pacing in a prospective trial with patients in both arms receiving β-blockade.[10] The accelerating interest in this costly problem will likely involve anesthesiologists and perhaps will include complex pacing prescriptions during the perioperative period.

Hypomagnesemia is common after cardiac surgery.[11,12] Magnesium supplementation has been used with varying success in CAGB patients to prevent AF.[13-16] Many of these studies were poorly designed and not randomized. This article by Levy (Abstract 5–44) et al suggests that even with normal magnesium levels that supplementation has value. This is consistent with an earlier study by Terzi.[17] Levy, in addition, unlike most anesthesiologists in the United States, delivered the magnesium for 4 days postoperatively. The results of this study are striking and suggest that we should all be more aggressive with magnesium supplementation in CABG patients. Further work is needed to both confirm this study and to ascertain whether these techniques are as effective when other prophylactic measures such as β-blockade are also used.

M. F. Trankina, MD

References

1. Aranki SF, Shaw DP, Adams DH, et al: Predictors of atrial fibrillation after coronary artery surgery. Current trends and impact on hospital resources. *Circulation* 94:390-397, 1996.

2. Kalman JM, Munawar M, Howes LG, et al: Atrial fibrillation after coronary artery bypass grafting is associated with sympathetic activation. *Ann Thorac Surg* 60:1709-1715, 1995.
3. Creswell LL, Damiano RJ Jr: Postoperative atrial fibrillation: An old problem crying for new solutions. *J Thorac Cardiovasc Surg* 121:638-641, 2001.
4. Mathew JP, Parks R, Savino JS, et al: Atrial fibrillation following coronary artery bypass graft surgery: Predictors, outcomes, and resource utilization. MultiCenter Study of Perioperative Ischemia Research Group. *JAMA* 276:300-306, 1996.
5. Mendes LA, Connelly GP, McKenney PA, et al: Right coronary artery stenosis: An independent predictor of atrial fibrillation after coronary artery bypass surgery. *J Am Coll Cardiol* 25:198-202, 1995.
6. Matsuura K, Takahara Y, Sudo Y, et al: Effect of Sotalol in the prevention of atrial fibrillation following coronary artery bypass grafting. *Jpn J Thorac Cardiovasc Surg* 49:614-617, 2001.
7. Seitelberger R, Hannes W, Gleichauf M, et al: Effects of diltiazem on perioperative ischemia, arrhythmias, and myocardial function in patients undergoing elective coronary bypass grafting. *J Thorac Cardiovasc Surg* 107:811-821, 1994.
8. Di Basi P, Scrofani R, Paje A, et al: Intravenous amiodarone vs propafenone for atrial fibrillation and flutter after cardiac operation. *Eur J Cardiothorac Surg* 9:587-591, 1995.
9. Maisel WH, Rawn JD, Stevenson WG: Atrial fibrillation after cardiac surgery. *Ann Intern Med* 135:1061-1073, 2001.
10. Gerstenfeld EP, Khoo M, Martin RC, et al: Effectiveness of bi-atrial pacing for reducing atrial fibrillation after coronary artery bypass graft surgery. *J Interv Card Electrophysiol* 5:275-283, 2001.
11. England MR, Gordon G, Salem M, et al: Magnesium administration and dysrhythmias after cardiac surgery. A placebo-controlled, double-blind, randomized trial. *JAMA* 268:2395-2402, 1992.
12. Fanning WJ, Thomas CS Jr, Roach A, et al: Prophylaxis of atrial fibrillation with magnesium sulfate after coronary artery bypass grafting. *Ann Thorac Surg* 52:529-533, 1991.
13. Parikka H, Toivonen L, Pellinen T, et al: The influence of intravenous magnesium sulphate on the occurrence of atrial fibrillation after coronary artery by-pass operation. *Eur Heart J* 14:251-258, 1993.
14. Casthely PA, Yoganathan T, Komer C, et al: Magnesium and arrhythmias after coronary artery bypass surgery. *J Cardiothorac Vasc Anesth* 8:188-191, 1994.
15. Nurozler F, Tokgozoglu L, Pasaoglu I, et al: Atrial fibrillation after coronary artery bypass surgery: Predictors and the role of MgSO4 replacement. *J Card Surg* 11:421-427, 1996.
16. Speziale G, Ruvolo G, Fattouch K, et al: Arrhythmia prophylaxis after coronary artery bypass grafting: Regimens of magnesium sulfate administration. *Thorac Cardiovasc Surg* 48:22-26, 2000.
17. Terzi A, Furlan G, Chiavacci P, et al: Prevention of atrial tachyarrhythmias after non-cardiac thoracic surgery by infusion of magnesium sulfate. *Thorac Cardiovasc Surg* 44:300-303, 1996.

6 Pediatric Anesthesia

QT Interval Lengthening in Premature Infants Treated With Doxapram
Maillard C, Boutroy M-J, Fresson J, et al (Maternité Régionale Universitaire, Nancy, France)
Clin Pharmacol Ther 70:540-545, 2001   6–1

Objective.—Doxapram, routinely used in premature infants treated for apnea of prematurity unresponsive to methylxanthines, has been related to cardiac conduction disorders. This study was designed to evaluate doxapram cardiac and general tolerance and its relationship to drug plasma concentrations in very premature infants.

Methods.—Forty infants (mean ± SEM, 28.9 ± 0.3 weeks of gestation) who were given intravenous doxapram, 0.5 to 1 mg/kg per hour, at 15.9 ± 2.4 days of life were evaluated prospectively. Electrocardiograms were

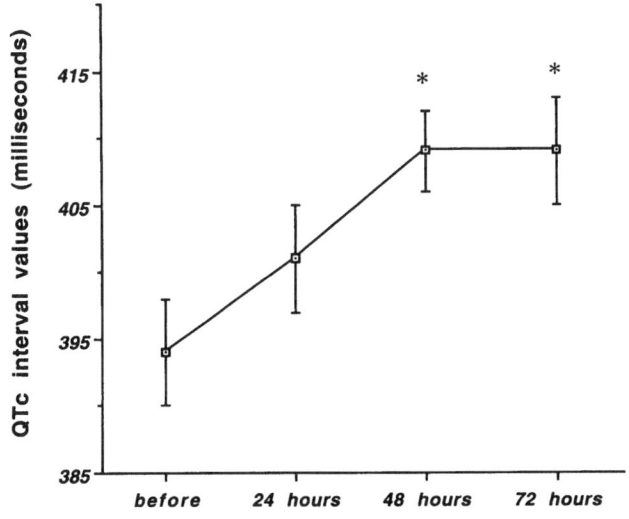

FIGURE 1.—Mean values (± SEM) for QTc interval duration (milliseconds) before and 24, 48, and 72 h after the first dose of doxapram (*asterisk*, P = .0065 vs before the first dose). QTc interval was significantly longer at 48 and 72 h than before onset of treatment. (Courtesy of Maillard C, Boutroy M-J, Fresson J, et al: Interval lengthening in premature infants treated with doxapram. *Clin Pharmacol Ther* 70:540-545, 2001.)

monitored before and during the first 3 days of treatment. QT interval corrected for heart rate (QTc) longer than 440 ms was regarded as clinically pertinent, given that it is considered a significant risk of conduction disorder leading to torsades de pointes and sudden death. Other side effects were recorded. Toxic plasma concentration of doxapram and ketodoxapram was set at >4 mg/L.

Results.—A statistically significant but moderate lengthening of QTc interval has been observed from 394 ± 4 ms before doxapram to 409 ± 4 ms at 48 and 72 hours of treatment ($P = .0065$) (Fig 1). For 6 patients, QTc interval became longer than 440 ms without any other rhythm or conduction disorder. Digestive disorders were observed in 20 infants but 9 presented with concomitant septicemia. No relationship was found between presence or absence of adverse effects and drug plasma concentrations.

Conclusion.—Our study enlightened the lengthening effect of doxapram on QTc interval in premature infants with a risk of exceeding the 440 ms threshold that is considered life-threatening. This finding emphasizes the need for electrocardiogram follow-up when using doxapram in neonates.

▶ Doxapram has been identified as yet another drug that increases the risk of QT interval lengthening and torsades de pointes and sudden death. Prolongation of the QT syndrome and doxapram use has also been described during anesthesia. ECG follow-up is needed when doxapram is administered to neonates.

M. Wood, MD, FRCA

Bronchospasm After Rapacuronium in Infants and Children
Meakin GH, Pronske EH, Lerman J, et al (Royal Manchester Children's Hosp, England; Children's Hosp of Austin, Texas; Univ of Toronto; et al)
Anesthesiology 94:926-927, 2001   6–2

Background.—In December 2000, the Paediatric Anaesthesia Conference discussion group invited its subscribers to report their experiences with the use of rapacuronium in children in the United States. The group did not request or encourage reports of specific side effects or responses to rapacuronium. A total of 19 cases of bronchospasm were reported, 12 of which were severe. Three of these cases were summarized.

> *Case 1.*—Boy, 12 years, weighing 64 kg had a diagnosis of acute appendicitis. He had a history of mild reactive airway disease characterized by occasional use of an albuterol inhaler, but he had no previous hospital stays. The last episode of wheezing had been 1 to 2 months before the present admission. A chest examination was unremarkable. A rapid sequence induction of anesthesia with 1 mg intravenous midazolam, 75 µg fentanyl, 200 mg propofol, and 100 mg rapacuronium was performed in the operating room.

The resident intubated the trachea, but when squeezing the reservoir he reported that the tube was not in the trachea and removed it. He reintubated the trachea but was unable to ventilate the lungs. There was no evidence of expired carbon dioxide on the capnograph. Albuterol and isoflurane were administered by inhalation along with a dose of vecuronium, and chest movement gradually became evident with bag compression. A capnogram trace then appeared. The oxygen saturation percentage at this time was in the low 80s. Chest compliance and oxygen saturation continued to improve with epinephrine 50 µg administered intravenously. Surgery proceeded when the patient's airways stabilized, and recovery was uneventful.

Case 2.—Girl, 4½ years, was seen in the emergency department with a prolonged seizure of sudden onset that had been treated with rectal diazepam. An anesthesiologist was consulted to intubate the trachea because of increasing respiratory distress. The girl's medical history included a mild upper respiratory tract infection without fever or anorexia. Findings on chest radiography were unremarkable. Her history included spina bifida, panhypopituitarism, choanal atresia, developmental delay, and reactive airway disease. Severe bronchospasm was noted immediately after a single dose of both propofol and rapacuronium, with falling oxygen saturations and difficult ventilation. The girl experienced asystole for 30 seconds, and the pulse returned after a single dose of epinephrine. Chest radiography revealed bilateral pneumothoraces. After treatment the child was stabilized and recovered.

Case 3.—Infant, 3 weeks old, was to undergo a pyloromyotomy. The infant was healthy and weighed 3.4 kg. The stomach was suctioned, and a rapid sequence induction was performed with 10 mg propofol, 7 mg rapacuronium, and 0.050 mg intravenous atropine. The trachea was intubated, but after two breaths no capnogram trace was evident. The tube was removed and the trachea reintubated, with still no capnogram trace. After confirming passage of the tube through the vocal cords with direct laryngoscopy, the lungs were ventilated for 60 to 90 seconds with 100% oxygen. During ventilation, bronchospasm was auscultated bilaterally. The chest appeared to move slightly with inflation. The pulse oximeter did not register any oxygen saturation during this time, and the heart rate slowed. A capnogram trace began to appear as bradycardia developed. Shortly afterward, the pulse oximeter registered a saturation of 99%. No rash was evident. Surgery then proceeded uneventfully.

Conclusions.—A total of 19 cases of bronchospasm after rapacuronium were reported. The details from some cases are incomplete, but overall these reports suggest an association between the administration of rapacuronium and the sudden development of severe, short-lived and self-limiting bronchospasm in children. Readers are encouraged to report all adverse events after rapacuronium administration to the manufacturer and to the US Food and Drug Administration.

Severe Bronchospasm and Desaturation in a Child Associated With Rapacuronium

Kron SS (Univ of Connecticut, Farmington)
Anesthesiology 94:923-924, 2001   6–3

Background.—Previously, the use of rapacuronium has been associated with occasional episodes of self-limited increased airway pressure, sometimes accompanied by mild oxygen desaturation and wheezing. This is the first report of severe bronchospasm and desaturation associated with rapacuronium administration.

> *Case Report.*—Girl, 10 years, had appendicitis diagnosed and was to undergo an appendectomy. Her history was negative with the exception of 1 week of abdominal pain and mild nausea but no vomiting. There was no history of previous anesthesia, environmental or drug allergies, recent upper respiratory tract infection, or reactive airway disease. There were no smokers in the household. The girl weighed 62 kg and was 138 cm tall. The physical examination was unremarkable with the exception of findings related to appendicitis, and her chest was clear. The patient was oxygenated, the usual monitors were applied, and 1 mg midazolam and 50 µg fentanyl were administered intravenously. A rapid sequence induction was performed with 150 mg propofol followed by 10 mg intravenous rapacuronium. Oxygen saturation was then noted to fall from 100% to about 95%, and ventilation by mask was applied for 45 seconds with 100% oxygen while cricoid pressure was applied. The girl's chest rose, but oxygen saturation improved only to 96%. An endotracheal tube was placed, followed by an immediate attempt at manual ventilation. However, breath sounds, chest movement, endotracheal tube fogging, end-tidal carbon dioxide, and gastric sounds were not detectable despite ventilating pressures up to 30 cm H_2O. Bag and mask ventilation was also unsuccessful. The patient was reintubated, but ventilation was still impossible. Approximately 2 minutes had elapsed since the initial intubation. The patient was noted to have truncal erythema and an oxygen saturation of 70%. Four doses of 100 µg albuterol aerosol were delivered via the endotracheal tube, and ventilation was attempted again with 8% sevoflurane in oxygen. Within the next minute, ventilation became possible with small tidal volumes and ventilating pressures between 20 and 30 cm H_2O. Oxygen saturation increased, and wheezing breath sounds were audible. A treatment of 2.5 mg nebulized albuterol was administered via the endotra-

cheal tube, and 50 mg Benadryl was given intravenously. During the next 5 minutes, manual ventilation became progressively easier. Surgery eventually resumed uneventfully. Postoperative chest radiography findings were negative, and the patient was discharged on the second postoperative day.

Conclusions.—There were no predisposing factors to a reactive airway in this patient. She responded quickly to β-adrenergic therapy and deepening anesthesia, and her symptoms resolved by the end of treatment.

▶ It is important to recognize that over the last 5 years, much of the anesthetic muscle relaxant literature was devoted to a new muscle relaxant, rapacuronium. Unfortunately, severe airway/respiratory problems in some patients led to its withdrawal from the market. These case reports (Abstracts 6–2 and 6–3) outline the problem.

M. Wood, MD, FRCA

Sensory Stimuli and Anxiety in Children Undergoing Surgery: A Randomized, Controlled Trial
Kain ZN, Wang S-M, Mayes LC, et al (Yale Univ, New Haven, Conn)
Anesth Analg 92:897-903, 2001   6–4

Background.—An estimated 50% to 75% of children undergoing surgery will experience extreme anxiety and distress during the perioperative period. This is an important phenomenon not only because of the postoperative maladaptive behaviors associated with extreme perioperative anxiety and distress, but also because of clinical outcomes and quality improvement efforts. In a recent report, a panel of 72 anesthesiologists reached a consensus on common low-morbidity clinical outcomes that are important to the patient. The outcomes that had the highest combined score were incisional pain, nausea, vomiting, preoperative anxiety, and discomfort caused by insertion of the intravenous line. The effectiveness of a behavioral intervention designed to reduce the perioperative anxiety of children undergoing anesthesia and surgery was evaluated.

Methods.—Children between the ages of 2 and 7 years who were scheduled for general anesthesia and surgery were randomly assigned to a control group (37 children) or to an intervention group (33 children). For patients in the intervention group, dimmed operating room lights and soft background music (Bach's "Air on a G String") were provided, and only the attending anesthesiologist interacted with the child during anesthesia induction. Children were evaluated in the preoperative holding area and during the induction of anesthesia by using two validated behavioral measures of anxiety and compliance, the modified Yale Preoperative Anxiety Scale and the Induction Compliance Checklist. Behavioral recovery was assessed with the Post Hospitalization Behavior Questionnaire.

Results.—Patients in the intervention group were significantly less anxious than those in the control group on entrance to the operating room and at introduction of the anesthesia mask. In addition, children in the intervention group were significantly more compliant during induction of anesthesia. However, there was no significant difference between the 2 groups in the incidence of postoperative behavioral changes.

Conclusions.—Children who were provided with low-level sensory stimuli and background music during anesthesia induction demonstrated significantly lower levels of anxiety and increased compliance with anesthesia induction compared with a control group.

▶ Dr Kain and coworkers have done some very nice work looking at anxiety and the effects of premedication in the perioperative period in children. It is the first time that real scientific principles have been applied to what can be a very sensitive area. This new work looks at ways of improving outcome after induction by reducing sensory stimuli in the operating room.

M. Wood, MD, FRCA

Severe Anaphylactic Reaction to Cisatracurium in a Child
Legros CB, Orliaguet GA, Mayer M-N, et al (Groupe Hospitalier Necker-Enfants Malades, Paris)
Anesth Analg 92:648-649, 2001   6–5

Background.—More than three quarters of cases of anaphylactic shock during anesthesia are attributable to muscle relaxants. Allergic reactions are less frequent in children than in adults. A new, nondepolarizing muscle relaxant, cisatracurium, induces fewer allergic reactions than other muscle relaxants. A case of anaphylactic reaction induced by cisatracurium in a child was described.

> *Case Report.*—Boy, 10 years, with American Society of Anesthesiologists physical status III was scheduled for decompressive craniectomy for treatment of intracranial hypertension. His medical history included asthma, left thoracotomy related to surgical correction of patent ductus arteriosus, meningitis, ectopic testicles, and psychomotor defect. In 9 previous surgical procedures, vecuronium was used without any adverse effect. The boy was not taking any daily medication and had no known allergies to medications. After preoperative medication with clorazepate dipotassic, anesthesia was induced with sevoflurane 8%, nitrous oxide 50% in oxygen, and sufentanil 25 µg, with cisatracurium (3.2 mg) administered for tracheal intubation. Anesthesia was maintained with desflurane (5%) and nitrous oxide 50% in oxygen. A moderate sinus tachycardia developed 10 minutes after induction, and blood pressure decreased to 60/30 mm Hg. A generalized erythema was noted, and the patient's breath sounds were decreased bilaterally

with wheezing. Anaphylactic shock was diagnosed. Desflurane and nitrous oxide were stopped. An IV line filled with Elohes was disconnected. Infusion with Elohes had not commenced when the anaphylactic reaction occurred. Blood pressure increased to 100/40 mm Hg after IV administration of 0.5 mg of epinephrine, which was repeated. An epinephrine infusion was started at 0.5 mg · h^{-1} along with an albumin infusion at 750 mL · h^{-1}. The patient also received 500 mg of hydrocortisone. His blood pressure stabilized to 90/50 mm Hg, and arterial oxygen saturation was 99%. The surgical procedure was canceled, and the patient was moved to the neurosurgical ICU, sedated, and mechanically ventilated for 12 hours. The boy was gradually weaned from epinephrine, which was discontinued 24 hours after onset of anaphylactic shock. His recovery was uneventful. Intradermal skin reaction testing yielded positive results for cisatracurium, Elohes, and other muscle relaxants.

Conclusions.—In this patient, who experienced an anaphylactic reaction to cisatracurium, other possible diagnoses were considered and included latex, Elohes, and sufentanil allergy. Latex allergy has been implicated in 17% of cases of intraoperative anaphylaxis in children and is the more frequent etiology in children. However, a latex test in this case was negative. The incidence of hydroxyethyl starch, including Elohes, is extremely low. In this case, although a line was connected, infusion with Elohes had not begun at the time of the anaphylactic reaction. It is possible that sufentanil was the cause of the anaphylactic response in this patient, but there are no reports of sufentanil allergy in the literature.

▶ Cisatracurium was introduced to supersede atracurium as a new nondepolarizing relaxant that is less likely to cause histamine release. This case report demonstrates that severe anaphylaxis can occur.

M. Wood, MD, FRCA

Caudal Ropivacaine in Infants: Population Pharmacokinetics and Plasma Concentrations
Hansen TG, Ilett KF, Reid C, et al (Princess Margaret Hosp for Children, Perth, Western Australia; Univ of Western Australia, Nedlands)
Anesthesiology 94:579-584, 2001   6–6

Background.—One of the most commonly performed regional anesthetic blocks in small children is the caudal epidural block with bupivacaine. Its primary use is as an adjunct to general anesthesia to provide good immediate postoperative analgesia and a smooth recovery. Occasionally, caudal epidural block with bupivacaine is used as the only anesthetic in infants at risk for complications from general anesthesia and tracheal intubation. Ropivacaine is a new, long-acting amino-amide local anesthetic. However, there are no data regarding its use in infants. The pharmacokinetics of caudal epidural block with ropivacaine in infants younger than 12 months were investigated.

Methods.—Two groups of infants, 1 aged 0 to 3 months (group 1, n = 15) and 1 aged 3 to 12 months (group 2, n = 15), were given a caudal bolus dose of 0.2% ropivacaine (2 mg/kg) before undergoing standardized general anesthesia. Serial blood samples were obtained for all infants for up to 12 hours and analyzed for total and free ropivacaine with high-performance liquid chromatography. Population pharmacokinetic modeling was used to obtain estimates of clearance, volume of distribution, and absorption rate constants for bupivacaine. An analysis of covariates on the kinetic parameters was performed.

Results.—The maximum free ropivacaine concentration was significantly higher in group 1 than in group 2 (99 µg/L vs 38 µg/L). This was also the case for the median free fraction of ropivacaine (10% vs 5%). The pharmacokinetic variables of the total population were best described by a one-compartment model with first-order absorption. Other pharmacokinetic values were mean clearance, 0.31 L · h^{-1} · kg^{-1}; volume of distribution, 2.12 L/kg; and absorption rate constant, 1.61 h^{-1}. Mean absorption and elimination half-lives were 0.43 and 5.1 hours, respectively. Significant covariates for clearance were age and percentage of free ropivacaine. The posterior Bayesian estimates of clearance were significantly higher in older children (38%) (Table 3).

Conclusions.—The concentrations of total and free plasma ropivacaine in infants after caudal ropivacaine were within the range of concentrations that have already been reported for older children and adults. Significant covariates of ropivacaine clearance were age and percentage of free ropivacaine.

TABLE 3.—Posterior Bayesian Estimates of Pharmacokinetic Parameters for Ropivacaine in All Infants (n = 30), Those Aged Less Than 3 Months (Group 1; n = 15), and Those Aged More Than 3 Months (Group 2; n = 15)

Parameter	Group	Mean*
CL/F (I · h^{-1} · kg^{-1})	All patients	0.34 (0.29, 0.39)
	Group 1 < 3 months	0.29 (0.22, 0.35)
	Group 2 > 3 months	0.39 (0.32, 0.47)†
V/F (I/kg)	All patients	2.21 (1.96, 2.45)
	Group 1 < 3 months	1.99 (1.70, 2.28)
	Group 2 > 3 months	2.42 (2.03, 2.81)
k$_a$ (h^{-1})	All patients	1.61 (1.39, 1.89)
	Group 1 < 3 months	1.47 (1.11, 1.81)
	Group 2 > 3 months	1.75 (1.44, 2.06)

*95% confidence interval.
†Two-tailed *t* test = 2.3; *P* = .029; power of test = 51%.
Abbreviations: CL, Clearance; F, bioavailability; V, volume of distribution; k$_a$, absorption rate, constant.
(Courtesy of Hansen TG, Ilett KF, Reid C, et al: Caudal ropivacaine in infants: Population pharmacokinetics and plasma concentrations. *Anesthesiology* 94:579-584, 2001. Copyright American Society of Anesthesiologists, Inc. Used with permission of Lippincott Williams & Wilkins, Inc.)

▶ I selected this article because the study was very carefully conducted, and unfortunately, detailed pharmacokinetic studies are not often performed in small infants. The data are important, and the authors are to be congratulated. Venous blood samples of 1.0 mL were obtained, proving that even in small infants with volume constraints, these studies can be done.

M. Wood, MD, FRCA

Anesthesia-Related Cardiac Arrest in Children: Initial Findings of the Pediatric Perioperative Cardiac Arrest (POCA) Registry
Morray JP, Geiduschek JM, Ramamoorthy C, et al (Univ of Washington, Seattle; Stanford Univ, Calif)
Anesthesiology 93:6-14, 2000   6–7

Background.—The risk of perioperative cardiac arrest is higher in children than in adults. Although a number of risk factors have been identified, it is sometimes difficult to identify the immediate cause of the arrest. Anesthesia-related cardiac arrest in children is an uncommon event. Data from the multi-institutional Pediatric Perioperative Cardiac Arrest Registry were used to analyze the causes and outcomes of anesthesia-related cardiac arrests in children.

Methods and Findings.—Since the registry's founding in 1994 through 1997, 289 arrests were reported by 63 participating institutions. One hundred fifty of these events were classified as anesthesia related. The incidence of anesthesia-related cardiac arrest was estimated at 1.4 per 10,000 instances of anesthesia. The associated mortality rate was 26%. Thirty-seven percent of arrests were medication related, and 32% were from cardiovascular causes (Table 2). Most of the medication-related arrests were related to cardiovascular depression from halothane, with or without other drugs.

One third of the children with anesthesia-related arrests were in American Society of Anesthesiologists (ASA) physical status category 1 or 2. The rate of medication-related arrests was 64% for this group, compared with 23% for children with ASA physical status 3 to 5 (Fig 1). Fifty-five percent of the anesthesia-related arrests were in infants younger than 1 year. On multivariate analysis, independent predictors of mortality were ASA physical status 3 to 5 (odds ratio [OR], 12.99) and emergency status (OR, 3.88).

Discussion.—This analysis of a large series of pediatric anesthesia-related cardiac arrests provides new information on the causes and outcomes of these rare events. Most such events occur in infants and in patients with severe underlying disease. Anesthesia-related arrests are more likely to be fatal in children with ASA physical status 3 to 5 and in those undergoing emergency surgery. The majority of anesthesia-related cardiac arrests are related to medications, especially halothane. The findings will help to guide preventive efforts.

TABLE 2.—Mechanism of Cardiac Arrest

Mechanism	Number of Arrests
Medication-related	55 (37%)
Inhalation agents	
Halothane alone	26 (46%)
Halothane plus an intravenous medication	11 (20%)
Sevoflurane alone	2 (4%)
Intravenous medications	
Single	5 (9%)
Combination	5 (9%)
Intravenous injection of local anesthetic	5 (9%)
Succinylcholine-induced hyperkalemia	1 (2%)
Cardiovascular	48 (32%)
Presumed CV, unclear etiology	18 (38%)
Hemorrhage, transfusion-related	8 (17%)
Inadequate/Inappropriate fluid therapy	6 (13%)
Arrhythmia	5 (10%)
Hyperkalemia	4 (8%)
Air embolism	2 (4%)
Pacemaker-related	2 (4%)
Vagel response	1 (2%)
Pulmonary hypertension	1 (2%)
Tetralogy hypercyanotic spell	1 (2%)
Respiratory	30 (20%)
Laryngospasm	9 (30%)
Airway obstruction	8 (27%)
Difficult intubation	4 (13%)
Inadequate oxygenation	3 (10%)
Inadvertent extubation	2 (7%)
Presumed respiratory, unclear etiology	2 (7%)
Inadequate ventilation	1 (3%)
Bronchospasm	1 (3%)
Equipment-related	10 (7%)
Central line	4 (40%)
Breathing circuit	2 (20%)
Peripheral intravenous catheter	1 (10%)
Other	3 (30%)
Multiple events	5 (3%)
Hypothermia	1 (<1%)
Unclear etiology	1 (<1%)

Abbreviation: CV, Cardiovascular.
(Courtesy of Morray JP, Geiduschek JM, Ramamoorthy C, et al: Anesthesia-related cardiac arrest in children: Initial findings of the Pediatric Perioperative Cardiac Arrest [POCA] Registry. *Anesthesiology* 93:6-14, 2000. Copyright American Society of Anesthesiologists, Inc. Used with permission of Lippincott-Raven Publishers.)

▶ This article reviews all the cases of perioperative cardiac arrest that occurred during a 4-year period at 63 institutions, the majority of which are university affiliated and almost half are pediatric hospitals. A total of 289 cases of cardiac arrest were reported, with 150 found to be anesthesia related. This careful review of causes and associated factors of cardiac arrest, and contributors to mortality provides important insight into cardiac arrest in the pediatric surgical population. Although two thirds of the patients who had cardiac arrests were ASA classification 3 to 5, indicating significant underlying illness, examining the one third otherwise healthy patients who had intraoperative arrests provides important information. Most notably, 64% were medication related, with almost three fourths of those being

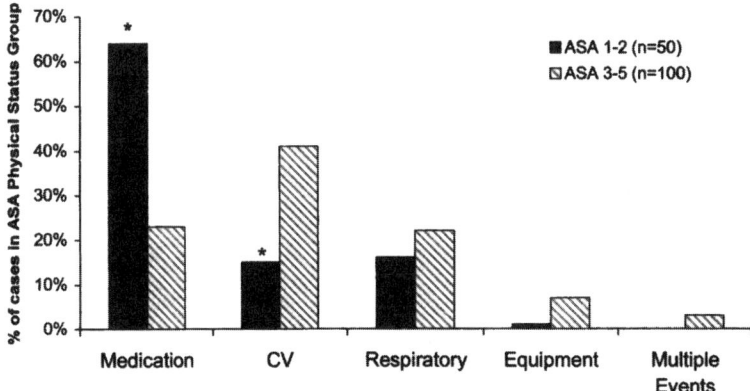

FIGURE 1.—Primary cause of anesthesia-related cardiac arrest in American Society of Anesthesiologists *(ASA)* physical status 1-2 and 3-5 patients. *Asterisk, P* < .01 compared with ASA physical status 3-5 patients. *Abbreviation:* CV, Cardiovascular. (Courtesy of Morray JP, Geiduschek JM, Ramamoorthy C, et al: Anesthesia-related cardiac arrest in children: Initial findings of the Pediatric Perioperative Cardiac Arrest [POCA] Registry. *Anesthesiology* 93:6-14, 2000. Copyright American Society of Anesthesiologists, Inc. Used with permission of Lippincott-Raven Publishers.)

related to administration of volatile anesthetic agents (primarily halothane). In general, the patients who had cardiac arrests related to the administration of halothane were infants (median age, 6 months), and the median halothane concentration was 2%. Of the 37 patients who had halothane-related arrests, 26 were receiving halothane at concentrations below 3%. These data are supportive of the concept that young patients (younger than 1 year) may be more susceptible to halothane-mediated cardiovascular depression than older children. All 3 of the deaths related to halothane occurred in patients with underlying cardiac disease. It remains to be seen whether the increasing use of sevoflurane will change the observed incidence of volatile anesthetic–related cardiac arrest in pediatric patients. Cardiac arrest related to injection of local anesthetic was reported in only 5 of the 150 cases. All of these patients recovered uneventfully.

A respiratory event as the cause for cardiac arrest was reported in only 20% of cases. This incidence is considerably lower than that in earlier reports and may be because of the near universal use of pulse oximetry and capnography in this series. These monitors may lead to an earlier diagnosis of respiratory problems, allowing correction of the problem before arrest. It is also possible that in earlier studies without routine use of pulse oximetry and capnography, cardiac arrest without other obvious causes might have been more commonly attributed to respiratory insufficiency. The most common respiratory problems in ASA 1 and 2 patients were laryngospasm and airway obstruction (in patients with underlying airway pathology). In patients who had cardiac arrest because of airway obstruction, no deaths occurred related to the arrest.

The ASA 1 and 2 patients differed significantly from the ASA 3 to 5 patients in several ways. First, the causes of arrests were different. Second, all deaths occurred in patients with significant underlying disease.

The mortality rate was 26% and was increased in patients with an ASA classification of 3 to 5 and in patients undergoing emergency surgical procedures. Although arrests were more common in the younger age group, age was not a predictor of mortality after arrest.

The purpose of projects such as this one is to identify both patient- and practice-related risk factors for cardiac arrest and to develop strategies to decrease the risk for intraoperative cardiac arrest, as well as to minimize morbidity or mortality related to perioperative arrest. The high proportion of arrests in otherwise healthy patients, especially infants, caused by volatile anesthetic agents is an important observation. It is likely that the vast majority of otherwise healthy children having surgery received a volatile agent, so that these data do not imply that these agents are dangerous in children. They do suggest that when using these agents, the development of "warning signs," as observed in 89% of these cases before arrest, should be responded to promptly and that in particular with younger children, we should pay close attention to anesthetic concentration—and duration of administration of high inspired agent concentration. The lack of mortality in otherwise healthy patients who have anesthesia-related perioperative cardiac arrest is reassuring that prompt recognition, diagnosis of the problem, and treatment will in most cases result in a good outcome. It is also encouraging that the improvements in monitoring over the years appear to have had a positive impact on our patient care.[1]

S. Black, MD

Reference

1. Morray J, Geiduschek J, Caplan R, et al: A comparison of pediatric and adult anesthesia malpractice claims. *Anesthesiology* 78:461-467, 1993.

Sevoflurane Mask Induction of Anaesthesia Is Associated With Epileptiform EEG in Children

Vakkuri A, Yli-Hankala A, Särkelä M, et al (Univ of Helsinki; Tampere Univ, Finland; Oulu Univ, Finland)
Acta Anaesthesiol Scand 45:805-811, 2001   6–8

Background.—Inducing and maintaining anesthesia for children and adults often involves the use of sevoflurane. Sevoflurane inhalation induction has been linked to epileptiform electroencephalographic (EEG) results in adults accompanied by increased heart rate and blood pressure levels. Children have been noted to have transient hyperdynamic cardiovascular responses to sevoflurane. A population of children was assessed for the presence of epileptiform EEG activity in association with transient hyperdynamic cardiovascular responses.

Methods.—Thirty-one children (ASA 1-2) who were scheduled for elective otolaryngologic surgery were assessed. All were older than 2 years and younger than 12 years. None had a history of cardiac, pulmonary, or neurologic disease; febrile convulsions or any other seizure activity; gastroesophageal reflux; or body mass index higher than 28. Premedication 30 minutes before anesthesia was oral midazolam 0.5 mg/kg to a maximum of 15 mg and atropine 0.03 mg/kg to a maximum of 1 mg. Patients were randomly assigned to a controlled ventilation (CV) group or a spontaneous breathing (SB) group for sevoflurane mask inhalation induction. Manual control of ventilation was started for the CV group when the children were unresponsive to verbal commands. End-tidal carbon dioxide ($ETCO_2$) level was documented and maintained between 4.3% and 5.3%. If a patient in the SB group had apnea develop, a 30-second waiting period without ventilation was accepted. If no spontaneous breathing resumed, slow controlled ventilation began. Their $ETCO_2$ rose to 6% to 6.7% to correspond to sevoflurane-induced ventilatory depression.

Results.—Twenty-five percent of the CV group and none of the SB group had suppression with spikes. Forty-four percent of the CV group and 20% of the SB groups had rhythmic polyspikes. Periodic epileptiform discharges occurred in 44% of the CV group and none of the SB group ($P < .01$). Thus, 88% of the CV group and 20% of the SB group had interictal epileptiform discharges ($P < .001$). After intubation, first $ETCO_2$ was 5.1% in the CV group and 5.6% in the SB group. The first end-tidal sevoflurane concentrations in the 2 groups were essentially equal. After endotracheal intubation, sevoflurane concentration was decreased to 2%, and all patients returned to a normal EEG pattern. The heart rate of those in the CV group increased from 96 to 120 beats/min at 2 minutes for a $P < .001$ within the group when compared with baseline and a $P < .05$ between the 2 groups. An initial increase (at 1 min) in mean arterial pressure occurred (88-97 mm Hg) that fell after 3 minutes. The SB group's heart rate increased from 106 to 133 beats/min at 2 minutes for a $P < .01$ within the group. A significant decline in mean arterial pressure (85-66

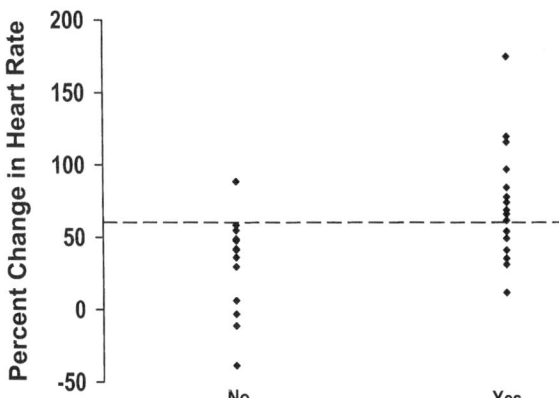

FIGURE 3.—Change (percentages from the baseline) in heart rate in patients without (*No*) and with (*Yes*) epileptiform EEG activity. *Dotted line* indicates a more than 60% change level used in the Fisher exact test. $P < .01$ between the groups. (Courtesy of Vakkuri A, Yli-Hankala A, Särkelä M, et al: Sevoflurane mask induction of anaesthesia is associated with epileptiform EEG in children. *Acta Anaesthesiol Scand* 45:805-811, 2001.)

mm Hg) occurred at 5 minutes. A heart rate increase exceeding 60% was linked to epileptiform EEG activity in all but 1 case (Fig 3).

Conclusions.—During sevoflurane inhalation induction, many children had epileptiform EEG activity corresponding to a hyperdynamic circulatory response. No jerking movements were noted during induction. Thus, the use of sevoflurane mask induction with a high inspiratory concentration from the start of induction carries the potential for triggering epileptogenic responses.

▶ This is a prospective trial of sevoflurane inhalation induction with CV or SB after loss of consciousness to examine the incidence of epileptiform activity. The authors postulate that the hyperdynamic response often seen with high inspired concentrations of sevoflurane may in some patients be caused by seizure activity. These results certainly lend credence to that theory. In patients with CV, almost 90% of patients had some epileptiform activity during the induction period. In SB patients (with higher ETCO$_2$ levels) the incidence of epileptiform activity was considerably lower (20%). Because the initial anesthetic concentration after intubation was the same between groups, this difference was not related to anesthetic depth but to the difference in ventilation. Of note are the qualitatively different hemodynamic responses (although the differences were not statistically significant). In the CV group with the high incidence of seizurelike activity, heart rate increase was greater and systemic blood pressure initially increased compared with the SB group, in whom heart rate increase was less and blood pressure decreased at all time points after induction of anesthesia. The authors also note that in all but 1 patient heart rate increased rather dramatically with the onset of the epileptiform activity. This study provides one possible mechanism for the observed hyperdynamic cardiovascular response sometimes seen with sevoflurane induction. It also raises an important clinical question regarding a potential adverse impact on cerebral homeostasis. No clinical recommendation regarding neurologic consequences of sevoflurane-induced epileptiform activity could be made based on this study. Some evaluation regarding cerebral metabolism, cerebral ischemic events, or neurologic/cognitive function would need to be made. Given the invasiveness and cost of some of these evaluations, such a study would be a daunting task.

S. Black, MD

Cardiovascular Effects of Sevoflurane, Isoflurane, Halothane, and Fentanyl-Midazolam in Children With Congenital Heart Disease: An Echocardiographic Study of Myocardial Contractility and Hemodynamics
Rivenes SM, Lewin MB, Stayer SA, et al (Baylor College of Medicine, Houston; Texas Children's Hosp, Houston)
Anesthesiology 94:223-229, 2001   6–9

Introduction.—The cardiovascular effects of halogenated anesthetic agents have not been well studied in children with congenital heart disease. Transthoracic echocardiography was used to compare systemic hemodynamics and effects on myocardial contractility of sevoflurane, isoflurane, halothane, and fentanyl-midazolam in children undergoing surgery for congenital heart defects.

Study Design.—Fifty-four pediatric patients undergoing surgery for congenital heart defects were randomly assigned to receive sevoflurane, isoflurane, halothane, or fentanyl-midazolam. Cardiovascular and echocardiographic data were recorded at baseline and at 1 and 1.5 minimum alveolar concentrations.

Findings.—The use of halothane for pediatric congenital heart surgery was associated with a significant decrease in mean arterial pressure, ejection fraction, and cardiac index. Fentanyl-midazolam caused a significant decrease in cardiac index, secondary to a decrease in heart rate. Sevoflurane maintained cardiac index and heart rate and had less hypotensive and negative inotropic effects than halothane. Isoflurane maintained cardiac index and ejection fraction and had less suppression of mean arterial pressure than halothane (Table 4).

Conclusions.—In a pediatric patients undergoing surgery for congenital heart defects, sevoflurane and isoflurane maintained systemic cardiac output, with little contractility change. Isoflurane also increased heart rate and lowered systemic vascular resistance. Fentanyl-midazolam maintained contractility but decreased heart rate and cardiac output. Halothane decreased contractility, cardiac output, mean arterial pressure, and systemic vascular resistance. It is not known whether use of halothane in this patient population is associated with a worse outcome. This information can be used to select anesthetic regimens for pediatric patients with congenital heart defects.

▶ In this well-controlled and clearly presented randomized prospective trial, the authors compare the cardiovascular effects of 3 different volatile anesthetic agents and fentanyl-midazolam in pediatric patients before repair of congenital heart defects. The authors used repeated transthoracic echocardiographic examinations along with measurement of heart rate, systemic blood pressure, and central venous pressure. It is a remarkably thorough evaluation of each agent's cardiovascular effects at different MAC levels (1 and 1.5 MAC). Isoflurane increased heart rate, decreased blood pressure and systemic vascular resistance, but preserved ventricular function. Halothane decreased blood pressure, ventricular function, and to a lesser extent sys-

TABLE 4.—Measured and Calculated Hemodynamic and Echocardiographic Variables

Agent	MAC	HR (beats/min)	MAP (mmHg)	EF (%)	SF (%)	SVI (ml/m²)	LVEDVI (ml/m²)	CI (l · min⁻¹ · m⁻²)	SVRI (dyne · s · cm⁻⁵ · m²)
Halothane	0	129 ± 22	77 ± 15	63 ± 9	40 ± 5	36 ± 16	44 ± 19	4.49 ± 1.87	1,425 ± 622
	1	130 ± 19	60 ± 11*	54 ± 12*	32 ± 7*†	28 ± 11*	38 ± 14	3.47 ± 1.17	1,331 ± 529
	1.5	129 ± 17	49 ± 12*	50 ± 13*	30 ± 8*†	26 ± 11*	39 ± 12	3.34 ± 1.36*	1,132 ± 503*
Sevoflurane	0	123 ± 32	67 ± 8	68 ± 11	44 ± 7	56 ± 41	37 ± 15	6.91 ± 4.32	1,014 ± 653
	1	126 ± 26	58 ± 13*	62 ± 9	39 ± 7	52 ± 31	36 ± 18	6.59 ± 4.04	883 ± 592
	1.5	128 ± 25	58 ± 13*	58 ± 10*	39 ± 9	46 ± 26	35 ± 14	5.78 ± 3.06	782 ± 390
Isoflurane	0	112 ± 27	69 ± 12	63 ± 7	39 ± 5	46 ± 22	46 ± 24	4.96 ± 2.74	1,377 ± 809
	1	125 ± 16*	54 ± 9*	62 ± 8	37 ± 4	39 ± 17	40 ± 17	4.82 ± 2.20	1,022 ± 601*
	1.5	128 ± 23*	50 ± 9*	59 ± 9	36 ± 5	39 ± 17	42 ± 19	4.59 ± 2.12	950 ± 513*
Fentanyl-midazolam	0	106 ± 22‡	66 ± 8	63 ± 6	40 ± 6	46 ± 34	54 ± 25	5.16 ± 4.39	1,261 ± 644
	1	87 ± 19*§	59 ± 11*	60 ± 7	39 ± 5	42 ± 30	47 ± 25	3.79 ± 3.05*	1,540 ± 806
	1.5	82 ± 18*§	56 ± 11*	59 ± 7	38 ± 7	43 ± 30	52 ± 24	3.67 ± 2.99*	1,559 ± 875

All values mean SD
*P < .05, one-way analysis of variance, different from 0 minimum alveolar concentration (MAC) within the same anesthetic group.
†P < .05, two-way analysis of variance, halothane versus sevoflurane and fentanyl-midazolam at 1 and 1.5 MAC.
‡P < .05, two-way analysis of variance, fentanyl-midazolam versus halothane at 0 MAC.
§P < .05, two-way analysis of variance, fentanyl-midazolam versus halothane, sevoflurane, and isoflurane at 1 and 1.5 MAC.
Abbreviations: HR, Heart rate; MAP, mean arterial pressure; EF, ejection fraction; SF, shortening fraction; SVI, stroke volume index; LVEDVI, left ventricular end-diastolic volume index; CI, systemic cardiac index; SVRI, systemic vascular resistance index.
(Courtesy of Rivenes SM, Lewin MB, Stayer SA, et al: Cardiovascular effects of sevoflurane, isoflurane, halothane, and fentanyl-midazolam in children wth congenital heart disease: An echocardiographic study of myocardial contractility and hemodynamics. Anesthesiology 94:223-229, 2001. Copyright American Society of Anesthesiologists, Inc. Used with permission of Lippincott-Raven Publishers.)

temic vascular resistance. Sevoflurane decreased blood pressure and left ventricular function, but significantly less than halothane. Fentanyl-midazolam decreased heart rate, systemic blood pressure, and cardiac index (because of decreased heart rate), while preserving left ventricular contractility. Although these results are hardly surprising, this study clearly defines these results. It confirms the effects of the individual agents on various parameters in the pediatric patient with heart disease. Sevoflurane as an agent for inhalation induction has potential advantages over halothane in some patients with congenital heart disease if avoiding myocardial depression is of clinical importance.

S. Black, MD

The Safety and Efficacy of Sevoflurane Anesthesia in Infants and Children With Congenital Heart Disease
Russell IA, Miller Hance WC, Gregory G, et al (Univ of California, San Francisco)
Anesth Analg 92:1152-1158, 2001   6–10

Background.—Although halothane has been used as the inhalation anesthetic of choice for pediatric patients, studies suggest that the use of sevoflurane may be preferable in those with heart disease. The safety of sevoflurane during induction and maintenance of anesthesia for cardiac surgery in pediatric patients was compared with that of halothane in a randomized, double-blind, open-label study.

Study Design.—A total of 180 prospectively enrolled pediatric patients scheduled for elective correction of congenital heart disease were studied. Each patient's history and findings from echocardiographic examination or cardiac catheterization were reviewed to confirm the diagnosis. Baseline arterial saturation, heart rate, and blood pressure were obtained. Patients were randomly assigned to inhalation anesthesia with either halothane or sevoflurane. Hemodynamics, arterial saturations, blood pressure, respiratory gases, ECGs, and echocardiograms were monitored during anesthesia. The primary outcome variables were severe hypotension, bradycardia, and oxygen desaturation.

Findings.—Pediatric cardiac surgery patients who received inhalation anesthesia with halothane had twice as many episodes of severe hypotension as those who received sevoflurane anesthesia (Table 3). These hypotensive episodes occurred despite an increased use of vasopressors in the patients in the halothane group. Multivariate regression analysis indicated that patients younger than 1 year were at increased risk of hypotension, and patients with preoperative cyanosis were at increased risk of developing oxygen desaturation.

Conclusions.—Inhalation anesthesia with sevoflurane may have hemodynamic advantages over inhalation anesthesia with halothane in pediatric patients undergoing surgery for congenital heart disease.

TABLE 3.—Outcomes

Variable	Halothane ($n = 89$)	Sevoflurane ($n = 91$)	P
Primary outcomes			
Incidences, n (%)			
Cardiovascular event	69 (78)	65 (71)	0.39
Severe bradycardia	5 (6)	3 (3)	0.49
Severe hypotension	67 (57)	64 (70)	0.51
Defibrillation/cardioversion	2 (2)	1 (1)	0.62
Arterial desaturation	7 (8)	5 (5)	0.56
Median no. episodes per patient			
Cardiovascular event	2	1	0.03
Arterial desaturation	0	0	0.56
Secondary outcomes			
Incidences, n (%)			
Moderate bradycardia	20 (22)	8 (9)	0.1
Moderate hypotension	87 (98)	86 (95)	0.44
Moderate tachycardia	89 (100)	89 (98)	0.50
Moderate desaturation	21 (24)	12 (13)	0.08
Emergent drug use	18 (20)	7 (8)	0.02
Atropine	4 (4)	1 (1)	0.21
Phenylephrine	9 (10)	6 (7)	0.43
Ephedrine	4 (4)	0 (0)	0.06
Epinephrine	1 (1)	0 (0)	0.49
Ventricular dysrhythmia	46 (52)	52 (58)	0.45
Junctional dysrhythmias	25 (28)	19 (21)	0.30
Induction characteristics			
Duration, min (mean ± SD)	3.4 ± 1.1	3.5 ± 1.1	0.75
Good acceptance, n (%)	48 (54)	52 (57)	0.76
Agitation, n (%)	36 (40)	35 (38)	0.88
Coughing, n (%)	5 (6)	4 (4)	0.75
Breath holding, n (%)	2 (2)	5 (5)	0.44
Salivation, n (%)	2 (2)	3 (3)	1.00
Obstruction, n (%)	5 (6)	7 (8)	0.77
Bronchospasm, n (%)	1 (1)	1 (1)	1.00

(Courtesy of Russell IA, Miller Hance WC, Gregory G, et al: The safety and efficacy of sevoflurane anesthesia in infants and children with congenital heart disease. *Anesth Analg* 92:1152-1158, 2001.)

▶ This is the second study included addressing the use of sevoflurane and halothane in patients with congenital heart disease undergoing cardiac surgical procedures. These authors conducted a randomized, prospective, blinded comparison of sevoflurane and halothane for inhalation induction followed by maintenance with the volatile agent supplemented with low-dose fentanyl (total dose, 10 µg/kg). The authors report a high, but similar incidence of hypotension with both techniques, with hypotension developing in more than 70% of patients. However, the number of episodes of severe hypotension per patient, the incidence of bradycardia, and the incidence of emergent drug administration were all higher in the patients anesthetized with halothane. There was no difference in the incidence of ventricular dysrhythmias as one might expect. Other predictors of intraoperative hypotension included an age of less than 1 year and the presence of congestive heart failure. The only predictor for development of intraoperative arterial oxygenation desaturation was preoperative cyanosis.

It might be expected that sevoflurane would have clinical advantages over halothane, especially in pediatric patients with cardiovascular disease. First, the lower blood solubility of sevoflurane would be expected to allow for more rapid titration of anesthetic depth, perhaps decreasing the incidence of anesthetic overdose. Second, the lower arrhythmia potential and lesser depression of cardiac function noted with sevoflurane might be expected to translate into a safer clinical profile as compared with halothane.

S. Black, MD

The Optimal Length of Insertion of Central Venous Catheters for Pediatric Patients

Andropoulos DB, Bent ST, Skjonsby B, et al (Texas Children's Hosp, Houston; Baylor College of Medicine, Houston)
Anesth Analg 93:883-886, 2001   6–11

Background.—Percutaneous central venous catheterization through the superior vena cava is often used for anesthesia during major surgery for

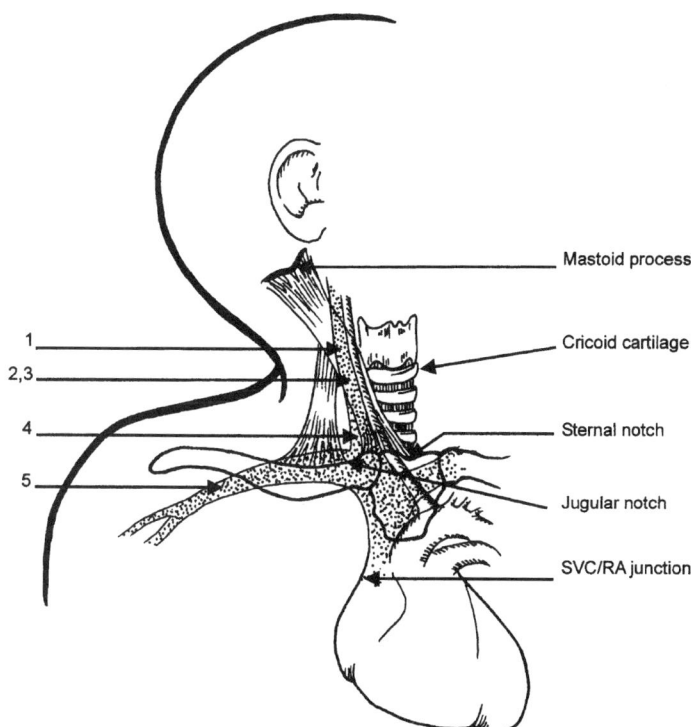

FIGURE 1.—Surface and deep landmarks for right internal jugular (RIJ) and subclavian venipuncture. Puncture sites: *1* = high approach to RIJ used in this study—midway between mastoid process and sternal notch. *2,3* = middle approach using apex of muscular triangle formed by the sternal and clavicular heads of the sternocleidomastoid muscle, or lateral to the cricoid cartilage. *4* = low approach using the jugular notch as a landmark. *5* = subclavian vein puncture site used in this study—1 cm lateral to the midpoint of clavicle for patient weighing <10 kg, 2 cm lateral if >10 kg. *Abbreviation: SVC/RA,* Superior vena cava/right atrium. (Courtesy of Andropoulos DB, Bent ST, Skjonsby B, et al: The optimal length of insertion of central venous catheters for pediatric patients. *Anesth Analg* 93:883-886, 2001.)

pediatric patients. The position of the central venous catheter (CVC) is often not examined until the postoperative chest radiograph, and a malpositioned CVC may remain for hours. A large series of CVC pediatric placements were reviewed to develop guidelines for the correct insertion and placement of a CVC in a pediatric patient.

Study Design.—A total of 456 CVC placements in pediatric patients undergoing surgery for congenital heart disease were reviewed. There were 330 insertions in the right internal jugular vein and 126 in the right subclavian vein (Fig 1). The first postoperative chest radiograph was used to localize the CVC. All data were collected prospectively and included patient height and weight. The distance from the CVC insertion site to the superior vena cava/right atrium junction was plotted versus patient height and weight. Regression lines, correlation coefficients, and confidence intervals were calculated.

Findings.—For right internal jugular or subclavian catheters in patients with a height of 100 cm or less: Initial length of insertion (cm) = (Height in cm/10) − 1. For patients with a height of more than 100 cm: Initial length of insertion (cm) = (Height in cm/10) − 2. The percentage of CVCs that would be placed correctly by using these formulas is 97%. Guidelines were also developed based on weight (Table 1). With these guidelines, the percentage of CVCs that would be placed correctly is 98%.

Conclusions.—With the use of the above guidelines, it should be possible to avoid the initial malpositioning of percutaneous CVCs in pediatric patients. The CVC position should still be confirmed as soon as possible by imaging, and any corrections should be performed to prevent complications.

TABLE 1.—Recommended Length of Central Venous Catheter *(CVC)* Insertion in Pediatric Patients Based on Weight

Patient Weight (kg)	Length of CVC Insertion (cm)
2-2.9	4
3-4.9	5
5-6.9	6
7-9.9	7
10-12.9	8
13-19.9	9
20-29.9	10
30-39.9	11
40-49.9	12
50-59.9	13
60-69.9	14
70-79.9	15
≥80	16

(Courtesy of Andropoulos DB, Bent ST, Skjonsby B, et al: The optimal length of insertion of central venous catheters for pediatric patients. *Anesth Analg* 93:883-886, 2001.)

▶ These authors make an excellent point: preoperatively placed CVCs often do not have their position confirmed until the postoperative period, and the rare complications associated with line placement may be increased with malpositioning. By studying a large series of pediatric patients, the authors have defined guidelines based on either height or weight for predicting proper placement length of the CVC from either right internal jugular vein or right subclavian vein cannulation. By their evaluation, these guidelines (formulas based on height, or specific insertion length based on weight ranges) resulted in proper placement in 97% of patients when using the height-based formulas, or 98% of patients when using the weight-based table. Before using these recommendations, please note that the skin insertion site for the internal jugular cannulation is somewhat higher than some anesthesiologists use and somewhat more lateral for subclavian vein cannulation. The authors recommend that if lower insertion sites for internal jugular vein cannulation (or more medial for subclavian vein cannulation) are used, that these distances should be subtracted from the insertion guidelines as recommended in this publication. As the authors recommend, proper positioning still needs to be confirmed with a chest x-ray in the perioperative period. Use of these simple guidelines, however, may result in a lower incidence of central line malposition.

S. Black, MD

7 Head Injury and Neuroanesthesia

Lack of Effect of Induction of Hypothermia After Acute Brain Injury
Clifton GL, Miller ER, Choi SC, et al (Univ of Texas, Houston; Virginia Commonwealth Univ, Richmond; Baylor College of Medicine, Houston; et al)
N Engl J Med 344:556-563, 2001   7–1

Background.—Small clinical studies have suggested that inducing hypothermia in patients with brain injury improves outcomes, but the results have not been definitive. A multicenter comparison of the effects of hypothermia with those of normothermia in patients with acute brain injury was reported.

Methods.—Three hundred ninety-two patients, aged 16 to 65 years, with coma after closed head injury were assigned randomly to treatment with hypothermia or normothermia. Treatment with hypothermia, in which body temperature was reduced to 33°C by surface cooling, was begun 6 hours after injury and maintained for 48 hours. The 2 treatment groups were comparable in mean age and injury type and severity. All other treatment was standard.

Findings.—The mean time between injury and randomization was 4.3 hours in the hypothermia group and 4.1 hours in the normothermia group. The mean time from injury to attainment of the target temperature in hypothermia recipients was 8.4 hours. Poor outcomes, including severe disability, vegetative state, or death, occurred in 57% of both groups (Table 4). The mortality rates were 28% and 27% in the hypothermia and normothermia groups, respectively. The patients treated with hypothermia had longer hospital stays and more complications than did patients in the normothermia group. Fewer patients receiving hypothermia had high intracranial pressure than those not receiving hypothermia.

Conclusions.—Treatment with hypothermia within 8 hours of severe head injury in patients with coma did not improve outcomes. Hypothermia treatment appeared to prolong hospitalization and increase the occurrence of complications.

▶ This study finally puts to rest the debate on whether hypothermia induction after acute brain injury might be beneficial. This was a multicenter study,

TABLE 4.—Rates of Poor Outcome and Death Six Months After Severe Brain Injury in Patients Treated With Induction of Hypothermia or Normothermia

Treatment Group	Total No.	No. (%) With Poor Outcome*	Relative Risk (95% CI)†	P Value	No. (%) Who Died	Relative Risk (95% CI)†	P Value
All patients‡	368		1.0 (0.8-1.2)	0.99		1.0 (0.7-1.4)	0.79
Hypothermia	190	108 (57)			53 (28)		
Normothermia	178	102 (57)			48 (27)		
Patients with Glasgow coma scores of 3-4 on admission	87		1.1 (0.8-1.4)	0.64		1.4 (0.4-2.4)	0.35
Hypothermia	50	39 (78)			22 (44)		
Normothermia	37	27 (73)			13 (35)		
Patients with Glasgow coma scores of 5-8 on admission	281		0.9 (0.7-1.2)	0.55		1.0 (0.6-1.5)	0.71
Hypothermia	140	69 (49)			30 (21)		
Normothermia	141	75 (53)			32 (23)		
Patients >45 years old	52		1.3 (1.0-1.7)	0.08		1.0 (0.3-2.0)	1.00
Hypothermia	26	23 (88)			10 (38)		
Normothermia	26	18 (69)			10 (38)		

*Poor outcome was defined as severe disability, vegetative state, or death and was adjusted for age and Glasgow coma score on admission.
†Values indicate the relative risk in the hypothermia group as compared with the normothermia group.
‡Data are presented for 368 patients because outcome data were missing for 7 patients and Glasgow coma score on admission, age, or both were missing for 17 patients.
Abbreviation: CI, Confidence interval.
(Reprinted by permission of *The New England Journal of Medicine*, courtesy of Clifton GL, Miller ER, Choi SC, et al: Lack of Effect of Induction of Hypothermia After Acute Brain Injury. *N Engl J Med* 344:556-563, 2001. Copyright 2001, Massachusetts Medical Society. All rights reserved.)

in which enrollment was stopped by the patient safety and monitoring board on the basis that no more patients needed to be enrolled to produce a conclusion.

M. Wood, MD, FRCA

Calcium Antagonists for Ischemic Stroke: A Systematic Review
Horn J, Limburg M (Univ of Amsterdam)
Stroke 32:570-576, 2001   7–2

Background.—At present, there is no effective, generally accepted, specific treatment for the early phase of an ischemic stroke. Cell death after an ischemic stroke results from a massive influx of calcium into hypoxic cells, which has prompted interest in the use of calcium antagonists to protect against cell death. Whether calcium antagonists have a neuroprotective effect or provide a survival advantage after an ischemic stroke is a matter of great debate. A systematic review of all clinical trials that examined the effectiveness of calcium antagonists for acute ischemic stroke was undertaken.

Methods.—With the assistance of the Cochrane Collaborative Stroke Group, the authors identified all randomized trials (published and unpublished) that involved the use of a calcium antagonist in patients with acute ischemic strokes. Only trials involving true randomization (randomization within 14 days of the ischemic stroke) and investigating the effects of a calcium antagonist (defined as a drug that primarily acts on voltage-sensitive calcium channels) were included in analyses. The primary outcome measures were death or a poor outcome at the end of follow-up; a poor outcome was defined as all-cause mortality or being dependent on others for activities of daily living. In addition, sensitivity analyses were performed to examine differences in outcomes based on the route of drug administration (oral vs IV), the time between stroke onset and the start of treatment, publication status, and trial methodology. A 5-credit system was created to assess methodological quality: 1 credit was awarded for randomization, for double-blinding, for clearly describing how randomization or double-blinding were performed, and for accounting for all patients. Good-, moderate-, and poor-quality trials were defined by scores of 5, 3-4, and 1-3, respectively.

Results.—Of the 47 trials identified, only 29 met the inclusion criteria (7665 patients). Of these 29 studies, 22 trials (6877 patients) could be used for analyses of poor outcomes. The length of follow-up in 10 trials was less than 3 months, in 5 trials, it was about 3 months, and in 14 trials, it was 6 to 12 months. Calcium antagonists did not have a statistically significant effect on outcomes at follow-up, either for the class of drugs as a whole (relative risk, 1.04; 95% CI, 0.98-1.09) or for individual drugs. On the basis of data from 7522 patients, calcium antagonists also did not have a statistically significant effect on survival at follow-up (relative risk, 1.07; 95% CI, 0.98-1.17). However, the 3 trials that included flunarizine showed a significantly greater risk of death when active treatment was initiated (relative risk, 1.3; 95% CI, 1.0-1.8). Overall, patients treated with calcium antagonists (particularly flunarizine) had more adverse events than did patients treated with placebo. Neither the route of administration nor the time between stroke onset and the start of treatment had a significant effect on the outcome. The effects of active drug versus placebo on outcomes also did not differ in the poor- or moderate-quality studies. In the good-quality studies, however, calcium antagonists had a significantly negative effect on the outcome. Outcomes also did not differ significantly between active drug and placebo groups in published trials; however, in unpublished trials, active treatment was associated with significantly worse outcomes.

Conclusions.—On the basis of this systematic review, no strong evidence exists to indicate a clinically important benefit of calcium antagonists after an acute ischemic stroke. To the contrary, in the few situations in which a statistically significant difference was seen between the active-drug and placebo groups, calcium antagonists had a negative effect on the outcome. A publication bias was apparent, in that unpublished trials were more likely than published trials to find a worse outcome with calcium antagonists, as were good-quality (vs poor- or moderate-quality) studies. Taken together, these findings do not support the use of calcium antagonists in patients with acute ischemic strokes.

▶ This article reports results from a meta-analysis of 29 randomized clinical trials of calcium antagonist use in patients with ischemic strokes. The results represent treatment of more than 7000 patients. The authors undertook the daunting task of reviewing the large and conflicting body of literature regarding use of these agents for cerebral protection. In addition, they attempted to quantify the "quality" of the studies included in the meta-analysis. They chose as their primary end point fatality or a poor outcome, which was defined as dependence in activities of daily living—certainly a very conservative description of a poor outcome. Their results show no benefit in terms of outcome by treatment with calcium channel blockers. Unlike other analyses, which have shown a benefit from administration of certain calcium channel blockers, at least when treatment was initiated early (within 12 hours) after the onset of symptoms, this review found no benefit associated with any individual drug or with early treatment groups.[1,2] They attribute this to inclusion of additional trials in this review as compared with others. Of particular concern is their observation that, in trials they deemed of good quality (ie, randomized, double-blind, clearly defined randomization and blinding, and all patients accounted for) as well as in trials not published, treatment with calcium channel blockers had an adverse impact on the long-term outcome. In procedures associated with a known risk of cerebral ischemia in the perioperative period (eg, valve replacement), use of the calcium channel blocker nimodipine was also associated with a worse outcome, in this case, primarily related to increased hemorrhagic complications.[3] Although nimodipine as prophylaxis for delayed neurologic deficits after aneurismal subarachnoid hemorrhaging remains a routine treatment, studies such as these suggest that, in the vast majority of clinical scenarios, use of calcium channel blockers to lessen ischemic neurologic injury is not warranted.

S. Black, MD

References

1. TRUST Study Group: Randomized, double-blind, placebo-controlled trial of nimodipine in acute stroke. *Lancet* 336:1205-1209, 1990.
2. Horn J, Limburg M, Vermeulen M: VENUS-Very early nimodipine use in stroke: Final results from a randomized-controlled trial. *Cerebrovasc Dis* 9:127S, 1999.
3. Legault C, Furberg CD, Wagenknecht LE, et al: Nimodipine neuroprotection in cardiac valve replacement. Report of an early terminated trial. *Stroke* 27:593-598, 1996.

Autoregulation of Cerebral Blood Flow in Patients Resuscitated From Cardiac Arrest

Sundgreen C, Larsen FS, Herzog TM, et al (Univ Hosp of Copenhagen)
Stroke 32:128-132, 2001   7–3

Introduction.—Changes in arterial blood pressure normally have only a minor influence on cerebral blood flow (CBF), but patients resuscitated from cardiac arrest may have impaired CBF autoregulation. Eighteen patients who had been resuscitated from cardiac arrest were examined for CBF autoregulation within the first 24 hours after resuscitation.

Methods.—The patients were 15 men and 3 women with a median age of 69 years. Six had been resuscitated in-hospital and 12 out-of-hospital. The mean estimated time to return of spontaneous circulation was 8 minutes. Patients were studied for a mean of 382 minutes after the index event. Six healthy volunteers also were studied. Relative changes in CBF were determined by transcranial Doppler mean flow velocity (V_{mean}) in the middle cerebral artery during a stepwise rise in mean arterial pressure (MAP) by use of norepinephrine infusion. To assess CBF autoregulation, MAP was plotted against the V_{mean}, and a lower limit of autoregulation was identified by double regression analysis based on the least-squares method.

Results.—In resuscitated patients, V_{mean} increased from a median of 33 to 37 cm/s during a norepinephrine-induced rise in MAP from 78 to 106 mm Hg. Impaired CBF autoregulation was observed in 8 patients. The lower limit of autoregulation was identified in 5 of the 10 patients with preserved CBF autoregulation (Table 2). The mean lower limit of CBF autoregulation was 76 mm Hg in the healthy volunteers and 114 mm Hg in patients with preserved autoregulation.

Discussion.—Because cerebral autoregulation is either absent or right shifted in a majority of patients in the acute phase after cardiac arrest, MAP may need to be kept at a higher level than commonly accepted to secure cerebral perfusion. These findings are supported by previous clinical

TABLE 2.—Lower Limit of Cerebral Autoregulation in the 5 Patients in Whom a Lower Limit of Cerebral Autoregulation Could Be Identified and in 6 Control Subjects

	Patient	Lower Limit, mm Hg
Patients	5	80
	8	114
	11	109
	15	118
	16	120
Median		114*
Range		80-120
Control subjects	A	76
	B	78
	C	79
	D	41
	E	64
	F	105
Median		76*
Range		41-105

Lower limit indicates calculated value of lower limit of autoregulation. See text for details.
*P < .01.
(Courtesy of Sundgreen C, Larsen FS, Herzog TM, et al: Autoregulation of cerebral blood flow in patients resuscitated from cardiac arrest. *Stroke* 32:128-132, 2001. Reproduced with permission of *Stroke.* Copyright 2001, American Heart Association.)

and experimental studies in which maintenance of a high MAP after resuscitation was associated with a favorable outcome.

▶ Increasing evidence suggests that maintenance of systemic blood pressure is an important factor in preventing secondary injury to patients who have had neurologic injury—either from head trauma or anoxic cerebral injury.[1] These studies have demonstrated that maintaining MAP at higher than conventional levels (eg, cerebral perfusion pressure above 70 mm Hg rather than above 50 mm Hg) is associated with fewer episodes of cerebral ischemia after the initial injury. It has been shown consistently in animal models and in human beings that after a global cerebral ischemic event, an initial period of cerebral hyperperfusion is followed by a period of cerebral hypoperfusion.[2] In this study, cerebral autoregulation was evaluated in patients after resuscitation from cardiac arrest on average 5 hours after resuscitation—likely during a period of potential cerebral hypoperfusion. The authors found an absence of cerebral autoregulation in 44% of patients and altered cerebral autoregulation in 28% of their patients after cardiac arrest. In the patients with altered autoregulation, the lower limit of autoregulation was right shifted, such that the average lower limit of autoregulation was above MAP of 110 mm Hg. Since most patients after cardiac arrest are managed with MAP below 110 mm Hg, most of these patients (72% in this study) would have decreases in CBF with any decrease in systemic blood pressure. Although markers for cerebral ischemia were not measured in this study, it certainly raises concern that patients after cardiac arrest might be at high risk for cerebral ischemia when their blood pressure is within a range generally considered acceptable.

Maintaining induced hypertension after cardiac arrest would be a management strategy likely associated with a high risk of cardiovascular complications. In this study, not unexpectedly, the majority of patients required vasopressors, inotropic agents, or both, to maintain their blood pressure within the usually accepted range. To further increase their blood pressure might be expected to result in a significant increased risk for further myocardial ischemia, congestive heart failure, or development of pulmonary edema. Although this study generates important clinical questions, it would first be necessary to evaluate the impact of impaired autoregulation and blood pressure changes on evidence of secondary neurologic injury as well as outcome. If this evaluation suggested that increases in blood pressure might have potential neurologic benefits, then careful trials must be conducted to examine the impact of strategies to elevate perfusion pressure on overall management outcome.

S. Black, MD

References

1. Robertson CS, Valadka AP, Hannay HJ, et al: Prevention of secondary insults after severe head injury. *Crit Care Med* 27:2086-2095, 1999.
2. Beckstead JE, Tweed WA, Lee J, et al: Cerebral blood flow and metabolism in man following cardiac arrest. *Stroke* 9:569-573, 1978.

Secondary Insults in Severe Head Injury—Do Multiply Injured Patients Do Worse?
Sarrafzadeh AS, Peltonen EE, Kaisers U, et al (Humboldt-Univ Berlin)
Crit Care Med 29:1116-1123, 2001   7–4

Introduction.—Patients with traumatic brain injuries are at risk of "secondary insults," which may result in the deterioration of the neurologic outcome, and prognosis may be worsened by the presence of multiple injuries, especially in the thoracic or abdominal region. Patients with severe head injuries (SHIs) were studied prospectively for the occurrence of secondary insults and the influence of extracranial injuries (ECIs) on cerebral oxygenation and outcome.

Methods.—Eligible patients were aged 6 to 75 years and had a Glasgow Coma Scale score of 3 to 7 on admission to the emergency department. The Abbreviated Injury Scale was used to characterize patients for mechanisms of trauma and distribution of injuries. Eighty of the 119 patients studied had closed severe head injuries: 44 with and 36 without associated ECIs (Injury Severity Score >29 and <30, respectively). A control group included 39 patients with ECIs and no head injuries. Patients with head injuries were monitored for intracranial pressure, mean arterial blood pressure, cerebral perfusion pressure, end-tidal CO_2 level, brain tissue PO_2 level, and jugular bulb oxyhemoglobin saturation level. Surgery was delayed for non–life-threatening ECI. Mean arterial blood pressure was monitored in control subjects.

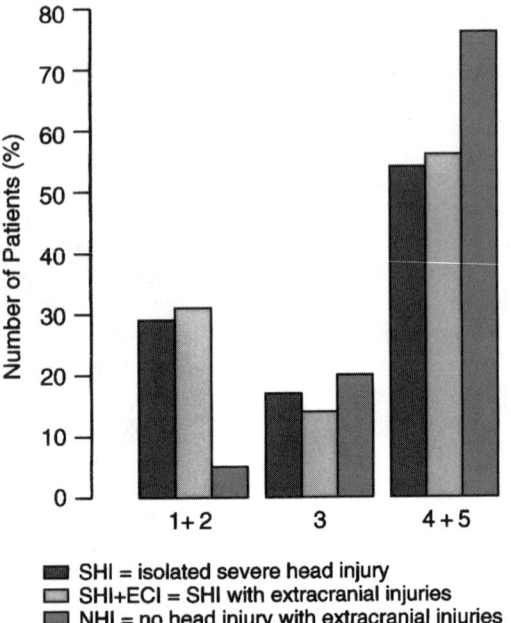

SHI = isolated severe head injury
SHI+ECI = SHI with extracranial injuries
NHI = no head injury with extracranial injuries

FIGURE 3.—Clinical outcome after 1 year in severely head-injured (SHI) patients with isolated severe head injury, SHI patients with associated extracranial injuries (SHI + ECI), and patients with exclusively extracranial injuries (NHI) according to the Glasgow Outcome Scale (GOS): GOS 1, dead; GOS 2, vegetative; GOS 3, severely disabled; GOS 4, moderately disabled; GOS 5, good outcome. In SHI patients, 1-year outcome was similar ($P = .301$), whereas NHI patients had a better outcome ($P = .046$). (Courtesy of Sarrafzadeh AS, Peltonen EE, Kaisers U, et al: Secondary insults in severe head injury—Do multiply injured patients do worse? *Crit Care Med* 29(6):1116-1123, 2001.)

Results.—Secondary insults, including elevated intracranial pressure, hypotension, and hypoxemia, occurred at comparable rates in patients with SHIs with and without associated ECIs. The duration of intracranial hypertension and arterial hypotension was significantly correlated with a poor outcome, independent of the Injury Severity Score. Among patients with SHIs only, 54% had moderate or good outcomes at 1 year, 29% were dead or in a vegetative state, and 17% were severely disabled; among patients with SHIs and ECIs, these categories were 56%, 31%, and 14%, respectively. Compared with both SHI groups (Fig 3), patients without head injuries had fewer secondary insults and better outcomes.

Conclusion.—In patients with SHIs, the incidence of secondary insults was not increased in the presence of ECIs when cerebral perfusion pressure and cerebral oxygenation were continuously monitored. The 1-year outcome in the setting of targeted management was mainly dependent on the head injury alone and independent of the presence of ECI.

▶ This is a prospective trial of 80 patients with SHIs and 39 patients with traumatic injuries not involving the head. The authors found that the presence of multiple ECIs did not worsen the outcome in patients with SHIs compared with those with isolated head injuries. The results contradict conventional wisdom—that patients with head injuries with significant ECIs fair worse. Studies such as the one by Chestnut et al,[1] which report higher morbidity and mortality rates after head injuries in multiple injured patients, are numerous. However, many predate current recommendations for management of patients with head injuries. The management protocol in this series emphasizes monitoring and control of intracranial dynamics. In addition, surgical intervention for non–life-threatening ECIs was delayed (usually to approximately 10 days after the injury) until the neurologic condition was stable. The authors also recorded incidences of secondary insults (as detected by brain tissue Po_2 or jugular venous oxygen saturation monitoring). They found that not only were long-term outcomes similar but also that the incidences of secondary insults were similar between those patients with isolated head injuries and those patients with multiple injuries. The authors concluded that their results suggest that secondary injuries are major contributors to morbidity and mortality rates after head injuries and that a management protocol improved outcomes in both patients with isolated brain injuries as well as patients with multiple injuries. The lack of difference demonstrated in this study could result from the small study size. Before it can be concluded that significant ECI does not lead to increased morbidity and mortality rates after a traumatic brain injury, a larger trial needs to be completed.

S. Black, MD

Reference

1. Chestnut RM, Marshall SB, Piek J, et al: Early and late systemic hypotension as a frequent and fundamental source of cerebral ischemia following severe head injury in the Traumatic Coma Databank. *Acta Neurochir Suppl (Wien)* 59:121-125, 1993.

Adult Respiratory Distress Syndrome: A Complication of Induced Hypertension After Severe Head Injury
Contant CF, Valadka AB, Gopinath SP, et al (Baylor College of Medicine, Houston; Univ of Houston)
J Neurosurg 95:560-568, 2001   7–5

Background.—The development of adult respiratory distress syndrome (ARDS) complicates the treatment of patients with severe head injury because therapies that are protective for the lungs can reduce cerebral blood flow (CBF) or increase intracranial pressure (ICP) (Fig 1). Previously, these authors compared the effects of managing patients with severe head injury by either an ICP-targeted strategy or a CBF-targeted strategy, and observed a significant increase in ARDS in the patients in the CBF-targeted management group. In this follow-up study, risk factors for the development of ARDS in this population were identified, and the effects of ARDS on outcome were examined.

Treatment Conflicts

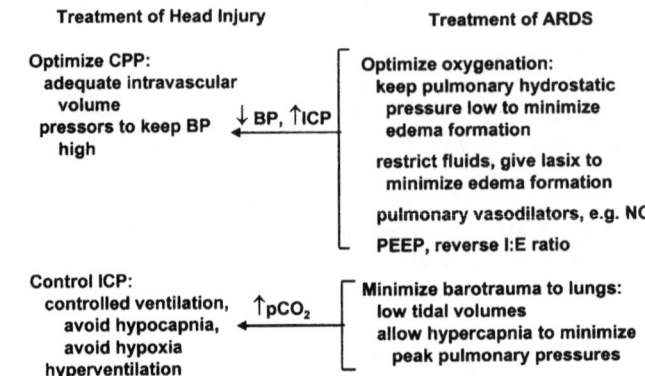

FIGURE 1.—Chart demonstrating that the development of acute respiratory distress syndrome (*ARDS*) complicates the management of severe head injury. Hypoxia is an important cause of secondary injury to the brain. The management strategies intended to improve oxygenation and to protect the lung from barotrauma, however, can reduce blood pressure (*BP*), increase intracranial pressure (*ICP*), and result in hypercarbia. *Abbreviations: I:E,* Inspiration/expiration; *NO,* nitric oxide; *CPP,* cerebral perfusion pressure; *PEEP,* positive end-expiratory pressure; pCO_2 = $PaCO_2$. (Courtesy of Contant CF, Valadka AB, Gopinath SP, et al: Adult respiratory distress syndrome: A complication of induced hypertension after severe head injury. *J Neurosurg* 95:560-568, 2001.)

Study Design.—The original study was a randomized clinical trial of ICP-targeted versus CBF-targeted management for patients with severe head injury. Chest radiography and arterial blood gases were used to identify patients with ARDS. Neurologic outcome was determined at 3 and 6 months by physicians blinded as to treatment. In this study, injury severity, physiologic data, and treatment data were compared for the 18 patients who developed ARDS versus the remaining 171 patients in the study group who did not develop ARDS. Logistic regression modeling was used to identify factors associated with the development of ARDS.

Findings.—There were no significant differences between the patients who developed ARDS and those who did not in either demographic characteristics or injury characteristics. The incidence of ARDS was almost 5 times higher among patients in the CBF-targeted management group, than in the ICP-targeted management group. Patients who developed ARDS were more likely to have received mannitol, barbiturates, dopamine, epinephrine, phenylephrine, and higher doses of morphine and vecuronium. They also had higher fluid intakes than those who did not develop ARDS. Patients who developed ARDS had higher intracranial hypertension. Long-term outcome was significantly worse among the patients who developed ARDS. Logistic regression analysis indicated that use of epinephrine, dopamine dose, history of drug abuse, and treatment protocol were independent predictors of the development of ARDS.

Conclusions.—Although this study was not originally designed to examine the risk factors for ARDS, a reanalysis of these data suggests that the risk factors for the development of ARDS in a patient population with severe head injury are primarily treatment related. Patient-related factors included a history of drug abuse and a midline shift on admission CT. Treatment-related factors were associated with the goals of the CBF-targeted management strategy, including greater fluid intake and increased use of pressor agents. The development of ARDS in these patients was associated with more severe intracranial hypertension, which may have offset the beneficial effects of this treatment regimen, resulting in worsened outcomes for these patients.

▶ Outcome after severe closed head injury remains poor in the majority of patients. Some recent work has suggested that management strategies aimed at maintaining an elevated cerebral perfusion pressure may have some benefits in terms of decreasing the incidence of secondary insults after head injury.[1] However, outcome data have been less encouraging.[2] In this study, the impact of management strategy (cerebral perfusion pressure [CPP]-guided treatment versus ICP-guided management) on the development of ARDS after severe head injury was evaluated. The primary difference in the treatment strategies was the lower limit of acceptable CPP in the ICP-guided treatment (50 mm Hg) as opposed to the CPP-guided treatment (70 mm Hg), and the avoidance of hyperventilation in the CPP-guided treatment. The results suggest that induced hypertension to maintain a CPP of 70 mm Hg is associated with a higher incidence of ARDS in patients with severe head injuries. Treatment and physiologic variables associated with the maintenance of an elevated systemic blood pressure (such as fluid balance, use of vasopressors, central venous pressure) were all significantly higher in patients who developed ARDS. Although the patients with ARDS did not have a higher incidence of secondary cerebral insults (as detected by jugular venous oxygen destaturations), the incidence of refractory intracranial hypertension was higher. Of note, patients with ARDS had a significantly worse outcome. They were more than twice as likely to die or be in a vegetative state.

The observed relationship between the development of ARDS and more severe intracranial hypertension could be caused by a number of factors. It is possible (and has been demonstrated in other studies[3]) that more severe head injury is related to a greater risk for pulmonary complications. It is also possible that the development of ARDS impaired the ability to manage the intracranial injury. It is probable that the observed worse outcome is indeed related to the development of ARDS. In fact, one fourth of the patients who developed ARDS died as a direct result of their pulmonary pathology. As outlined by the authors, the goals of management in head injury patients with elevated ICP are often in conflict with the management goals in ARDS. Perhaps the potential benefit of improved cerebral perfusion seen in patients managed with relatively high systemic blood pressure is in part offset by the development of ARDS.

S. Black, MD

References

1. White JRM, Zareen F, Bull C, et al: Predictors of outcome in severely head injured children. *Crit Care Med* 29:534-540, 2001.
2. Robertson CS, Valadka AB, Hannay HG, et al: Prevention of secondary insults after severe head injury. *Crit Care Med* 27:2086-2095, 1999.
3. Braton SL, Davis RL: Acute lung injury in isolated traumatic brain injury. *Neurosurgery* 40:707-712, 1977.

Predictors of Outcome in Severely Head-Injured Children
White JRM, Farukhi Z, Bull C, et al (Children's Natl Med Ctr, Washington, DC; Johns Hopkins Hosp, Baltimore, Md)
Crit Care Med 29:534-540, 2001   7–6

Introduction.—More than 30% of all admissions to pediatric ICUs (PICUs) are for serious head injuries. Even so, reliable predictive variables have yet to be identified. Those variables in the acute care period associated with survival and PICU length of stay (LOS) in children with severe traumatic brain injury were retrospectively determined.

Study Design.—A total of 136 pediatric patients with severe, nonpenetrating head injury and a Glasgow Coma Scale score of no more than 8 at admission to the PICU from 1991 through 1995 were studied. Chart reviews were performed to obtain injury severity, physiologic variables,

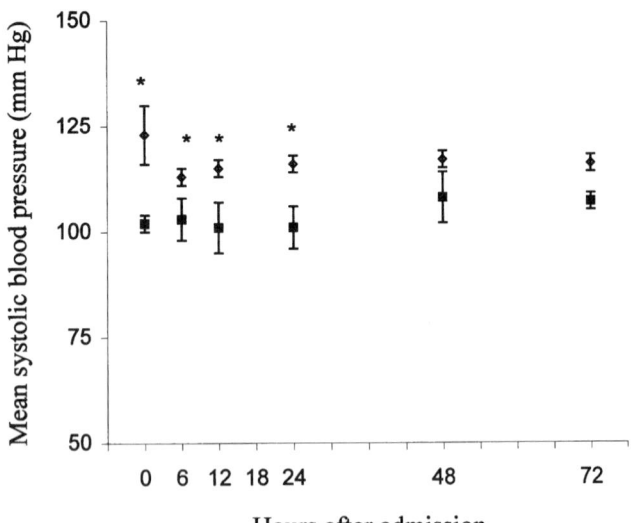

Hours after admission

FIGURE 2.—Mean systolic blood pressure as a function of the time interval after admission in survivors (*diamonds*) versus nonsurvivors (*squares*). Mean systolic blood pressure is higher among survivors than nonsurvivors at 0, 6, 12, and 24 hours. *Asterisk, P < .05*. Survivors had their highest mean systolic blood pressure at admission (*P < .05*). All points represent mean ± SEM. (Courtesy of White JRM, Farukhi Z, Bull C, et al: Predictors of outcome in severely head-injured children. *Crit Care Med* 29(3):534-540, 2001.)

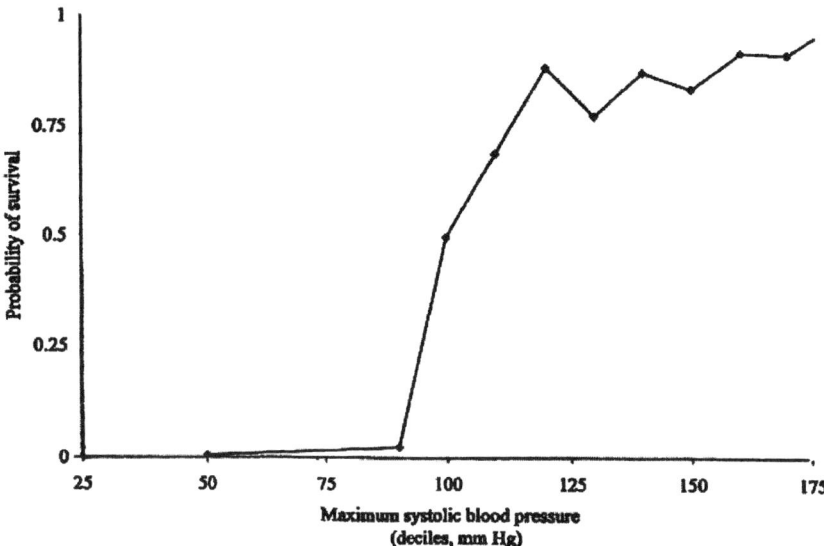

FIGURE 3.—Adjusted probability of survival as a function of maximum systolic blood pressure. The greatest probability of survival occurs when the maximum systolic blood pressure is 135 mm Hg, after which the probability curve plateaus. (Courtesy of White JRM, Farukhi Z, Bull C, et al: Predictors of outcome in severely head-injured children. *Crit Care Med* 29(3):534-540, 2001.)

CT findings, hospital course, and Glasgow Coma Scale score for the first 72 hours after admission. End points included survival, LOS, and day at which Glasgow Coma Scale score was at least 14.

Findings.—The mortality rate was 24%. Survival was independently predicted by Glasgow Coma Scale score at 6 hours after admission and maximum systolic blood pressure (Fig 2). The odds of survival increased almost 20-fold when maximum systolic blood pressure was at least 135 mm Hg (Fig 3). By discharge, 67% of these patients had an age-appropriate Glasgow Coma Scale score. The average hospital cost for survivors was $8798. Only mannitol use was independently associated with increased cost. For the survivors, the average PICU LOS was 2 days. The 6-hour Glasgow Coma Scale score and mannitol use were independently associated with a prolonged LOS.

Conclusions.—Among severely head-injured children, supranormal maximum systolic blood pressure was associated with increased survival. The Glasgow Coma Scale score at 6 hours was predictive of mortality. The use of mannitol was associated with extended LOS in the PICU and higher hospital costs, but conferred no survival advantage. Blood pressure targets and the use of mannitol should be reevaluated in children with severe traumatic head injury.

▶ Trauma and head injury remain a major cause of morbidity and mortality in children. Although some innovations in care have occurred during the past decades, morbidity and mortality from head injury remain high. This study covers a 4-year period at one institution. During that time, the management of head injury consisted of aggressive monitoring, maintenance of normal cerebral perfusion pressure ($\geq$50 mm Hg in infants and $\geq$70 mm Hg in children), and use of routine hyperventilation (only in the first 2 years of the review period). Intracranial hypertension was treated with barbiturates, mannitol, hypertonic saline, sedation, and hyperventilation. With this management protocol, survival to discharge was 76%, with 67% of survivors having an "age-appropriate" Glasgow Coma Scale score at the time of discharge. Long-term outcome was not defined further. The authors attempted to identify variables associated with survival. As other recent reports have shown, higher systemic blood pressure, especially in the first 6 to 12 hours after injury, was associated with a higher survival rate. This finding was independent of vasopressor use or severity of injury. This suggests that the higher perfusion pressure itself is beneficial, rather than simply being a marker for the use of a specific vasoactive agent or for a less severe injury. Many studies, similar to this one, have demonstrated that the Glasgow Coma Scale score on admission is not predictive of outcome. In this evaluation, the Glasgow coma score at 6 hours after injury was highly predictive of survival, with all pediatric patients with a Glasgow Coma Scale score of more than 8 surviving to discharge. This is a relatively early, reliable predictor of patients who will survive. The CT scan findings were also predictive of survival, with cerebral edema, subdural hematoma, subarachnoid hemorrhage, and diffuse axonal injury being predictive of mortality. Finding reliable predictors of outcome should prove to have important implications for planning therapeutic maneuvers in patients with head injury.

The use of mannitol was associated with no difference in outcome, but with a longer PICU stay and a higher cost. The reason for this is unclear, as this finding is independent of injury severity or outcome. However, the authors conclude that since mannitol increases cost without improving outcome, hypertonic saline as an alternative effective osmotic therapy for intracranial hypertension should be considered as the preferred treatment. Results from this study and others suggest that maintenance of normal to supranormal blood pressure in the early hours after head injury is critical in improving neurologic recovery and preventing further injury. The role of hyperventilation and mannitol in the routine treatment of head injury, mainstays for many years, will likely continue to decrease as a consequence of these and similar results.

S. Black, MD

A Comparative Study Between a Calcium Channel Blocker (Nicardipine) and a Combined α-β-Blocker (Labetalol) for the Control of Emergence Hypertension During Craniotomy for Tumor Surgery

Kross RA, Ferri E, Leung D, et al (Cornell Univ, New York; Univ of Ferrara, Italy)
Anesth Analg 91:904-909, 2000   7–7

Introduction.—Therapy designed to prevent the occurrence of hypertension during neurosurgery can reduce the risk of postoperative bleeding and cerebral edema. At the study institution, a combination of enalaprilat and labetalol is used to maintain systolic blood pressure (SBP) at less than 140 mm Hg. An IV infusion of nicardipine offers an alternative for patients with contraindications to β-adrenergic blocking drugs. The combination of the calcium channel blocker nicardipine and enalaprilat was compared with enalaprilat–labetalol for efficacy and adverse effects in patients undergoing craniotomy for tumor surgery.

Methods.—The randomized, open-label clinical trial included 42 patients, none of whom had hypertension or were being treated with angiotensin-converting enzyme inhibitors, calcium channel blockers, or β-blockers. Enalaprilat (1.25 mg IV) was administered at dural closure, followed by either multidose nicardipine (2 mg IV) or labetalol (5 mg IV) to maintain the SBP below 140 mm Hg. No narcotic was administered in the operating room after incision. Drug failure was defined as the occurrence of SBP greater than 140 mm Hg and lasting more than 2 minutes after initiation of the study therapy.

Results.—The success rate for control of SBP was 99% with enalaprilat–labetalol and 90% with enalaprilat–nicardipine. Marginally fewer treatment failures occurred with labetalol than with nicardipine (Table 2). The number of doses administered to control blood pressure was significantly greater with labetalol than with nicardipine (mean, 11 vs 5). Adverse effects (ie, bradycardia, tachycardia, and hypotension) occurred in 9 patients in the nicardipine group but in only 2 patients in the labetalol group (both experienced bradycardia). Mean costs of the study drug per patient were lower with labetalol ($5.23 vs $23.65).

Conclusion.—Nicardipine and labetalol have some important pharmacologic differences, but both are capable of controlling emergence hypertension after a craniotomy.

▶ Strict control of postoperative blood pressure is an often-stated goal in the management of patients undergoing neurosurgery. Patients who have undergone craniotomy for resection of mass lesions may have transiently impaired cerebral autoregulation in the area of resection (or perhaps under retractor sites). Likewise, abnormal vascularity may remain in the tumor bed. These problems may result in severe postoperative cerebral edema or intracerebral hemorrhage should hypertension develop in the early postoperative period. Fortunately, these dire complications are quite rare. A number of different strategies have been tried, including prophylactic and therapeu-

TABLE 2.—Failures by Test Drug

	OR	PACU	Total
Nicardipine	6	4	10
Labetalol	2	2	4

Abbreviations: OR, Operating room; *PACU*, postanesthesia care unit.
(Courtesy of Kross RA, Ferri E, Leung D, et al: A comparative study between a calcium channel blocker (nicardipine) and a combined α-β-blocker (labetalol) for the control of emergence hypertension during craniotomy for tumor surgery. *Anesth Analg* 91(4):904-909, 2000.)

tic use of a variety of antihypertensive agents, greater reliance on narcotics in the anesthetic maintenance, and local scalp infiltration.

This study compares labetalol with nicardipine when added to routine enalaprilat for control of postoperative blood pressure. As many studies have demonstrated good results using labetalol alone,[1] the indication for routine use of an angiotensin-converting enzyme inhibitor in addition to the study drugs is not clearly identified. Nonetheless, the study does provide a valid comparison of the 2 agents. The total narcotic dose was rather low, which could contribute to the high dose requirements observed in this study for both agents. The efficacy of IV nicardipine was slightly lower than that for labetalol, and the incidence of complications (ie, hypotension, tachycardia, and bradycardia) were slightly higher with nicardipine. Fortunately, no morbidity occurred as the result of either drug treatment. Although nicardipine was quite effective in this study, these results would suggest that labetalol is the better choice, except in those patients in whom contraindication exists for its use.

S. Black, MD

Reference

1. Muzzi DA, Black S, Losasso TJ, et al: Labetalol and esmolol in the control of hypertension after intracranial surgery. *Anesth Analg* 70:68-71, 1990.

A Comparison of Superficial Versus Combined (Superficial and Deep) Cervical Plexus Block for Carotid Endarterectomy: A Prospective, Randomized Study
Pandit JJ, Bree S, Dillon P, et al (Univ of Michigan, Ann Arbor)
Anesth Analg 91:781-786, 2000   7–8

Introduction.—A regional block for carotid endarterectomy may be performed with use of a superficial cervical plexus block or a combination of superficial and deep cervical plexus blocks, often with a supplemental injection of lidocaine as a local anesthetic. Serious complications are possible, however, with a deep cervical plexus block, and there is a risk of epidural, subarachnoid, or vertebral artery injection of local anesthetic. Such complications might be avoided by use of superficial block alone. Outcomes were compared in 40 patients undergoing carotid endarterectomy who were randomly assigned to a superficial or a combined cervical plexus block.

Methods.—Twenty patients had a superficial block with an injection of approximately 30 mL of 0.375% bupivacaine at the midpoint of the sternocleidomastoid muscle. The maximum dose, 1.4 mg/kg, was planned to allow for expected supplementation by surgeons during the operation. For the 20 patients in the combined block group, the deep element of the block was performed with use of a single-injection technique at the C4 level. The superficial part was performed as in the previous patient group. About one third of the total dose (30 mL 0.375% bupivacaine) was placed deep, and two thirds was placed superficially. Surgeons unaware of the type of block administered additional 1% lidocaine when considered necessary for patient discomfort.

Results.—Median supplemental lidocaine requirements were 100 mg in the superficial block group and 115 mg in the combined block group, which was not a statistically significant difference (Fig 1). The median time to first postoperative analgesia was 150 minutes in the superficial block group and 45 minutes in the combined block group. Although this difference was large, it was not statistically significant. The number of patients needing postoperative analgesia was similar: 11 in the deep block group and 8 in the superficial block group.

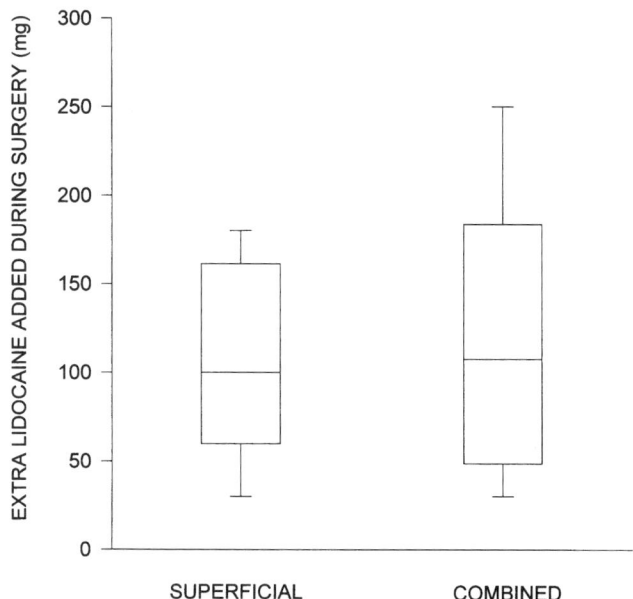

FIGURE 1.—Box plot of supplementary lidocaine requirements during carotid endarterectomy for superficial and combined blocks. The *horizontal line* represents the median dose, the *lower* and *upper limits of the box* represent the interquartile range, and the *error bars* represent the range. (Courtesy of Pandit JJ, Bree S, Dillon P, et al: A comparison of superficial versus combined (superficial and deep) cervical plexus block for carotid endarterectomy: A prospective randomized study. *Anesth Analg* 91(4):781-786, 2000.)

Conclusion.—Both a superficial block and a combined deep and superficial block are effective techniques for carotid endarterectomy. The 2 patient groups did not differ in the main end point of amount of supplemental lidocaine used intraoperatively. In addition, the superficial and combined block groups did not differ significantly in pain scores or postoperative analgesia requirements.

▶ Over the last 15 years, regional anesthesia for carotid endarterectomy has become increasingly popular. This likely results from a number of issues. First, some form of neurologic monitoring is recommended by most for patients undergoing carotid endarterectomy. A simple neurologic examination of an awake patient is accepted by all as adequate intraoperative monitoring of neurologic status. It certainly requires less additional equipment and personnel than the alternatives, such as intraoperative electroencephalography or evoked potential monitoring. Second, performing carotid endarterectomy with use of regional anesthesia has been shown in a number of studies to be less expensive than performing it with use of general anesthesia. However, other studies have shown similar cost effectiveness for general anesthesia when use of the ICU postoperatively is not routine but only as indicated by the patient's clinical course.[1] Finally, in nonrandomized trials, the incidence of postoperative hypertension and, perhaps, cardiac events has been suggested to be less when regional anesthesia is used. Even though no prospective randomized trial has been published to date that indicates that regional anesthesia is superior to general anesthesia, regional anesthesia is being used increasingly for these procedures when possible.[2,3]

The technique used for regional anesthesia for carotid endarterectomy generally includes some combination of local infiltration, deep cervical plexus block, and superficial cervical plexus block. In this randomized, prospective trial of 40 patients, the authors compared combined superficial and deep cervical plexus blocks with a superficial cervical plexus block alone. They found no difference in intraoperative variables, such as dose of supplemental lidocaine, analgesics, or sedatives given intraoperatively. Likewise, they found no difference in postoperative variables, such as the dose and timing of postoperative analgesia. Of note, the dose of supplemental lidocaine was reported to be as high as 25 mL of 1% lidocaine. Perhaps addition of a mandibular nerve block might have decreased the requirement for supplemental infiltration by the surgeon. The authors note that the deep cervical plexus block is associated with a high rate of unilateral diaphragmatic dysfunction—which may be detrimental to patients with severely compromised pulmonary function—and a low incidence of other complications such as vertebral artery injection. They conclude that the use of the deep cervical plexus block is may not be warranted.

S. Black, MD

References

1. Godin MS, Bell WH, Schwedler M, et al: Cost effectiveness of regional anesthesia in carotid endarterectomy. *Am Surg* 55:656-658, 1989.
2. Corson JD, Chang BB, Leopold PW, et al: Perioperative hypertension in patients undergoing carotid endarterectomy: Shorter duration under regional block anesthesia. *Circulation* 74:1S-4S, 1986.
3. Becquemin JP, Paris E, Valverde A, et al: Carotid surgery. Is regional anesthesia always appropriate? *J Cardiovasc Surg* 32:592-598, 1991.

Transcranial Doppler Ultrasonography as a Screening Technique for Detection of a Patent Foramen Ovale Before Surgery in the Sitting Position

Stendel R, Gramm H-J, Schröder K, et al (Freie Universität Berlin)
Anesthesiology 93:971-975, 2000   7–9

Introduction.—Advantages of the sitting position for neurosurgical procedures in the posterior fossa and the cervical spine include optimum access to midline lesions and improved cerebral venous drainage. Venous air embolism is fairly common in such cases, however, and paradoxical air embolism has been reported to occur in 14% of patients. A risk factor of paradoxical air embolism is a patent foramen ovale (PFO). The sensitivity and specificity of contrast-enhanced transcranial Doppler US (c-TCD) and contrast-enhanced transthoracic echocardiography (c-TTE) in detecting a PFO were compared, and contrast-enhanced transesophageal echocardiography (c-TEE) was used as the reference standard.

Methods.—The prospective study included 92 patients scheduled for neurosurgical procedures in the sitting position. All were studied with c-TCD, c-TEE, and c-TTE 1 day before surgery and anesthesia. Studies were performed during the Valsalva maneuver after IV echo-contrast medium (D-Galactose) was administered.

TABLE 1.—Diagnostic Characteristics of Contrast-Enhanced Transcranial Doppler US (c-TCD), Contrast-Enhanced Transthoracic Echocardiography (c-TTE), and Contrast-Enhanced Transesophageal Echocardiography (c-TEE) in Detecting a Patent Foramen Ovale (PFO) Before Operations in the Sitting Position

	c-TCD	c-TTE	c-TEE
PFO (%)	22 (23.9)	10 (10.8)*	24 (26.0)
Sensitivity	0.92	0.42*	1
Specificity	1	1	1
Positive predictive value	1	1	1
Negative predictive value	0.97	0.83	1

Note: c-Tee was defined as the gold standard (n = 92, chi-square test).
*$P < .05$.

(Courtesy of Stendel R, Gramm H-J, Schröder K, et al: Transcranial Doppler ultrasonography as a screening technique for detection of a patent foramen ovale before surgery in the sitting position. *Anesthesiology* 93:971-975, 2000. Copyright American Society of Anesthesiologists, Inc. Used with permission of Lippincott-Raven Publishers.)

Results.—A PFO was detected in 24 patients (26%) by c-TEE, in 22 patients by c-TCD, and in only 10 patients by c-TTE. For most patients with a posterior fossa lesion and a PFO, the operative position was changed to the prone or park bench position. No change in positioning was ordered for patients with PFO and cervical disk herniation. The difference in sensitivity between c-TCD and c-TEE was not significant, but the difference between c-TTE and c-TEE was statistically significant (Table 1). No complications occurred during any of the studies, and no side effects were associated with the echo-contrast medium. The negative predictive value was 0.97 for c-TCD and 0.83 for c-TTE. Intraoperative venous air embolism occurred in 35% of cases of cervical foraminotomy and in 75% of posterior fossa cases as detected by c-TEE.

Conclusion.—c-TCD was found to be a highly sensitive and specific method for detecting a PFO. This noninvasive technique may be more suitable than the semi-invasive and uncomfortable c-TEE for routine screening for a PFO. c-TTE is not reliable in detecting a PFO.

▶ Venous air embolism continues to be a frequently observed intraoperative problem during sitting neurosurgical procedures. It is also reported less frequently during any number of other surgical procedures in which a pressure gradient favors gas entrainment rather than bleeding (eg, joint replacement, laparoscopic procedures, and genitourinary procedures). Complications from venous air embolism are caused primarily by hemodynamic compromise caused by gas emboli in the right ventricle and pulmonary vasculature and paradoxical air emboli, which cause cerebral and/or coronary ischemia. Paradoxical air embolism occurs in the majority of cases via a PFO, which have been demonstrated to be present in up to 25% to 30% of patients with no known cardiac disease. Consequently, many authors over the last decade have recommended that patients scheduled to have surgical procedures with a known high risk of venous air embolism should be screened for the presence of a PFO.

Early studies using c-TEE to preoperatively detect PFO before sitting neurosurgical procedures had varying success. Many demonstrated PFO in well under the expected 25% of patients, and, in other studies, patients in whom a PFO was not detected preoperatively had paradoxical air embolism diagnosed via intraoperative c-TEE after development of venous air embolism.[1] This, in all likelihood, was caused by the alteration in atrial pressure gradients developing such that right-to-left shunting occurred only after significant venous air embolism developed intraoperatively. The Valsalva maneuver is designed to cause reversal of the normal atrial pressure gradient to reveal right-to-left shunting at the atrial level. In recent years, improvements in contrast echocardiography have been demonstrated in numerous studies, allowing a very high sensitivity and specificity in detection of PFO by c-TEE with the Valsalva maneuver.

This study compares the accepted standard technique for PFO detection (c-TEE) with c-TTE and c-TCD. Both c-TTE and c-TCD have the advantage of being noninvasive and not uncomfortable to the patient. c-TTE is slightly invasive and is uncomfortable. Serious complications from c-TEE are rare but have occured and have been fatal. This study demonstrates very encouraging results: c-TCD may prove to be an acceptable alternative screening method for PFO in patients undergoing procedures who are at high risk of venous air embolism.

S. Black, MD

Reference

1. Black S, Muzzi DA, Nishimura RA, et al: Preoperative and intraoperative echocardiography to detect right-to-left shunt in patients undergoing neurosurgical procedures in the sitting position. *Anesthesiology* 72:436-438, 1990.

Haemodynamic Stability During Moderate Hypotensive Anaesthesia for Spinal Surgery: A Comparison Between Desflurane and Isoflurane

Beaussier M, Paugam C, Deriaz H, et al (St Antoine Univ Hosp, Paris)
Acta Anaesthesiol Scand 44:1154-1159, 2000   7–10

Introduction.—Agents used to produce moderate arterial hypotension during spinal surgery help to control local bleeding. Both isoflurane and desflurane are suitable for this purpose and allow a good preservation of cardiac index. Desflurane, however, is most often used to treat acute hypertensive responses to surgery rather than to obtain hemodynamic stability during induced hypotension. Desflurane and isoflurane were compared for their capability to maintain haemodynamic stability in spinal procedures requiring moderate levels of controlled arterial hypotension.

Methods.—Twenty patients were included in the open-label trial; 10 were randomly assigned to desflurane and 10 were randomly assigned to isoflurane for maintenance of anesthesia. The inhaled agents were started within 2 minutes after tracheal intubation. All patients received standardized fentanyl dosing, volume loading, and blood pressure monitoring. A target systolic blood pressure (SBP) range of 80 to 100 mm Hg was maintained during the study period. Any SBP reading outside this range was defined as a haemodynamic event (HE).

TABLE 3.—Number of Haemodynamic Events (HE) During the Study Period, From Prone Positioning (T_0) to the End of Surgery (T_{end})

	Desflurane	Isoflurane
Number of HE	24	57*
SBP>140 mmHg	0	2
120<SBP<140 mmHg	0	4
100<SBP<120 mmHg	17	33
80>SBP>70 mmHg	6	16
SBP<70 mmHg	1	2

*$P < .05$.
Abbreviation: SBP, Systolic blood pressure.
(Courtesy of Beaussier M, Paugam C, Deriaz H, et al: Haemodynamic stability during moderate hypotensive anaesthesia for spinal surgery: A comparison between desflurane and isoflurane. *Acta Anaesthesiol Scand* 44:1154-1159, 2000.)

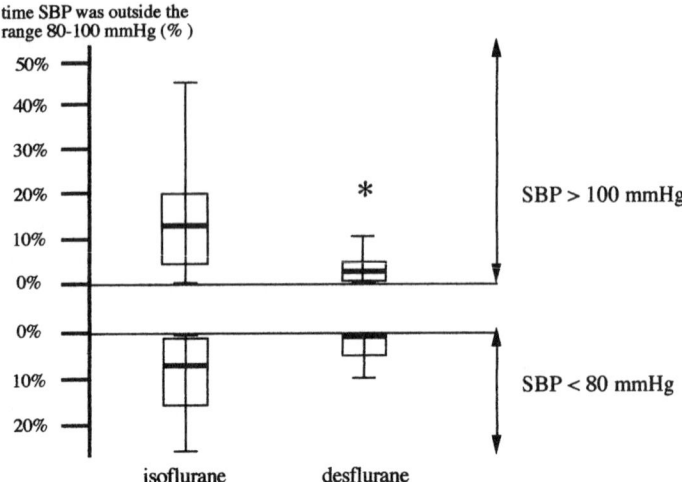

time SBP was outside the
range 80-100 mmHg (%)

FIGURE 1.—Time SBP was outside the range of 80 to 100 mm Hg during the period between prone positioning (T_0) and the end of surgery (T_{end}). Results in medians (*thick lines*) and interquartiles (*box*) with ranges (*thin lines*). *P < .05. *Abbreviation: SBP*, Systolic blood pressure. (Courtesy of Beaussier M, Paugam C, Deriaz H, et al: Haemodynamic stability during moderate hypotensive anaesthesia for spinal surgery: A comparison between desflurane and isoflurane. *Acta Anaesthesiol Scand* 44:1154-1159, 2000.)

Results.—Patients were all undergoing procedures without a high risk of blood loss, and a bloodless surgical field was obtained in all cases. The 2 groups did not differ significantly in patient demographic data, preoperative systolic and diastolic blood pressure and heart rate, or in total doses of thiopental, fentanyl, and vecuronium. However, during the period from prone positioning to the end of surgery, the number of HEs was statistically greater in the isoflurane group (Table 3) than in the desflurane group. The mean time that SBP was outside the defined range was 21.2% with isoflurane versus 5.1% with desflurane (Fig 1). Surgeons rated bleeding as similar between the 2 groups.

Conclusion.—During spinal surgery requiring moderate hypotension, a fresh gas flow of 1 L/min desflurane was more efficient than isoflurane in maintaining haemodynamic stability.

▶ This prospective, randomized open-label study compares the hemodynamic profile of moderate, induced hypotension during lumbar spine surgery. The authors chose a SBP range of 80 to 100 mm Hg as their desired blood pressure range. No patient had a history of hypertension, and, indeed, all patients' preoperative blood pressure before induction of anesthesia was within the normal range. With use of relatively low-flow anesthesia, desflurane was more effective at keeping SBP within the desired range as compared with isoflurane. This is not particularly surprising, given the lower solubility of desflurane. The authors also point out the greater number of HEs in the isoflurane group. These HEs consisted mainly of minor deviations of blood pressure outside the desired range (ie, SBP between 100 and 120 mm Hg or between 70 and 80 mm Hg). This likely represents an efficacy issue rather than a safety issue. Of note, the initial desflurane concentrations were at a significantly higher minimum alveolar concentration equivalent than for isoflurane. Perhaps the anesthesiologists were more comfortable using a higher dose of desflurane, given its lower solubility and the likelihood that a dose change could be accomplished more rapidly. This could, in an open label-study, contribute to the greater success with desflurane.

Use of moderate, induced hypotension during spine surgery remains controversial. Although some studies demonstrate lower intraoperative blood loss, other studies fail to demonstrate a difference in estimated blood loss, and, importantly, few studies demonstrate any decrease in the requirement for an intraoperative transfusion. As a consequence, the utility of this technique is questionable.[1,2] Nonetheless, it is still used widely. One important additional consideration is the impact of a hypotensive technique on spinal cord blood flow. Studies comparing different agents for use during spine surgery have demonstrated important differences in spinal cord perfusion between agents used for hypotension.

S. Black, MD

References

1. Mandel RJ, Brown MD, McCollough NC, et al: Hypotensive anesthesia and autotransfusion in spinal surgery. *Clin Ortho* 154:27-33, 1981.
2. Nuttall GA, Horlocker TT, Santrach PJ, et al: Predictors of blood transfusions in spinal instrumentation and fusion surgery. *Spine* 25:596-601, 2000.

The Recovery of Cognitive Function After Remifentanil–Nitrous Oxide Anesthesia Is Faster Than After an Isoflurane–Nitrous Oxide–Fentanyl Combination in Elderly Patients
Bekker AY, Berklayd P, Osborn I, et al (New York Univ; New York Methodist Hosp, Brooklyn)
Anesth Analg 91:117-122, 2000   7–11

Introduction.—Anesthetics with rapid clearance are desirable in elderly patients for whom postoperative confusion is a common and significant complication. Remifentanil, an ultrashort-acting synthetic opioid, does not accumulate in the body and may allow rapid emergence. The recovery of cognitive function was compared in 2 groups of patients undergoing spinal surgery: one randomized to remifentanil–nitrous oxide anesthesia (remi group) and the other to an isoflurane–nitrous oxide–fentanyl combination (iso/fent group).

Methods.—Study participants were 60 patients age 65 years or older who were scheduled for lumbar laminectomy. All underwent induction with 3.6 ± 1.2 mg/kg IV thiopental and endotracheal intubation with 1.4 ± 0.5 mg/kg succinylcholine. Patients in the iso/fent group were maintained with 0.5% to 1.5% isoflurane, 70% N_2O, and up to 7 µg/kg fentanyl; the remi group received 48 ± 11 µg/kg remifentanil and 70% N_2O. Cognitive ability was assessed preoperatively, 15, 30, and 60 minutes after arrival in the postanesthesia care unit, and at 12 to 24 hours postoperatively.

Results.—The time to spontaneous ventilation did not differ between the 2 groups, but the time to eye opening, extubation, and verbalization were significantly shorter for the remi group. Postoperatively, 21 patients in the remi group and 7 in the iso/fent group were treated for nausea with prochlorperazine and ondansetron. Antihypertensive drugs and morphine or meperidine for pain were used by a similar number of patients in each group. Although postoperative Mini-Mental State Examination scores were significantly lower in the iso/fent group at 15, 30, and 60 minutes, the scores were equivalent in the 2 groups after 12 hours.

Conclusion.—A remifentanil-based anesthetic shortened the time to recovery of cognitive function in elderly patients, but postoperative pain, the perioperative use of vasoactive drugs, and duration of postanesthesia care unit stay were similar in the remi and iso/fent groups. Antiemetics were needed by more patients in the remifentanil group.

▶ In this study, the recovery profile after lumbar spine surgery in elderly patients was compared after either a remifentanil–nitrous oxide anesthetic or an isoflurane–nitrous oxide–fentanyl anesthetic. Time to eye-opening, spontaneous ventilation, extubation, and verbalization were compared. With the exception of time to spontaneous ventilation, these times were statistically significantly shorter after remifentanil–nitrous oxide administration. Whether the shorter times of 2.5 to 5.5 minutes faster are truly clinically significant is questionable. Certainly, after neurosurgical procedures, the sooner the patient is awake and found to be neurologically intact, the less stress experienced by the surgical and anesthetic teams. Other intraoperative variables that were different included a greater requirement in the volatile anesthetic group for antihypertensive agents and a numerically (but not statistically) greater requirement for treatment of hypotension in the remi group. This is certainly consistent with effective blocking of the sympathetic response to surgery that is seen with relatively high-dose narcotic techniques, as described here.

Postoperatively, the remi group had a quicker return to normal cognitive function, as accessed by the Mini-Mental State Examination, than did the patients receiving a volatile anesthetic. This, however, did not translate into the patients being ready for recovery room discharge any sooner. The requirement for postoperative analgesic medication was not different between groups. It must be stressed that both groups received IM ketorolac and local anesthetic infiltration at the wound. Other more extensive procedures (eg, intra-abdominal or thoracic surgery or major joint replacement) done with a similar remifentanil technique might be expected to cause greater problems with postoperative pain management.

Similar studies done in other patient populations have had varying results. Although some show faster early awakening, others fail to demonstrate any faster emergence and recovery with the use of remifentanil.[1,2] This may well be caused, as the authors suggest, by the use of additional agents (eg, benzodiazepines, volatile agents, or propofol) along with remifentanil and nitrous oxide. Avoidance of preoperative anxiolysis may not be appropriate in all patients. Some anesthesiologists may also be uncomfortable with not adding additional agents to ensure amnesia intraoperatively. Finally, some procedures may require administration of longer acting narcotics intraoperatively to prevent development of severe pain immediately on emergence from a remifentanil–nitrous oxide anesthetic.[1] Perhaps the greatest advantage of the technique, as described here, is the slightly faster and more predictable emergence after remifentanil–nitrous oxide in those patients in whom a clear mental state is important in their early postoperative management.

S. Black, MD

References

1. Guy J, Hindman BJ, Baker KZ, et al: Comparison of remifentanil and fentanyl in patients undergoing craniotomy for supratentorial space-occupying lesion. *Anesthesiology* 86:514-524, 1997.
2. Schutter J, Albrecht S, Breivic H, et al: A comparison of remifentanil and alfentanil in patients undergoing major abdominal surgery. *Anaesthesia* 52:307-317, 1997.

Hemodynamic and Catecholamine Responses to Laryngoscopy and Tracheal Intubation in Patients With Complete Spinal Cord Injuries
Yoo KY, Lee J, Kim HS, et al (Chonnam Natl Univ, Gwangju, South Korea)
Anesthesiology 95:647-651, 2001 7–12

Background.—Laryngoscopy and endotracheal intubation often cause hypertension and tachycardia in patients undergoing general anesthesia. Although the mechanisms of action for these effects is unknown, these hemodynamic responses may be caused by a reflex sympathetic discharge after stimulation of the upper respiratory tract. If so, then these hemodynamic responses may be different in patients with spinal cord injuries compared with healthy patients. Thus, the cardiovascular responses to laryngoscopy and endotracheal intubation were compared in healthy patients and in patients with differing levels of complete spinal cord injury.

Methods.—The research subjects were 54 patients with traumatic complete spinal cord injury who were scheduled for surgery (spinal or nonspinal) requiring general anesthesia and 20 age-matched, nondisabled patients (control subjects; 18 men and 2 women; mean age, 38 years). The patients included 22 with quadriplegia (injury above C7; 19 men and 3 women; mean age, 40 years), 8 with high-level paraplegia (HP group; injury between T1 and T4; 6 men and 2 women; mean age, 42 years); and 24 with low-level paraplegia (LP group; level of injury below T5; 22 men and 2 women; mean age, 37 years). For all patients, the spinal cord injury had occurred 4 weeks or more before the scheduled surgery. A radial artery cannula connected to a pressure transducer was used to record blood pressure and to obtain blood samples for plasma epinephrine and norepinephrine (NE) measurements. These data, plus heart rate (HR) and heart rhythm, were measured at baseline and at intervals up to 5 minutes after intubation. Anesthesia was induced with 5 to 7 mg/kg IV thiopental plus 0.12 mg/kg IV vecuronium after full preoxygenation. Intubation was achieved within 15 seconds for all research subjects, and anesthesia was maintained with 50% nitrous oxide and 1% isoflurane in oxygen. Differences in hemodynamic and catecholamine responses to intubation were compared among the 4 groups.

Results.—At baseline, the 4 groups did not differ significantly in hemoglobin concentrations, HR, or systolic arterial pressure (SAP). After the induction of anesthesia, SAP fell significantly in all 4 groups. After endotracheal intubation, SAP increased significantly in all groups, except in the patients with quadriplegia, in whom SAP remained unchanged. In the other 3 groups, SAP peaked within 30 seconds and lasted for 2 minutes after intubation, after which SAP decreased to or went below levels at baseline; the decrease was significantly quicker in the HP group than in the LP and control groups. HR also increased significantly after the induction of anesthesia in all 4 groups. After endotracheal intubation, HR continued to increase in all 4 groups, but the increase was significantly greater in the HP group than in the control or quadriplegic groups. Compared with the control group, patients with quadriplegia were significantly less likely to experience hypertension and more likely to experience hypotension. Again compared with control subjects, the HP group was significantly more likely to experience tachycardia. None of the 4 groups differed significantly, however, in the incidence of bradycardia. Endotracheal intubation did not cause a significant increase in plasma epinephrine levels in any of the 4 groups. However, intubation caused a significant increase in plasma NE levels in all 4 groups. Compared with the change in the control group, the increase was greater in the LP group, less in the quadriplegic group, and of the same magnitude in the HP group.

Conclusions.—Hemodynamic and plasma NE responses to endotracheal intubation are different in patients with spinal cord injuries than in control subjects and also differ according to the level of spinal cord injury

TABLE 4.—Hemodynamic and Catecholamine Responses to Intubation in Patients With Spinal Cord Injuries and in Control Patients

	Control (n = 20)	QP (n = 22)	HP (n = 8)	LP (n = 24)
Hemodynamic				
SAP	↑ ↑	—	↑ ↑	↑ ↑
HR	↑ ↑	↑ ↑	↑ ↑ ↑	↑ ↑
Catecholamine				
Norepinephrine	↑ ↑	↑	↑ ↑	↑ ↑ ↑
Epinephrine	—	—	—	—

Abbreviations: QP, Quadriplegic patients; *HP,* high-level paraplegic patients; *LP,* low-level paraplegic patients; *n,* number of patients; *SAP,* systolic arterial pressure; *HR,* heart rate; ↑, minimal increase; ↑ ↑, moderate increase; ↑ ↑ ↑, marked increase; —, no change.

(Courtesy of Yoo KY, Lee J, Kim HS, et al: Hemodynamic and catecholamine responses to laryngoscopy and tracheal intubation in patients with complete spinal cord injuries. *Anesthesiology* 95:647-651, 2001. Copyright American Society of Anesthesiologists, Inc. Used with permission of Lippincott-Raven Publishers.)

(Table 4). These findings lend credence to the belief that the circulatory responses are affected by differences in sympathetic innervation.

▶ These authors carefully studied the hemodynamic and catecholamine response to laryngoscopy and intubation in patients with chronic spinal cord injuries and compared that response to the response in control patients without neurologic injuries. The authors noted statistically significant differences in the hemodynamic responses of patients with varying levels of cord injuries (as compared with control subjects) that may well be clinically significant also. In addition, they speculated on the mechanisms responsible for the alteration in hemodynamic and catecholamine responses to intubation present after a spinal cord injury. They suggested that the lack of pressor response but the preservation of chronotropic response in the patients with quadriplegia is caused by complete loss of sympathetic tone to the vasculature and heart; control of HR after chronic (but not acute) spinal cord injuries may be maintained by alterations in vagal nerve activity alone. The HP groups' preserved pressor response and exaggerated tachycardic response may be caused by enhanced sympathetic activity to the heart and vasculature above the level of the lesion to compensate for the loss of sympathetic tone below the injury. Finally, the preserved cardiovascular response and increased catecholamine response in the LP group were attributed to enhanced sympathetic activity below the level of the lesion and alteration in end organ responsiveness to the increased catecholamine levels.

The anesthetic technique (ie, thiopental and vecuronium without other agents) for induction and intubation is one known to be associated with significant tachycardia and hypertension. The clinical implications of the observed differences in hemodynamic responses may well be of importance in those patients with other illnesses, such as coronary artery or cerebrovascular disease, which might predispose them to morbidity if transient hemodynamic alterations occur. Of particular note are the patients with quadriplegia with preserved tachycardic responses, but absent pressor responses. In addition, the patients with quadriplegia were more likely to have hypotension develop sooner. Attempts to blunt the tachycardic response with, for example, β-blockers might lead to excessive and unexpected degrees of hypotension in this group. Also, the HP group had increased tachycardic responses, preserved pressor responses, and earlier decreases in blood pressure after completion of laryngoscopy, which might put them at risk of both complications from excessive tachycardia and excessive hypotension as a consequence of overzealous treatment to prevent or treat the tachycardia. As clinicians caring for these patients, we may consider not so much altering the agents we use but perhaps monitoring more intensively and adjusting doses and the timing of therapy.

S. Black, MD

Threshold-Level Repetitive Transcranial Electrical Stimulation for Intraoperative Monitoring of Central Motor Conduction

Calancie B, Harris W, Brindle GF, et al (Univ of Miami, Fla)
J Neurosurg: Spine 95:161-168, 2001   7–13

Background.—Intraoperative electrophysiologic monitoring of spinal cord function during spinal surgery can help to minimize postoperative neurologic deficits. These authors have previously reported the use of threshold-level repetitive transcranial electrical stimulation (TES) for intraoperative monitoring of central motor conduction. Their experience with an additional 160 surgical procedures was reported.

Study Design.—A total of 160 surgical patients, aged 8 to 89 years, who underwent procedures in which neural function was considered to be at risk were studied. Anesthesia was induced with intravenous propofol and remifentanil, supplemented with inhaled nitrous oxide. Neuromuscular block was avoided. Electromyography (EMG), somatosensory evoked response (SSEP), and TES were monitored during the procedures.

Findings.—Muscle response to threshold-level repetitive TES could be achieved in almost all cases. Cortical SSEP responses could not be achieved in about 25% of cases (Table 1). TES responses accurately predicted postoperative motor status (Table 2). SSEP was almost as accurate for predicting postoperative sensory status. There were instances of deficit that were not predicted by one or the other form of monitoring. There were no adverse events attributed to TES-based monitoring.

Conclusions.—Intraoperative threshold-level repetitive TES-based monitoring of central motor conduction has been shown to be a safe, simple, and accurate method for minimizing motor deficit during surgery involving the spinal cord. It adds little additional cost or time into an intraoperative setting in which EMG and SSEP monitoring are already in place.

▶ Although SSEP monitoring remains the standard and most common form of neurologic monitoring used during spine surgical procedures placing

TABLE 1.—Number of Cases in Which There Was Either No Significant Change or Deterioration in Intraoperative SSEP Waveforms and Thresholds for TES-Evoked Muscle Responses*

TES	No. of Patients	
	No Change (SSEP)	Worse (SSEP)
no change	87	22
worse	13	23

*Values reflect a comparison with baseline status.
Abbreviations: SSEP, Somatosensory evoked response; *TES*, transcranial electrical stimulation.
(Courtesy of Calancie B, Harris W, Brindle GF, et al: Threshold-level repetitive transcranial electrical stimulation for intraoperative monitoring of central motor conduction. *J Neurosurg: Spine* 95:161-168, 2001. Copyright, Williams & Wilkins.)

TABLE 2.—Comparisons of Intraoperative SSEP or TES Findings With Postoperative Clinical Findings*

| | No. of Patients | | | |
Type of Monitoring	True Positive	True Negative	False Positive	False Negative
SSEP (sensory)	20	36	4	3
TES (motor)	29	51	0	0

*True positive = significant deterioration in intraoperative records, combined with new (or worsened) postoperative clinical deficit specific to modality; *True negative* = no significant change in intraoperative records, combined with no worsening of postoperative clinical status specific to modality; False positive = significant deterioration in intraoperative records but no detectable worsening of postoperative clinical status specific to modality; False negative = no significant change in intraoperative records, combined with new (or worsened) postoperative clinical deficit specific to modality.

Abbreviations: SSEP, Somatosensory evoked response; *TES,* transcranial electrical stimulation.

(Courtesy of Calancie B, Harris W, Brindle GF, et al: Threshold-level repetitive transcranial electrical stimulation for intraoperative monitoring of central motor conduction. *J Neurosurg: Spine* 95:161-168, 2001. Copyright, Williams & Wilkins.)

neurologic function at risk, isolated motor deficits and false negatives continue to occur. As a consequence, a reliable form of motor pathway monitoring that can be carried out under an acceptable general anesthetic regimen is being sought by many investigators. This is the second report from these authors describing their results with repetitive TES and muscle monitoring for spine surgery. Their technique is unique in that their monitoring end point is a change in threshold stimulation level required for each muscle monitored, rather than the nature (amplitude and latency) of the response generated. Because they historically have also used EMG monitoring during these procedures, avoidance of muscle relaxants intraoperatively is a routine part of their anesthetic management. The anesthetic regimen consists of propofol, remifentanil, and nitrous oxide. As yet, they have had no cases of intraoperative recall. In addition, all patients were routinely monitored with SSEP. The authors report a higher success rate for obtaining responses they could monitor with TES than with SSEP. They also report a higher sensitivity and specificity with TES and muscle monitoring than with SSEP. Their conclusion is that motor tract monitoring with TES as described here should be added to, rather than replace, intraoperative SSEP and EMG monitoring during spine surgery.

The possible problems associated with TES need to be considered. Thus far, complications reported relate to muscle contraction of the jaw causing tongue, tooth, and jaw injuries. These are not insignificant, and one must also consider the impact of movement in patients stabilized in a pin fixation device during cervical spine surgery. Seizures and serious skin injury are also possible, but likely rare complications. Concern regarding a possible increased incidence of intraoperative recall cannot be addressed as yet because of the relatively small size of the series to date. The cost of the monitoring is related not only to the additional equipment (monitors, electrodes), but also to the cost of the anesthetic technique required as compared with the use of longer acting narcotics with volatile agent supplementation. Still, the ability to reliably monitor motor pathways offers considerable potential benefit to patients at risk for intraoperative spinal cord injury.

S. Black, MD

Monitoring of Intraoperative Motor Evoked Potentials to Increase the Safety of Surgery in and Around the Motor Cortex

Kombos T, Suess O, Ciklatekerlio Ö, et al (Free Univ of Berlin)
J Neurosurg 95:608-614, 2001   7–14

Background.—Several studies in recent years have substantiated the need for intraoperative functional mapping and monitoring during surgery in and around the motor cortex. Recently the clinical use of monopolar stimulation of the motor cortex has been described. The monopolar high-frequency stimulus elicits motor-evoked potentials (MEPs), which can act as a monitoring parameter for qualitative and quantitative analysis during surgery of the motor cortex. Previously there has been little or no experience with intraoperative monitoring of MEPs in patients undergoing craniotomy under general anesthesia. The clinical relevance of monitoring MEPs during surgery in and around the motor cortex was evaluated. The correlation between intraoperative changes in MEPs and postoperative neurologic condition was also analyzed.

Methods.—This prospective study involved 70 patients who underwent MEP monitoring during craniotomy for lesions near the motor cortex after induction of general anesthesia without the aid of muscle relaxants. The motor pathways were monitored during the entire surgical procedure by repetitive high-frequency anodal monopolar stimulation. MEPs were evaluated throughout surgery to determine latency, potential duration, and amplitude. Recorded alterations in these parameters were then correlated with surgical maneuvers and postoperative neurologic deterioration.

Results.—Latency, potential duration, and amplitude had a broad interindividual range of variation. In 8 patients a correlation was observed between individual intraoperative changes in the potentials and surgical maneuvers or postoperative neurologic deterioration. A spontaneous shift in latency of more than 15% or a sudden reduction in the amplitude of the

---

TABLE 3.—Individual Variations in MEPs as Related to Reference Values

Recording Site	Latency Period	MEP Duration	MEP Amplitude
thenar muscle	−1.4 to 2.9%	−12.1 to 20.2%	−20.9 to 35.2%
forearm flexor	−2.4 to 2.8%	−10.1 to 21.7%	−32.8 to 31.9%
quadriceps muscle	−1.5 to 1.8%	−9.1 to 26%	−16.6 to 41.6%

(Courtesy of Kombos T, Suess O, Ciklatekerlio Ö, et al: Monitoring of intraoperative motor evoked potentials to increase the safety of surgery in and around the motor cortex. *J Neurosurg* 95:608-614, 2001.)

potential greater than 80% was considered a warning criterion. Postoperative neurologic deterioration was evident in all patients when there was an irreversible change in latency or a complete loss of potentials (Table 3).

Conclusions.—Repetitive stimulation of the motor cortex was found to be a reliable means for monitoring the motor pathways. Changes in the latency and amplitude of MEPs had prognostic value and served as warning criteria.

▶ MEP monitoring has been described most extensively for monitoring intraoperative spinal cord integrity. This report details early experience with electrical stimulation of the motor cortex during intracranial surgery. Traditional transcranial electric or magnetic stimulating techniques could not be easily used—if at all—to monitor the motor cortex on the operative side during a craniotomy. The authors have developed an apparently small stimulating monopolar electrode that could be placed, after opening the dura, over the motor cortex. By their account, it did not interfere with the surgical procedure and was only rarely dislodged during the course of the operation. Of note, intraoperative variability—even comparing each patient to his or her own baseline recordings—of all monitored variables was very high. However, the authors were able to identify changes in MEPs that reliably correlated with postoperative neurologic changes, both deterioration and improvement. Of concern are the 5 cases of false-negative findings with MEP monitoring. The authors attributed the neurologic deterioration in all 5 patients noted within the first "several" hours postoperatively to postoperative problems—either edema or infection. Although this may be true, larger series are required to confirm that intraoperative motor pathway monitoring during intracranial surgery in the vicinity of the motor cortex is adequately sensitive and specific.

The anesthetic technique—total intravenous anesthetic without muscle relaxation—is one many anesthesiologists might find uncomfortable. However, the other technique described for intraoperative monitoring during surgery on or near the motor cortex includes intraoperative awake neurologic exam. This intraoperative course is challenging for the patient, surgeon, and anesthesiologist. If a reliable method to monitor motor pathway integrity during craniotomy under general anesthesia could be found, the number of patients who might benefit from intraoperative motor monitoring would greatly increase.

S. Black, MD

8 Critical Care Medicine

Adult Critical Care Medicine

Early Goal-Directed Therapy in the Treatment of Severe Sepsis and Septic Shock

Rivers E, for the Early Goal-Directed Therapy Collaborative Group (Case Western Reserve Univ, Detroit; et al)
N Engl J Med 345:1368-1377, 2001   8–1

Introduction.—Previous studies have evaluated the impact of goal-directed therapy for ICU patients with severe sepsis and septic shock. Some authors have called for studies of earlier intervention in an attempt to reduce mortality. The effects of early goal-directed therapy—beginning before ICU admission—in patients with severe sepsis and septic shock were evaluated.

Methods.—The prospective randomized trial included 263 patients with severe sepsis or septic shock seen at 1 emergency department over a 4-year period. One group received 6 hours of goal-directed therapy, including central venous catheterization; the other group received standard therapy. The patients were then transferred to the ICU, where care was provided without knowledge of the patients' group assignment. The 2 groups were compared for their incidence of multiorgan dysfunction, mortality, and resource utilization.

Results.—The 2 groups were similar in their baseline characteristics. In-hospital mortality was significantly reduced in the goal-directed therapy group: 30.5% versus 46.5%. During the first 3 ICU days, patients receiving early goal-directed therapy had higher mean central venous oxygen saturation and a lower lactate level than those receiving standard therapy. Patients in the goal-directed therapy group also had lower Acute Physiology and Chronic Health Evaluation II scores, suggesting less severe organ dysfunction.

Conclusion.—For patients seen in the emergency department with severe sepsis or septic shock, early goal-directed therapy significantly improves mortality and other outcome indicators. Early therapy identifies patients at high risk for cardiovascular collapse, allowing restoration of the balance between oxygen delivery and demand.

▶ The authors of this study should be commended for excellent work. This study demonstrates that the early identification of patients (in this case when they hit the ER) at risk for cardiovascular collapse can be treated and in effect their mortality improved versus standard care (hang on and let's get them to where they should be and then start treating them aggressively). This is also a great example of multidisciplinary team work (ER faculty, residents and nurses and also critical care clinicians that included faculty, fellows, and residents providing 24 h/d coverage). Also of interest was that central venous catheters were placed instead of pulmonary artery catheters, and the right atrial venous saturation used as a surrogate marker of mixed venous saturation. Obviously, many of us would probably not follow this particular algorithm, but in the chaos of the ER this is a very efficient approach. Patients who have sepsis, severe sepsis, and septic shock all demonstrated reductions in mortality with early goal-directed therapy. Do we now couple the results of this study with the study using Xigris and reduce mortality in patients with severe sepsis even more?

J. D. Lang, Jr, MD

The Effects of Vasopressin on Hemodynamics and Renal Function in Severe Septic Shock: A Case Series
Holmes CL, Walley KR, Chittock DR, et al (Univ of British Columbia, Vancouver, Canada)
Intensive Care Med 27:1416-1421, 2001   8–2

Introduction.—The mortality rate for septic shock continues to be greater than 50%. Recent reports have indicated that vasopressin may be useful as a rational therapy for septic shock. The literature does not indicate whether vasopressin for septic shock is safe and titratable, and whether there are any adverse effects. All cases of septic shock treated in a 14-bed mixed medical-surgical ICU of a tertiary referral hospital between August 1997 and March 1999 were reviewed retrospectively.

Methods.—The following data were extracted from medical records of patients with septic shock who received vasopressin for 4 hours or more: age, gender, Acute Physiology and Chronic Health Evaluation (APACHE) II score 24 hours before the start of vasopressin, source of sepsis, hospital mortality, hemodynamic data (mean arterial pressure [MAP], systolic pulmonary arterial pressure, cardiac index), hourly urine output, dose of vasopressin used each hour, and dosage of other vasoactive agents. Pressor dose was defined as the total units of dopamine (μg·kg·min ÷ 3) plus norepinephrine (μg/min) plus epinephrine (μg/min). Values at baseline (T0) were compared with those at 4 (T4), 24 (T24), and 48 (T48) hours of infusion of vasopressin.

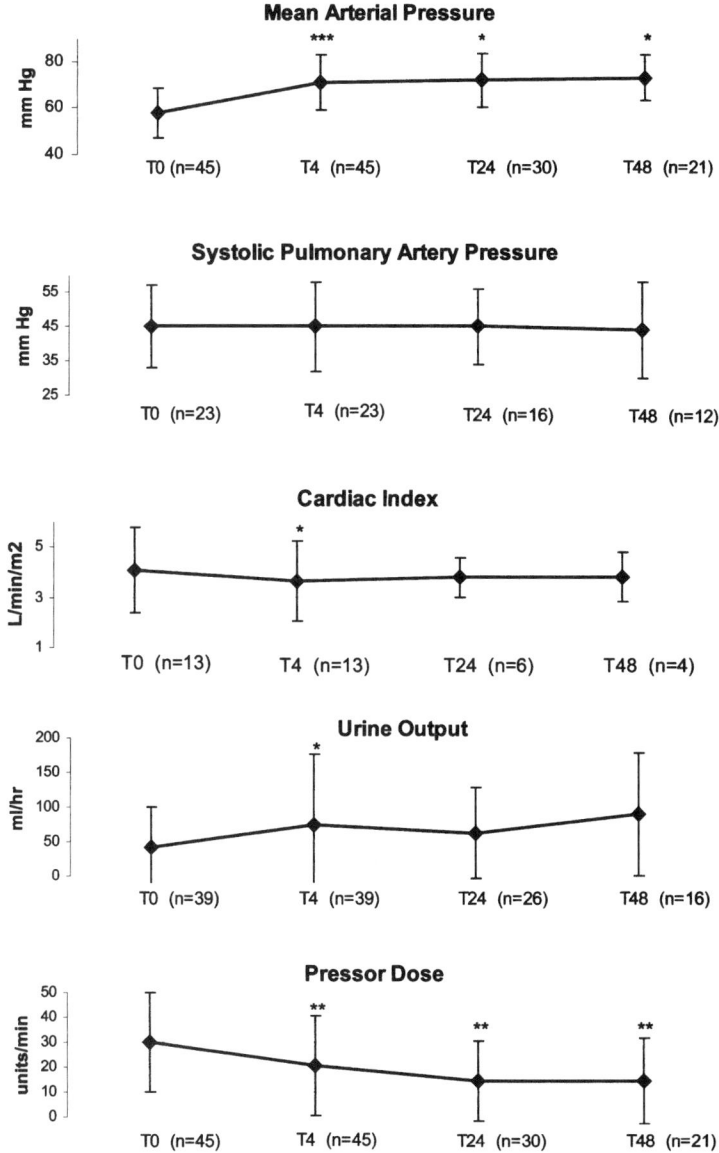

FIGURE 1.—Hemodynamics, urine output and pressor dose in 45 patients who had severe septic shock and who received vasopressin infusion (*n* number of subjects still alive and on vasopressin infusion in whom measurements were made). Anuric patients were excluded from urine output measurements, *P* (see text for test used) for each time period versus baseline (TX vs TO), *pressor dose*: dopamine ($\mu g \cdot kg \cdot min$)/3 + norepinephrine ($\mu g \cdot min$) + epinephrine ($\mu g \cdot min$). *Asterisk*, P < .05; *double asterisk*, P < .005; *triple asterisk*, P < .0001. (Courtesy of Holmes CL, Walley KR, Chittock DR, et al: The effects of vasopressin on hemodynamics and renal function in severe septic shock: A case series. *Intensive Care Med* 27:1416-1421. Copyright 2001, Springer-Verlag.)

Results.—The mean age of 50 patients was 60 years. The mean APACHE II score was 27. The MAP increased by 18% from T0 to T4 and remained stable at T24 (P = .006) and T48 (P = .008). The systolic pulmonary artery pressure remained unchanged at a mean of 45 mm Hg. The mean cardiac index decreased by 11% at T4 (P = .03). The urine output increased 79% at T4 (P = .005); further increases were not significant at T24 or T48. The mean pressor dosage decreased by 33% at T4 (P = .001), by 53% at T24 (P = .002), and by 48% at T48 (P = .01) (Fig 1). The hospital mortality rate was 85%. Six patients had cardiac arrests; all except one occurred at a vasopressin dosage of 0.05 U/min or more.

Conclusion.—Vasopressin infusion increased MAP and urine output and reduced catecholamine requirements in patients with severe septic shock. Dosages of more than 0.04 U/min were not associated with increased effectiveness and may have produced a higher rate of adverse events.

▶ As happens many times in medicine, a therapy is being revisited. This time a prominent group from British Columbia has shared with us their retrospective findings of vasopressin used as "rescue therapy" in patients with septic shock. This study has obvious limitations, but it is a nice effort to characterize some of the effects of vasopressin at varying dosages on global measurements in patients with refractory septic shock. There seems to be a physiologic rationale for its potential efficacy: (1) vasopressin concentrations are decreased in noncardiac shock[1]; (2) vasopressin has vasodilatory effects on the pulmonary vasculature (not observed in this study); (3) it causes dilation of the renal afferent arteriole and constriction of the efferent arteriole; (4) it increases atrial natriuretic peptide concentrations; and (5) its agonism of oxytocin results in a natriuresis. Of concern were the increased cardiac events in patients receiving dosages greater than 0.03 U/min, potentially resulting from coronary artery vasoconstriction. A prospective, randomized, controlled trial comparing this agent with others is needed. Serial measurements of variables such as mixed venous saturation, lactate, intramucosal pH, and the effects on the expression of various inflammatory mediators (eg, tumor necrosis factor-α, interleukin-6, interleukin-10) would be informative, in addition to clinical outcomes measurements.

J. D. Lang, Jr, MD

Reference

1. Landry D, Levin R, Gallant E, et al: Vasopressin deficiency contributes to the vasodilatation of septic shock. *Circulation* 95:1122-1125, 1997.

Inhaled Nitric Oxide Down-regulates Intrapulmonary Nitric Oxide Production in Lipopolysaccharide-induced Acute Lung Injury

Koh Y, Kang JL, Park W, et al (Univ of Ulsan, Seoul, Korea; Ewha Womans Univ, Seoul, Korea)
Crit Care Med 29:1169-1174, 2001   8–3

Background.—Patients with severe acute respiratory distress syndrome (ARDS) commonly receive inhaled nitric oxide (NO) to increase oxygenation. Aan effort was made to determine whether inhaled NO affects the intrapulmonary production of NO, reactive oxygen species, and nuclear factor-κB in a lipopolysaccharide (LPS)-induced model of acute lung injury.

Methods.—Twenty male rabbits weighing 2.5 to 3.5 kg were studied in the prospective investigation. Rabbits were randomly assigned to receive saline solution or LPS, 5 mg/kg body weight, given intravenously with or without NO inhalation.

Findings.—The LPS increased the lung leak index, neutrophil and NO levels in bronchoalveolar lavage fluid, and NO levels produced by resting. It also stimulated alveolar macrophages. Inhaled NO reduced the lung leak index, neutrophil and NO levels in lavage fluid, and NO levels produced by resting. Alveolar macrophages were also stimulated. In addition, inhaled NO blocked the activities of reactive oxygen species and nuclear factor-κB binding to DNA in lavage cells and alveolar macrophages.

Conclusions.—In this animal study, inhaled NO attenuated LPS-induced acute lung injury, possibly by reducing lung NO production. The mechanism underlying this may partly involve the activities of reactive oxygen species, nuclear factor-κB, or both.

▶ A clinically relevant study demonstrating the effects of inhaled NO on cell signaling. After 5 mg/mL of LPS was given intravenously, inhaled NO (10 ppm) attenuated the endogenous production of NO. Of significant interest was that the production of superoxide radical (as per a decrease in chemiluminescence) was significantly decreased in the group given LPS plus inhaled NO. NF-κB was also significantly decreased in this group, indirectly hinting that cytokines such as TNF-α may be decreased by inhaled NO as well. The overall net effect was a decrease in lung leak. As we all know, inhaled NO has been disappointing in the adult patient with ARDS, but in other disorders suffered by adults, such as ischemia-reperfusion and maybe "early-onset" lung injury (within minutes to 1 to 2 hours), inhaled NO may exert this anti-inflammatory effect. With inhaled prostaglandins being more commonly used in the adult population because of its reduced cost, the enthusiasm once exhibited by investigators mesmerized by NO is waning. However, data like this should re-invigorate investigations with this interesting biomolecule.

J. D. Lang, Jr, MD

Peritoneal Lavage With Oxygenated Perfluorochemical Preserves Intestinal Mucosal Barrier Function After Ischemia-Reperfusion and Ameliorates Lung Injury

Ohara M, Unno N, Mitsuoka H, et al (Hamamatsu Univ, Japan)
Crit Care Med 29:782-788, 2001   8–4

Background.—Peritoneal lavage with oxygenated perfluorochemical (PFC) may protect the intestinal mucosa and prevent translocation of enteric bacteria or endotoxins after superior mesenteric artery occlusion and reperfusion.

Methods.—In this prospective, randomized, controlled study, male Sprague-Dawley rats were subjected to ischemia by clipping of the superior mesenteric artery. The clip was released to produce reperfusion. Abdominal cavity lavage was done by inflow and outflow of oxygenated PFC solution during ischemia.

Findings.—Rats undergoing peritoneal lavage with oxygenated PFC had a significantly better survival rate after intestinal ischemia-reperfusion injury (IIR). The PFC group had a significantly lower frequency of bacterial translocation and endotoxin concentration in superior mesenteric venous blood. In addition, luminal acidosis was relieved in the PFC group. Lavage with PFC preserved the intestinal mucosal architecture and inhibited interstitial edema and inflammatory cell infiltration in the lungs.

Conclusions.—Peritoneal lavage with oxygenated PFC appears to protect the intestinal mucosa and to maintain barrier function after IIR. Preserving the intestinal mucosa will alleviate lung injury after IIR.

▶ In this rat model, the use of an oxygenated perfluorocarbon solution (Fluosol-DA) administered via peritoneal lavage attenuated intestinal and pulmonary injury via ischemia-reperfusion as per histologic evaluation, reductions in endotoxin concentrations, lung weight:dry analysis, and luminal pH changes. Mortality rate was reduced in the rats receiving Fluosol-DA. This study brings to light an interesting route of treatment. But is it a practical one? Also, various strategies employing perfluorocarbon solutions have been undertaken. Will this ever find a niche? Or is it nothing more than a physiologic curiosity looking for an indication?

J. D. Lang, Jr, MD

Septic Shock and Respiratory Failure in Community-acquired Pneumonia Have Different TNF Polymorphism Associations

Waterer GW, Quasney MW, Cantor RM, et al (Univ of Western Australia, Perth; Univ of Tennessee, Memphis; Univ of California, Los Angeles; et al)
Am J Respir Crit Care Med 163:1599-1604, 2001   8–5

Background.—Community-acquired pneumonia (CAP) is a significant health problem throughout the world. In the United States, CAP is the leading cause of death from infection and the sixth leading cause of death overall. The severity of CAP at presentation can vary widely, ranging from fulminant septic shock (SS) at the most severe end of the spectrum to virtually asymptomatic disease at the other end. As antibiotic resistance has increased, particularly in *Streptococcus pneumoniae*, attention has focused on the need to develop nonantibiotic strategies for both prevention and treatment. This approach will require a better understanding of the determinants of individual immune responses to CAP. It is likely that genetic factors have a role in its variable presentation. This study was conducted to determine whether the LTα+250 (TNFβ+250) and TNFα−308 gene polymorphisms are associated with different presentations of CAP.

Methods.—A total of 280 patients with CAP admitted from November 1, 1998, to January 31, 2000, were enrolled in this prospective investigation. SS was defined according to the criteria of the American College of Chest Physicians/Society of Critical Care Medicine. Type 1 respiratory failure was defined as an oxygen saturation on room air of less than 90% with a normal PCO_2.

Results.—SS was present in 31 of the 280 patients, while 80 patients had type 1 respiratory failure. Patients with at least 1 AA (TNF high secretor) genotype had an 18% risk for SS compared with 6.8% for non-AA patients. Patients with GG homozygotes (TNF low secretors) at both loci had only a 2.9% risk for SS. SS was found to be associated with the LTα+250 (TNFβ+250):TNFα−308 A:G haplotype but not the A:A haplotype, a finding that suggested that LTα+250 is a marker rather than a causative polymorphism. Carriage of the G:G haplotype was found to provide a significant protective effect against the development of SS. Type 1 respiratory failure was not associated with the LTα+250 AA genotype. In the absence of SS, there was a significant trend toward greater type 1 respiratory failure in patients with the LTα+250 GG genotype.

Conclusion.—The identification of different genotype associations for septic shock and type 1 respiratory failure has important implications for the development of immunotherapy in both CAP and sepsis and for the definition of the systemic inflammatory response syndrome.

▶ We are at the threshold of molecular medicine playing a large role in patient prognostication, but also with therapeutic strategies as well. This study provided insight into the genetic milieu and how patients with CAP would behave. But as is usual, the complexity of the human body continues to keep us off balance, as in this study, type 1 respiratory failure (T1RF) occurred more commonly in patients with the TNF hyposecretor genotype (LTα+250GG) and not the TNF hypersecretors. However, TNF hypersecretors (LTα+250AA) did develop the greatest proportion of SS. At this point, reasons for the disparity in clinical correlate between T1RF and septic are sheer speculation. The point to be made here is the progress in molecular medicine and its potential impact in critical care medicine.

J. D. Lang, Jr, MD

Comparison of Two Methods for Weaning Patients With Chronic Obstructive Pulmonary Disease Requiring Mechanical Ventilation for More Than 15 Days

Vitacca M, Vianello A, Colombo D, et al (Scientific Int of Gussago, Italy; Ospedale Civile, Padova, Italy; INRCA Casatenovo, Italy; et al)

Am J Respir Crit Care Med 164:225-230, 2001   8–6

Background.—Patients with chronic obstructive pulmonary disease (COPD) and acute respiratory failure often need endotracheal intubation and mechanical ventilation. Difficulties may occur during weaning, resulting in a need for tracheostomy. The relative efficacies of 2 weaning protocols—inspiratory pressure support ventilation (PSV) and spontaneous breathing (SB) trials—were compared in patients with COPD requiring mechanical ventilation for more than 15 days.

Methods.—Fifty-two of 75 patients failing an initial T-piece trial at admission were enrolled in the prospective, multicenter, controlled study. By random assignment, 26 patients received PSV and 2 had SB.

Findings.—The weaning success rates in the PSV and SB groups were 73% and 77%, respectively. Mortality rates were 11.5% and 7.6%, respectively; duration of ventilatory assistance, 181 and 130 hours; and stay in long-term weaning units (LWU), 33 and 35 days. These differences were not significant. Total hospital stay was also comparable in the 2 groups. When compared retrospectively with an "uncontrolled clinical practice" in weaning of historical control patients, the 2 current protocols were superior in the overall 30-day weaning success rate and time spent under mechanical ventilation by surviving and weaned patients. In addition, LWU and hospital stays were significantly shorter.

Conclusions.—SB trials and decreasing PSV levels are equally effective in difficult-to-wean patients with COPD. The use of a well-defined protocol, regardless of mode, appears to yield better outcomes than uncontrolled clinical practice.

▶ A nicely designed study focusing on the COPD population confirming most of our suspicions that mode per se is not the answer but that strategy and protocols are what is truly pivotal in patient weaning success.

J. D. Lang, Jr, MD

Nitric Oxide and Nitrotyrosine in the Lungs of Patients With Acute Respiratory Distress Syndrome

Sittipunt C, Steinberg KP, Ruzinski JT, et al (Univ of Washington, Seattle; Univ of Alabama, Birmingham)

Am J Respir Crit Care Med 163:503-510, 2001   8–7

Background.—Patients with inflammatory lung diseases such as acute respiratory distress syndrome (ARDS) have nitric oxide (NO) end products, specifically nitrate and nitrite, present in bronchoalveolar lavage

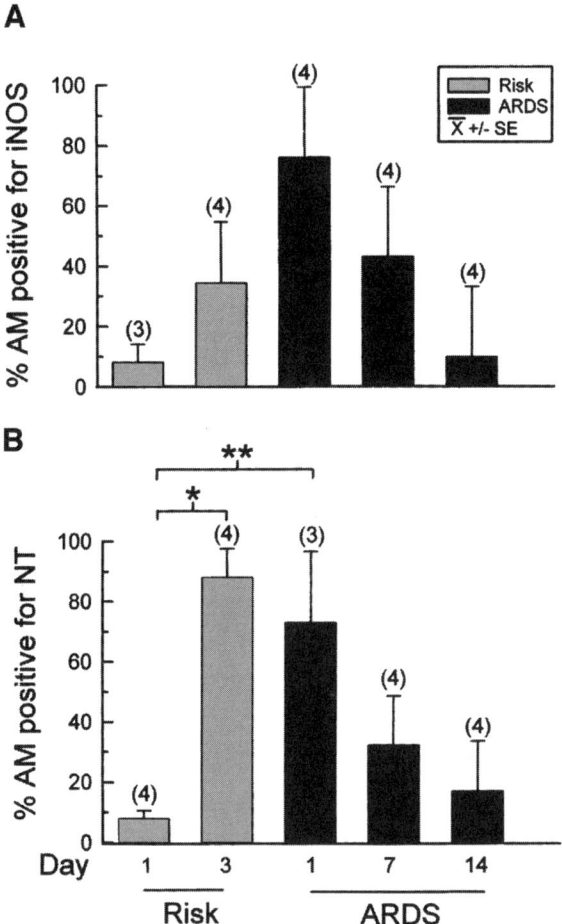

FIGURE 6.—Measurement of iNOS and nitrotyrosine-positive alveolar macrophages (AM) in cytospin preparations of ARDS BAL cells. **A,** iNOS-positive alveolar AM (% of total AM). **B,** Nitrotyrosine positive AM (% of total AM). *P = .02 for risk day 1 vs risk day 3. **P = .034 for risk day 1 vs ARDS day 1. (Courtesy of Sittipunt C, Steinberg KP, Ruzinski JT, et al: Nitric oxide and nitrotyrosine in the lungs of patients with acute respiratory distress syndrome. *Am J Respir Crit Care Med* 163:503-510, 2001. Official Journal of the American Thoracic Society. Copyright American Lung Association.)

(BAL) fluid. These reactive nitrogen intermediates cause damage to macromolecules by oxidation of redox-active complexes or nitration of aromatic amines. Levels of these NO end products were measured in BAL fluid before and after ARDS developed in patients to see if these products are linked to the expression of inducible NO synthase (iNOS) enzyme in BAL cells and with the nitration of BAL proteins.

Methods.—Nineteen patients at risk for ARDS underwent BAL along with 41 patients who had ARDS. These procedures were carried out 1, 3, 7, 14, and 21 days after the onset of risk factors. Total nitrite and protein-associated nitrotyrosine concentration was determined for each sample. Immunocytochemical studies were used to identify iNOS and nitrotyrosine.

Results.—The BAL fluid from patients at risk for ARDS had nitrate and nitrite concentrations significantly higher than those found in normal subjects 1 and 3 days after onset; the samples from patients with ARDS had elevated concentrations throughout the period of the ARDS. Most of the products were nitrate in the ARDS patients. Although patients at risk and those with ARDS had essentially equal nitrate plus nitrite concentrations, on day 21 after ARDS onset the levels were the lowest. As long as 14 days after the onset of ARDS, nitrotyrosine was detectable in all BAL samples from ARDS patients but not in those from normal volunteers. Neither iNOS nor nitrotyrosine residues were detectable in samples from normal volunteers. Patients with ARDS also had alveolar macrophages positive for iNOS and nitrotyrosine, and these remained positive for up to 14 days (Fig 6). The concentrations were significantly higher on days 3 and 7 in ARDS patients who died, although the BAL nitrate and nitrite did not predict ARDS onset.

Conclusions.—The products of NO accumulate in the lungs of patients both before and after ARDS onset, and this development is linked to iNOS expression in alveolar macrophages as well as nitrotyrosine formation in soluble proteins and BAL leukocytes. High nitrate plus nitrite concentrations seem to accompany higher mortality rate, although they were not predictive. Thus for patients before and after the onset of ARDS, the pathways depending on NO in the lungs play an important role.

▶ This study documents the participation of NO-mediated reactions in patients with ARDS versus healthy controls. It has been known for years that NO production, especially iNOS, is upregulated in patients with septic shock and is a significant contributor to the loss of tone observed in these patients. It is also well established through laboratory investigations that the NO-mediated pathways significantly alter oxidative and nitrosative stress in a way that is generally unfavorable for those studied. However, the true consequences of reaction products such as 3-nitrotyrosine are truly unknown. Recent data in patients with ARDS receiving inhaled NO (iNO) have demonstrated increases in 3-nitrotyrosine formation in bronchoalveolar lavage samples in patients receiving iNO versus those not receiving iNO. Mortality rate analysis was not an aim of the study. In a separate study, patients receiving iNO were found to have a significant degree of plasma protein nitration. The clinical significance these findings, nevertheless interesting, warrants much more detailed investigation. For instance, we have found hypercapnia significantly upregulates NO production, iNOS expression, and the formation of 3-nitrotyrosine in the laboratory.[1] In addition, the flux of radiolabeled albumin, indicating barrier dysfunction, was greatest under hypercapnic conditions as well. One could draw the conclusion that in patients with ARDS, NO-derived products are increased—but if one uses permissive hypercapnia the production would then be greater.

J. D. Lang, Jr, MD

Reference

1. Lang JD Jr, Chumley P, Eiserich JP, et al: Hypercampia induces injury to alveolar epithelial cells via a nitric oxide-dependent pathway. *Am J Physiol Lung Cell Mol Physiol* 279:L994-L1002, 2000.

Factors Associated With Reintubation in Intensive Care: An Analysis of Causes and Outcomes
Beckmann U, Gillies DM (John Hunter Hosp, Newcastle, Australia)
Chest 120:538-542, 2001   8–8

Background.—Reintubation studies generally offer information related to unsuccessful extubation or self-extubation and have tried to identify risk factors that lead to the need for reintubation. A database analysis offered the opportunity to identify actual and latent problems and to trace causes, adverse outcomes, and contributing or limiting factors.

Methods.—Data were obtained from the Australian Incident Monitoring Study in Intensive Care and analyzed.

Results.—Of the more than 11,000 incidents reported, 241 involved re-intubation. A total of 98 were related to accidental extubation; 143 incidents were not. Most (n = 114) involved an oral endotracheal tube, 20 a nasal endotracheal tube, and 9 a tracheostomy. Only 8% of these occurred on weekends or public holidays, 33% occurred during the weekday night shift, and 59% occurred during the weekday day shift. All incidents occurred in the ICU except for 1 case. Most patients were older than 14 years (n = 118), with the rest distributed as follows: 10 patients between ages 1 and 14 years, 10 patients between ages 28 days and 1 year, and 5 patients less than age 28 days. The prominent precipitating events were tube malposition (17%), securing or taping problems (17%), pilot tube or cuff problems (16%), blocked or kinked airway (14%), failed extubation (14%), and poor planning for the extubation process (6%). One fourth of incidents involved hypoxia, 12% had hypercarbic respiratory failure, 7% aspirated, 7% had sputum retention, and 6% had cardiac arrhythmias. Fifty-two percent of patients had major physiologic complications; 16% required a prolonged hospital stay. Among the factors contributing most to the need for reintubation were judgment or problem recognition error (62%), high level of activity on the unit (20%), difficult patient habitus (26%), and lack of cooperation on the part of the patient (14%). Adverse outcomes were limited by rechecking the patient and the equipment, seeking skilled assistance, applying previous experience, and using protocol.

Conclusions.—Reintubation that was not in response to accidental extubation still resulted in significant physiologic complications and lengthened hospital stay. Trained, experienced staff who followed correct procedures and rechecked patients and equipment helped to limit or avoid adverse outcomes.

▶ This is an unusual study focusing on incidents deemed significant during the reintubation of patients not related to accidental extubation. The design of the study has many flaws but does reveal a rather appealing database linking multiple ICUs within Australia. The events reported and consequences of such events were assigned in a rather subjective way using a tickbox list. The reporters varied between nurses, physicians, and other so-called "professionals." The reintubation data lack a denominator; therefore the conclusions are unfortunately descriptive. The data are consistent, however, with other data supporting prolonged ICU stays and increased complication rates as a result of reintubations not related to accidental extubations, which in most cases are associated with a higher complication rate. Once more, the study is rather weak, but the mechanisms in place within the Australian system are impressive and do seemingly allow for excellent peer review within a particular institution and for comparisons between some or all other institutions if necessary.

J. D. Lang, Jr, MD

Effect of Postpyloric Feeding on Gastroesophageal Regurgitation and Pulmonary Microaspiration: Results of a Randomized Controlled Trial
Heyland DK, Drover JW, MacDonald S, et al (Queen's Univ, Kingston, Ont, Canada)
Crit Care Med 29:1495-1501, 2001   8–9

Background.—The most frequent cause of infection acquired in the ICU is pneumonia. Both the ICU stay and the patient's risk of dying are increased when pneumonia develops. For critically ill patients, upper gastrointestinal tract abnormalities contribute significantly to the pathogenesis of nosocomial pneumonia. Tracheal secretions can be contaminated by gastric colonization, which leads to pneumonia. When duodenogastric reflux—which is evidenced by conjugated bilirubin found in stomach secretions—occurs, gram-negative bacteria will likely be isolated from the stomach and trachea of mechanically ventilated patients. Delivering enteral feedings directly to the small bowel may decrease the risk of aspiration, although this remains unproved in critically ill patients. Even noncritically ill patients show aspiration is not wholly eliminated. Whether feeding into the small bowel produces less gastroesophageal regurgitation and pulmonary aspiration, as detected by the presence of technetium 99, was evaluated.

Methods.—The randomized trial focused on 33 patients in the ICU (mean age 59.2 years, 42.4% female) who were to remain ventilated for more than 72 hours; did not have esophageal, gastric, or small bowel surgery in the preceding week; and did not have either overt or clinically significant gastrointestinal bleeding. The patients' mean Acute Physiology

TABLE 2.—Relation between Tube Position and Gastroesophageal Regurgitation (GER)

Tube Position	No. of Patients	% Positive GER*	% Positive Aspiration†	% Positive Reflux‡
Stomach	21	31.2	5.8	NA
D1	8	27.1	4.1	58.3
D2	3	11.1	1.8	57.4
D4	1	5.5	0	100.0

*$P = .004$.
†$P = .09$.
‡$P = NS$.
Abbreviations: Reflux, duodenogastric reflux; *NA*, not applicable; *D1*, first part of duodenum; *D2*, second part of duodenum; *D4*, fourth part of the duodenum. There were no tubes in the third part of the duodenum.
(Courtesy of Heyland DK, Drover JW, MacDonald S, et al: Effect of postpyloric feeding on gastroesophageal regurgitation and pulmonary microaspiration: Results of a randomized controlled trial. *Crit Care Med* 29:1495-1501, 2001.)

and Chronic Health Evaluation II score was 22.5. Patients received either gastric (n = 21) or postpyloric enteral feedings (n = 12), with ^{99}Tc added to the feedings for 6 hours of each of the first 3 days. Hourly samples were drawn from the oropharynx and trachea, and radioactivity was measured.

Results.—Twenty-nine of the patients had at least 1 episode of gastroesophageal regurgitation (all those receiving postpyloric feedings and 81% of those in the gastric group). Age and sex were not factors. Those fed into the stomach had more episodes of gastroesophageal regurgitation (39%) than those in the postpyloric group (24.9%). The gastric group had higher levels of radioisotope, but the difference did not reach statistical significance. Aspiration occurred in 45.5% of patients at least once, with 52.4% of the gastric group and 33% of the postpyloric group having this symptom. The gastric group had more episodes and the level of radioisotope tended to be higher in them, but neither of these results was statistically significant. Aspiration was more likely to occur in patients who had gastroesophageal regurgitation (Table 2).

Conclusions.—Feeding beyond the pylorus tended to reduce the frequency of gastroesophageal regurgitation and the occurrence of aspiration.

▶ As we all know, pneumonia is the most frequent ICU-acquired infection, with a significant attributable mortality rate. Gastric colonization of pathogenic organisms plays a significant role in the development of nosocomial pneumonia. Strategies to decrease aspiration have proven to reduce pneumonia rates. This study, although very small, nicely demonstrates the high rate of gastroesophageal regurgitation and patients' predisposition to have microaspiration if fed by a gastric protocol. The more distal the placement of the 12F feeding tube the less gastroesophageal regurgitation occurred. However, there is a paucity of data supporting this. Most studies have been very small, thus differences in pneumonia occurrence were not statistically significant. Our current ICU uses gastric protocols in certain patient populations, but with the use of sucralfate, the head elevated to 45°, and the nasogastric tube removed if at all possible. Certain other institutions also acidify the feeds to reduce the colonization rate.

J. D. Lang, Jr, MD

Bronchoscopy With Bronchoalveolar Lavage Via the Laryngeal Mask Airway in High-Risk Hypoxemic Immunosuppressed Patients
Hilbert G, Gruson D, Vargas F, et al (Pellegrin Hosp, Bordeaux, France)
Crit Care Med 29:249-255, 2001   8–10

Introduction.—Severe hypoxemia is an accepted contraindication to fiberoptic bronchoscopy (FOB) in patients who are not intubated. In these high-risk patients, the physician may choose to perform intubation with mechanical ventilation to guarantee adequate gas exchange during FOB, or refrain from FOB and use empiric treatment. The feasibility and safety of laryngeal mask airway (LMA)-supported FOB with bronchoalveolar lavage (BAL) were prospectively examined in immunosuppressed patients with suspected pneumonia and severe hypoxemia.

Methods.—Forty-six patients with suspected pneumonia and a ratio of PaO_2 to fraction of inspired oxygen (PaO_2/FIO_2) of 125 or less were admitted to a medical ICU. After administration of 0.3 mg·kg^{-1} of etomidate, the patients underwent manual ventilation while receiving 1.0 FIO_2. After the patients were given 2.5 mg·kg^{-1} of propofol, followed by an infusion of 9.1 ± 2.3 mg·kg^{-1}·h^{-1} of propofol, the LMA (size 3 or 4) was placed and connected to a bag-value unit to permit manual ventilation with 1.0 FIO_2. The FOB was introduced through a T-adapter that was attached to the LMA. The BAL was performed with 150 mL of sterile 0.9% saline solution via sequential instillation and aspiration of 50-mL aliquots.

Results.—Three patients had transient laryngospasm during passage of the bronchoscope through the LMA. This resolved with deepening of the anesthesia. There were no significant changes in mean blood pressure, heart rate, PaO_2/FIO_2, or $PaCO_2$ values as a result of LMA-supported FOB with BAL. Seven patients (15%) had hypotension (mean blood pressure, <60 mm Hg) maintained for 120 ± 40 seconds, necessitating plasma expanders in 3 patients. Oxygen desaturation to below 90% occurred in 6 patients (13%) during BAL. The lowest arterial oxygen saturation (SaO_2) during the procedure was significantly higher, compared with the initial SaO_2 (94% vs 90%). Tracheal intubation was not needed during the 8-hour procedure. The overall diagnostic yield for BAL was 65%. Treatment was modified in 33 (72%) patients because of the BAL findings.

Conclusion.—The use of LMA seems to be a safe and effective alternative to intubation for accomplishing FOB with BAL in immunosuppressed patients with suspected pneumonia and severe hypoxemia.

▶ The use of noninvasive positive pressure ventilation (PPV) versus intubation plus PPV has been demonstrated to decrease the mortality in selected patient populations, such as those with chronic obstructive pulmonary disease. These authors hypothesized that by circumventing intubation, the associated morbidity and mortality would be lessened in this vulnerable cohort. This study demonstrated that the transition from noninvasive PPV to BAL for diagnostic purposes by way of the LMA was relatively safe. There was a decreased intubation rate (50%-75%) when compared with their previous experience assessing continuous positive airway pressure (CPAP) for respiratory failure in neutropenic patients who required intubation.[1] Advantages of the LMA include ease of placement, a decreased stress response, and a decreased incidence of upper airway bleeding complications (for this patient population). Disadvantages include the increased risk of aspiration and the theoretic ease of dislodgement occurring when bronchoscopy and BAL are being performed. I think this study offers another alternative to bronchoscopy and BAL in critically ill patients, but not a definitive approach demonstrating superiority over another.

J. D. Lang, Jr, MD

Reference

1. Hilbert G, Gruson D, Valentino R: Non-invasive continuous positive airway pressure in neutropenic patients with acute respiratory failure requiring ICU admission. *Crit Care Med* 28:3185-3190, 2000.

Systemic Inflammatory Response After Bronchoalveolar Lavage in Critically Ill Patients

Bauer TT, Arosio C, Montón C, et al (Univ of Barcelona)
Eur Respir J 17:274-280, 2001   8–11

Introduction.—Bronchoscopic bronchoalveolar lavage (BAL) may be followed by a systemic inflammatory response that may be caused by a proinflammatory cytokine release. Pneumonia may be a predisposing condition, with systemic cytokines acting as possible mediators. Systemic cytokine levels were examined after bronchoscopically guided BAL in mechanically ventilated patients, with and without pneumonia.

Methods.—Systemic levels of interleukin (IL)-1 , IL-6, and tumor necrosis factor-α (TNF-α) were evaluated before and at 12 hours and 24 hours after bronchoscopically guided BAL in 30 patients receiving mechanical ventilation. The median patient age was 67 years (range, 54-76 years). The median Simplified Acute Physiology Score II was 33 (12-56). Twenty patients had pneumonia and 10 did not (controls). The ratio of PaO_2 to the fraction of inspired oxygen (PaO_2/FIO_2), the body temperature, the mean arterial pressure, and the cardiac frequency were recorded. Most patients (28/30; 93%) received antibiotic therapy before BAL.

Results.—The PaO_2/FIO_2 ratio was lower at 12 hours than at baseline in patients with pneumonia (baseline, median 192 [range, 65-256]; 12 hours, 160 [66-190], $P < .001$) and in ventilated controls (baseline, 293 [205-473]; 12 hours 226 [153-330], $P = .011$). There was a return to baseline

TABLE 3.—Comparison of Clinical and Cytokine Data Between Patients With Pneumonia and Recovery of a Potentially Pathogenic Micro-organism (*PPM*) in Bronchoalveolar Lavage (*BAL*), and Patients With Pneumonia and Sterile BAL Cultures

	Before BAL	12 h	24 h
PPM recovered (n = 11)*			
Mean arterial blood pressure, mmHg	88 (67-110)	77 (65-108)	82 (73-100)
Axilliary body temperature, °C	36.2 (35.6-37.6)	37.0 (35.8-38.6)	36.8 (36.2-38.0)
Cardiac frequency beats·min^{-1}	95 (80-145)	100 (75-125)	105 (70-135)
TNF-α, pg·mL^{-1}	39 (13-88)	41 (0-64)	37.5 (15-63)
IL-1β, pg·mL^{-1}	2 (0-12)	3 (0-14)	4 (0-122)
IL-6, pg·mL^{-1}	297 (47-4300)	359 (53-3778)	194 (23-924)
BAL sterile or no PPM (n = 7)*			
Mean arterial blood pressure, mmHg	68 (57-107)	70 (57-110)	73 (62-112)
Axilliary body temperature, °C	37.2 (35.8-38.0)	36.4 (35.8-38.0)	36.8 (35.0-38.8)
Cardiac frequency beats·min^{-1}	85 (60-115)	90 (50-105)	85 (80-110)
TNF-α, pg·mL^{-1}	22 (10-47)	25 (14-44)	23.5 (0-48)
IL-1β, pg·mL^{-1}	0 (0-13)	2 (0-31)	4 (0-43)
IL-6, pg·mL^{-1}	78 (9-1424)	53 (16-1487)	43 (11-596)

Data are represented as median (range).
*Microbiological results were not available in 2 of 20 (10%) patients with pneumonia. No significant differences were observed for the comparison between time points or between patients with and without recovery of a PPM.
Abbreviations: TNF-α, Tumor necrosis factor-α; *IL*, interleukin.
(Courtesy of Bauer TT, Arosio C, Montón C, et al: Systemic inflammatory response after bronchoalveolar lavage in critically ill patients. *Eur Respir J* 17:274-280, 2001.)

levels at 24 hours (pneumonia, 194 [92-312], *P* = .991; controls, 309 [173-487], *P* = .785). There were no other changes in clinical variables. The systemic TNF-α levels before BAL (pneumonia, 35 [10-88] pg·mL^{-1}; controls, 17 [0-33] pg·mL^{-1}) did not increase at 12 hours (pneumonia, 35 [0-64] pg·mL^{-1}, *P* = .735; controls, 16 [0-21] pg·mL^{-1}, *P* = .123 comparison with baseline) or at 24 hours (pneumonia, 31 [0-36] pg·mL^{-1}, *P* = .464; controls, 19 (0-43) pg·mL^{-1}, *P* = .358). No changes were observed in IL-1β (baseline: pneumonia, 0 [0-13] pg·mL^{-1}; controls, 1 [0-32] pg·mL^{-1}) or IL-6 levels (baseline: pneumonia, 226 [9-4300] pg·mL^{-1}; controls, 53 [0-346] pg·mL^{-1}) (Table 3).

Conclusion.—No deterioration of clinical variables and no increase in systemic cytokine release were seen after BAL in critically ill patients. The potential cytokine release may be too insignificant in relation to the pre-existing inflammatory response, to produce clinically significant findings. Antibiotic treatment may have been a major confounding factor.

▶ Approximately 30% of patients in the ICU show signs and symptoms of systemic inflammatory response syndrome after bronchoscopic procedures. Severe consequences are rare, nevertheless, the causation is important. This study demonstrated reductions in the PaO$_2$/FIO$_2$ ratio in both groups, but to a greater degree in the patients with preexisting pneumonia. This ratio was lowest at 12 hours and increased to baseline measurements by 24 hours. No measurable changes in cytokines were noted, but this was probably because concentrations were so significantly increased to start with. Patients undergoing elective outpatient bronchoscopy have demonstrated increases in cytokines, such TNF-α. Certain limitations of the study were obvious. Nearly all patients received antibiotics, and certain patients received corticosteroids as well, thus potentially blunting the inflammatory response and eliminating the potential to culture organisms. But this does reflect the real world. The take-home message is that patients do not seem to have untoward consequences from either hypoxemia or inflammation resulting from BAL.

J. D. Lang, Jr, MD

Alveolar Fluid Clearance Is Impaired in the Majority of Patients With Acute Lung Injury and the Acute Respiratory Distress Syndrome
Ware LB, Matthay MA (Univ of California, San Francisco)
Am J Respir Crit Care Med 163:1376-1383, 2001   8–12

Introduction.—Experimental trials have demonstrated that intact alveolar epithelial fluid transport function is important for resolution of pulmonary edema and acute lung injury (ALI). Alveolar fluid clearance has never been systematically characterized in a large series of patients with ALI or acute respiratory distress syndrome (ARDS) and was thus examined in 79 patients with ALI or ARDS.

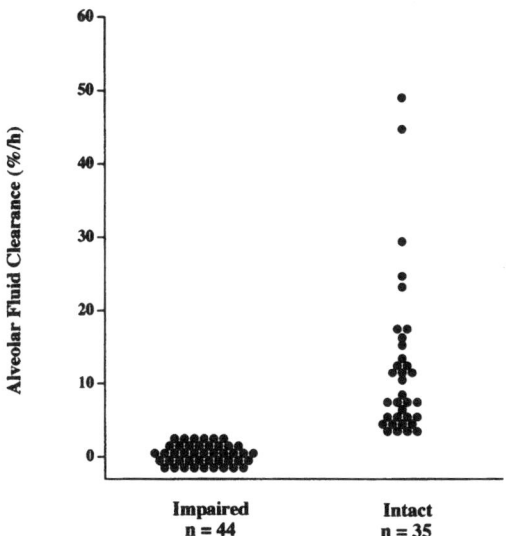

FIGURE 1.—Plot of rate of alveolar fluid clearance in 79 patients with acute lung injury or the acute respiratory distress syndrome, showing that the majority of patients had impaired alveolar fluid clearance. Alveolar fluid clearance was measured from serial protein concentrations in the pulmonary edema fluid samples obtained from 79 patients. Intact clearance was defined as ≥3%/h and impaired clearance as <3%/h. Each symbol (*solid circle*) represents the rate of alveolar fluid clearance in a single patient. n = number of subjects. (Courtesy of Ware LB, Matthay MA: Alveolar fluid clearance is impaired in the majority of patients with acute lung injury and the acute respiratory distress syndrome. *Am J Respir Crit Care Med* 163:1376-1383, 2001. Official Journal of the American Thoracic Society. Copyright American Lung Association.)

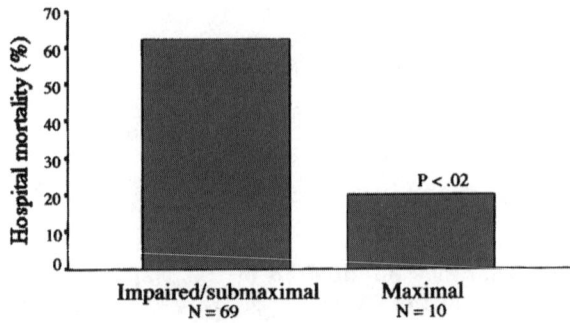

Alveolar Fluid Clearance

FIGURE 3.—Plot of hospital mortality of two groups of patients with acute lung injury or the acute respiratory distress syndrome; those with maximal alveolar fluid clearance (≥14%/h) and those with impaired or submaximal alveolar fluid clearance (<14%/h). Columns represent percent hospital mortality in each group. Hospital mortality of patients with maximal alveolar fluid clearance was significantly less (P < .02). N = number of patients. (Courtesy of Ware LB, Matthay MA: Alveolar fluid clearance is impaired in the majority of patients with acute lung injury and the acute respiratory distress syndrome. *Am J Respir Crit Care Med* 163:1376-1383, 2001. Official Journal of the American Thoracic Society. Copyright American Lung Association.)

Methods.—Pulmonary edema fluid and plasma were sampled serially during the first 4 hours after intubation. The net alveolar fluid clearance was determined from sequential edema fluid protein measurements.

Results.—The mean alveolar fluid clearance was 6% per hour. Of 79 patients, 56% had impaired alveolar fluid clearance (<3%/h), 32% had submaximal clearance (≥3%/h, <14%/h), and 13% had maximal clearance (≥14%/h) (Fig 1). These findings are in contrast to a recent report by these same investigators of 65 patients with hydrostatic pulmonary edema, in whom the mean alveolar fluid clearance was 13% per hour; only 25% had impaired clearance, and 75% had submaximal or maximal clearance. Patients with ALI who had maximal alveolar fluid clearance were more likely to be female (P = .03) and less likely to have sepsis (P = .01). Endogenous and exogenous catecholamines were not correlated with alveolar fluid clearance. Patients with maximal alveolar fluid clearance had significantly lower mortality (Fig 3) and a shorter period of mechanical ventilation.

Conclusion.—Unlike patients with hydrostatic pulmonary edema, alveolar fluid clearance in most patients with ALI and ARDS is impaired. Maximal alveolar fluid clearance is correlated with better clinical outcomes.

▶ Elucidated mechanisms to aid in the resolution of inflammatory-mediated lung injury are lacking. This study builds on the experimental data and characterizes what occurs in the adult patient population with ARDS (permeability pulmonary edema) and nicely contrasts that with patients who have cardiogenic pulmonary edema (hydrostatic pulmonary edema). For alveolar fluid clearance (AFC) to be maximal, an intact alveolar epithelial membrane must be present. Thus, one might reason that more alveolar injury was present in the patients with submaximal/impaired AFC. In the baseline comparison of these patients, there was a trend (but not statistically significant) for patients with maximal AFC ($\geq 14\%/h$) to have a slightly lower lung injury score, a smaller alveolar-arterial gradient, and a higher PaO_2/FIO_2 ratio. Also, sepsis as the cause of ARDS was much lower in these patients. Lastly, gender differences were significant in discriminating between maximal and submaximal/impaired AFC, with females having a predisposition for maximal AFC. Are females less prone to injury? Do females have superior compensatory and repair mechanisms? Is the number of subjects just too small and is this observation insignificant? Only future evaluation will tell. In addition, resolution of pulmonary edema occurs predominantly by vectorial Na^+ transport. Na^+ is transported across the alveolar epithelium mostly via the apical amiloride-sensitive sodium channels and the basolaterally located Na,K-ATPases. Upregulation of these increases active transport of Na^+ and hastens edema resolution. β-Adrenergic and dopaminergic agonism has been demonstrated to increase AFC further.[1] However, in this particular study that was not observed. I hope this study will stimulate other investigators to pursue additional lines of study to this intriguing observation.

J. D. Lang, Jr, MD

References

1. Sznajder JI: Strategies to increase alveolar epithelial fluid removal in the injured lung. *Am J Resp Crit Care Med* 160:1441-1442, 1999.

Mechanistic Scheme and Effect of "Extended Sigh" as a Recruitment Maneuver in Patients With Acute Respiratory Distress Syndrome: A Preliminary Study
Lim C-M, Koh Y, Park W, et al (Univ of Ulsan, Seoul, Korea)
Crit Care Med 29:1255-1260, 2001   8–13

Introduction.—Both experimental and human investigations show that opening of a degassed lung unit depends on the inflating pressure and on the time of pressure sustained, the so-called inflating pressure–time product (pressure $\times$ time). For a recruitment maneuver to be effective in a lung of a patient with acute respiratory distress syndrome (ARDS), it is likely that this physical term needs to be incorporated. A new form of sigh, an extended sigh (ES), was designed to achieve adequate pressure $\times$ time, yet prevent excessive airway pressure in the lung with ARDS. The ES was evaluated in 20 consecutive patients with ARDS as a recruitment maneuver in a prospective, uncontrolled clinical trial.

Methods.—The mean age of 18 males and 2 females was 59 years. After baseline settings of tidal volume (VT) of 8 mL/kg and positive end-expiratory pressure (PEEP) of 10 cm H_2O on volume control mode with the high pressure limit at 40 cm H_2O, the VT-PEEP values were changed to 6-15, 4-20, and 2-25; each step was 30 seconds (inflation phase). After

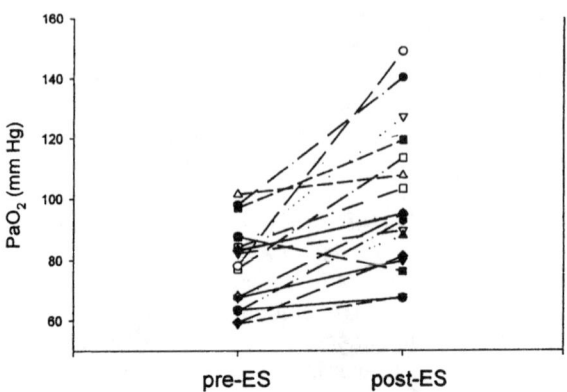

FIGURE 3.—Individual Pao$_2$ levels before (*pre-ES*) and after recruitment by extended sigh (*post-ES*). *Note: P < .001* compared with pre-ES. (Courtesy of Lim C-M, Koh Y, Park W, et al: Mechanistic scheme and effect of "extended sigh" as a recruitment maneuver in patients with acute respiratory distress syndrome: A preliminary study. *Crit Care Med* 29:1255-1260, 2001.)

VT-PEEP 2-25, the mode was changed to continuous positive airway pressure of 30 cm H$_2$O for 30 seconds (pause). The baseline setting was resumed after the reverse sequence of inflation (deflation phase). This ES was done twice with 1 minute of baseline ventilation between. The airway pressures and hemodynamic parameters were tracked during the ES. Arterial blood gases and physiologic parameters were ascertained before ES (pre-ES), at 5 minutes after 2 ES (post-ES), then every 15 minutes for 1 hour. It was estimated that the recruiting pressure × time of the inflation phase was 32.8 to 35.4 cm H$_2$O × 90 seconds.

Results.—Compared with the inflation phase, the inspiratory pause pressure of the deflation phase was lower at VT-PEEP 6-15 (mean, 28.9 cm H$_2$O vs 27.3 cm H$_2$O) and 4-20 (mean, 31.8 cm H$_2$O vs 31.1 cm H$_2$O; both P < .05). Compared with pre-ES, Pao$_2$ (mean, 81.5 mm Hg vs 104.8 mm Hg; P < .001) (Fig 3) and static respiratory compliance both rose post-ES

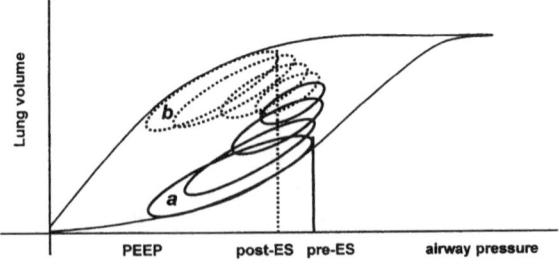

FIGURE 4.—A suggested effect of extended sigh (*ES*). A gradual inflation on a stepwise increase in end-expiratory pressure "recruits and splints" lung units that have a high opening and closing pressure (*solid loops*). With the resumption of baseline ventilation (*dashed loops*), the tidal pressure-volume loop may have been transferred from the initial position (*a*) toward the deflation limb (*b*). *Abbreviation: PEEP*, Positive end-expiratory pressure. (Courtesy of Lim C-M, Koh Y, Park W, et al: Mechanistic scheme and effect of "extended sigh" as a recruitment maneuver in patients with acute respiratory distress syndrome: A preliminary study. *Crit Care Med* 29:1255-1260, 2001.)

(mean, 27.9 mL/cm H_2O vs 30.2 mL/cm H_2O; $P = .009$). Improvement in these parameters was sustained, and major hemodynamic or respiratory complications were not observed throughout the evaluation period.

Conclusion.—A new form of sigh (ES) was presented that is able to achieve an augmented recruitment pressure × time by using a prolonged inflation on a gradually increased end-expiratory pressure (Fig 4). The ES may be a useful recruitment maneuver for patients with ARDS because of its sustained effect and absence of major complications.

▶ An interesting study emphasizing alveolar recruitment on the expiratory limb of the volume-pressure curve. No doubt most strategies or modes of ventilation have targeted as one of their objectives, improvements in oxygenation. That should not be discouraged, but one fascinating aspect of the recently published NIH ARDS Network trial was that the PaO_2/FIO_2 ratio was not different between the low and traditional tidal volume groups, yet a significant decrease in mortality was observed in the low tidal volume group. Although the ES does not allow the pressure × time product to go significantly above 35 cm H_2O pressure, the net effect of "ventilator-induced lung injury" or "biotrauma" was not tested. Positive effects on oxygenation may be short-lived, even overridden by excessive lung injury initiated by such a strategy. A way to enhance the relevance of the study would be to add other measurements such as alveolar fluid flux, bronchoalveolar lavage protein, several pro- and anti-inflammatory cytokines, and a transcriptional regulating protein such as NF-κB as a beginning.

J. D. Lang, Jr, MD

Predictors of Successful Extubation in Neurosurgical Patients
Namen AM, Ely EW, Tatter SB, et al (Wake Forest Univ, Winston-Salem, NC; Vanderbilt Univ, Nashville, Tenn; Johns Hopkins Univ, Baltimore, Md)
Am J Respir Crit Care Med 163:658-664, 2001   8–14

Introduction.—The ability to recognize a patient's readiness to wean and eventually become extubated successfully has been a priority since the introduction of mechanical ventilation. A respiratory care practitioner (RCP)-driven weaning protocol incorporating daily screens, spontaneous breathing trials (SBTs), and prompts to caregivers has been correlated with superior outcomes in patients receiving mechanical ventilation. The effectiveness of this approach was examined in 100 neurosurgical patients during a 14-month evaluation period in a randomized, controlled trial.

Methods.—All patients underwent daily screens of weaning parameters. Patients in the RCP intervention group who passed the screens underwent a 2-hour SBT. The decision to extubate was made by the primary neurosurgical team.

Results.—Forty-nine patients in the intervention group and 51 patients in the control group had similar demographic characteristics, illness severity, and neurologic injury. Forty-five patients in the control group and

42 patients in the intervention group passed at least one daily screen. Forty patients (82%) in the RCP passed SBTs; however, a median of 2 days passed before extubation was attempted, usually because of concerns about the patient's sensorium. Of 167 successful SBTs, extubation was not tried in 126 (75%) on the same day. The median time for mechanical ventilation was 6 days for both groups. Groups did not differ in outcome. Death, reintubation, and pneumonia occurred in 36%, 16%, and 9% of patients, respectively. Twenty-nine percent of patients required tracheostomies. Multivariate analysis revealed that Glasgow Coma Scale (GCS) score ($P < .0001$) and the ratio of partial pressure of arterial oxygen to fraction of inspired oxygen ($P < .0001$) were correlated with extubation success. The odds of successful extubation rose by 39% with each GCS score increment. A GCS score of 8 or higher at extubation was correlated with success in 85% of patients, compared with 33% for a GCS score below 8 ($P < .0001$).

Conclusion.—Implementation of a weaning protocol based on traditional respiratory physiologic parameters has practical limitations in neurosurgical patients because of concerns about neurologic impairment. Whether protocols combining respiratory parameters with neurologic measures lead to superior outcomes in neurosurgical patients requires further evaluation.

▶ This group of investigators has vast experience in the area of weaning, and the question of whether neurologic status is a valuable predictor of extubation success is very worthy of study. Intuitively, one would believe yes. Reasons generally articulated are airway protection and the ability of the patient to actively participate in pulmonary therapy. Interestingly, in this study, when patients passed daily respiratory screens followed by 2-hour SBTs, only 25% of the time did the neurosurgeon extubate the patient. This led to an extubation delay in the majority of patients. A GCS of at least 8 at the time of extubation was associated with a successful extubation in 75% of cases versus 36% when the GCS was 7 or less. This result contrasts with a previous study in which 80% of patients with a GCS of 8 or greater were successfully extubated.[1] An additional study arm that would have allowed for immediate extubation in patients meeting the daily respiratory screen and SBT criteria would have been ideal. Then a comparison between that arm, the neurosurgeon delay arm, and the control arm could have been interesting. The 2-day delay caused by the neurosurgeon could have resulted in increased rates of ventilator-associated pneumonia and other complications associated with prolonged ventilator days. In this study, there was a trend towards increased ICU and total hospital costs in the protocol group versus the control group. However, the point was proved that a protocol used for patients with predominantly cardiopulmonary ailments does not fare well in a more specialized critical care setting.

J. D. Lang, Jr, MD

Reference

1. Coplin W, Pierson D, Cooley K, et al: Implications of extubation delay in brain-injured patients meeting standard weaning criteria. *Am J Respir Crit Care Med* 161:1530-1536, 2000.

Right Heart Catheterization and Cardiac Complications in Patients Undergoing Noncardiac Surgery: An Observational Study
Polanczyk CA, Rohde LE, Goldman L, et al (Harvard Med School, Boston; Univ of California, San Francisco; Univ of California, Los Angeles)
JAMA 286:309-314, 2001   8–15

Background.—For patients who are undergoing elective noncardiac surgery, cardiac complications are the most common cause of death. Research has demonstrated that intraoperative hemodynamic changes are associated with increased complication rates, and this finding has led clinicians to consider right heart catheterization (RHC) for hemodynamic monitoring in selected patients who are undergoing high-risk procedures. However, the benefits of this strategy have not been conclusively demonstrated. The relationship between the use of perioperative RHC and postoperative cardiac complication rates was evaluated in patients who underwent major noncardiac surgery.

Methods.—A prospective observational cohort study was conducted at a tertiary care teaching hospital. The study group was composed of 4059 patients aged 50 years or older who underwent major elective noncardiac procedures with an expected length of hospitalization of 2 days or more. RHC was performed on 221 patients, and 3838 patients did not undergo RHC. The primary outcome measure was the combined end point of major postoperative cardiac events, including unstable angina, ventricular fibrillation, myocardial infarction, cardiogenic pulmonary edema, documented ventricular tachycardia or primary cardiac arrest, and sustained complete heart block.

Results.—There were major cardiac events in 172 patients (4.2%). A 3-fold increase in the incidence of major cardiac events was noted in patients who underwent perioperative RHC. Multivariate analyses resulted in adjusted odds ratios of 2.0 and 2.1 for postoperative major cardiac and noncardiac events, respectively, in patients who underwent RHC. A case-control analysis of 215 matched pairs of patients who did and did not undergo RHC indicated that patients who underwent perioperative RHC were also at increased risk of postoperative heart failure and major noncardiac events.

Conclusions.—There was no evidence of a reduction in complication rates associated with the use of this procedure. The effects of perioperative

RHC should be evaluated in randomized trials because of the morbidity and high costs associated with this intervention.

▶ Seems like another attempt to assassinate the pulmonary artery catheter with sophisticated statistical techniques and lack of a level 1 design. The patients receiving a pulmonary artery catheter in this study were deemed "sicker" or more at risk. Thus, the increases in some postoperative complications may have justified the use of RHC. These patients were simply more at risk in preoperative judgment, of their physicians and thus use of the pulmonary artery catheter may have prevented more adverse outcomes. The definitive answer of pulmonary artery catheter changing outcomes will be very difficult to quell. Has any monitor ever been held to the standard of benefiting outcomes? Even if disparaging evidence is demonstrated, a study powered to take into consideration variables such as differences in surgeons' skills, differences in surgical approach and technique, pulmonary artery catheter operator and interpreter differences, length of case, and type of anesthestic probably cannot be overcome. On more than 1 occasion, the use of the pulmonary artery catheter has been shown to change the therapeutic decisions made after it was placed, and in 1 case it improved survivabilty in the cohort that underwent the change. Evidence is beneficial; however, it is currently lacking in the ultimate form, and most intensivists who truly understand the pitfalls and utility of this catheter have a very strong conviction about its application to their patients. Until other affordable and easily applied and interpretable technologies (echocardiography) are available, the use of the pulmonary artery catheter will continue, as it should for selected patients chosen by experienced practitioners of critical care.

J. D. Lang, Jr, MD

Long-term Infusion of Atrial Natriuretic Peptide (ANP) Improves Renal Blood Flow and Glomerular Filtration Rate in Clinical Acute Renal Failure
Swärd K, Valson F, Ricksten S-E (Sahlgrenska Univ, Göteborg, Sweden)
Acta Anaesthesiol Scand 45:536-542, 2001   8–16

Background.—In patients with acute renal dysfunction, short-term infusion of atrial natriuretic peptide (ANP) enhances renal blood flow (RBF) and glomerular filtration rate (GFR). The effects of long-term ANP infusion on RBF and GFR in patients with acute renal impairment needing pharmacologic circulatory support after cardiac surgery were investigated.

Methods.—Eleven patients were enrolled in the study. Long-term infusion was defined as infusion for more than 48 hours. Urinary clearance of chromium-ethylene diamine tetra-acetic acid (Cr-EDTA) and para-aminohippuric acid(PAH) and central hemodynamic measurements were obtained for 2 to 3 consecutive 30-minute periods during infusion, 1 hour after ANP cessation, and immediately after ANP infusion was reinstituted.

Findings.—During ANP infusion, mean urine flow (UF) was 6.4 mL · min⁻¹; GFR, 19.9 mL · min⁻¹; RBF, 408 mL · min⁻¹; and renal vascular resistance (RVR), 0.286 mm Hg · min · mL⁻¹. When ANP infusion was stopped, UF, GFR, and RBF declined significantly by 28%, 32%, and 31%, respectively. RVR increased by 93%, and the filtration fraction was unchanged. After ANP infusion was begun again, all renal variables returned to baseline. The number of ANP treatment days was not significantly associated with the percentage decline in GFR or RBF during ANP withdrawal. Withdrawal of ANP did not affect central hemodynamic factors.

Conclusions.—In patients with acute renal impairment, ANP infusion improves RBF and GFR after cardiac surgery. The renal vasodilatory effect is maintained during long-term infusion and appears to be safe hemodynamically.

▶ ANP is an agent of significant appeal for patients at risk of renal failure. At the study doses of 50 ng/kg/min, it improved renal hemodynamics and did not detrimentally affect global hemodynamics. In addition, there is emerging evidence that ANP also attenuates inflammation-mediated injury, perhaps in scenarios such as postcardiopulmonary bypass or in patients with sepsis. I think the study demonstrates strong potential, but ANP must be subjected to the scrutiny of a randomized, controlled, double-blinded study before it can be implemented routinely for this particular patient population. There is an ongoing study assessing the hemodynamic/anti-inflammatory effect of ANP in patients with adult respiratory distress syndrome as well (sponsored by Suntory Pharmaceuticals, Inc.). Currently, routine use of the promising agent is cost prohibitive.

J. D. Lang, Jr, MD

Effects of Prophylactic Fenoldopam Infusion on Renal Blood Flow and Renal Tubular Function During Acute Hypovolemia in Anesthetized Dogs
Halpenny M, Markos F, Snow HM, et al (Univ College Cork, Wilton, Ireland; St James's Hosp, Dublin)
Crit Care Med 29:855-860, 2001   8–17

Introduction.—Fenoldopam mesylate is a selective dopamine agonist that may preserve renal function and reduce tubular oxygen consumption during states of hypoperfusion, including hypovolemic shock. The effects of fenoldopam (0.1 µg·kg⁻¹·min⁻¹) on renal blood flow, urine output, creatinine clearance, and sodium clearance in pentobarbital-anesthetized canines that had undergone partial exsanguination to acutely reduce cardiac output were examined in a prospective, randomized, controlled experiment.

Methods.—Eight female beagle dogs underwent measurements of arterial blood pressure, heart rate, cardiac output, renal blood flow, urine

TABLE 1.—Heart Rate, Mean Arterial Blood Pressure (*MAP*), Cardiac Index (*CI*), Total Peripheral Vascular Resistance (*TPR*), Urine Output, Plasma Creatinine Concentration (*Creat*), Creatinine Clearance (*CrCl*), Renal Blood Flow (*RBF*), Fractional Excretion of Sodium (*FENa*), Lithium Clearance (*LiCl*), Plasma Osmolality (*P Osmo*), Urine Osmolality (*U Osmo*), Arterial pH, Renal Vascular Resistance (*RVR*), and Filtration Fraction (*FF*) During Four Time Periods of the Experiment

	Group	Control Period (60 Mins)	Infusion Period (60 Mins)	Hypovolemia Period (90 Mins)	Transfusion Period (60 Mins)
Heart rate, beats/min	Fenoldopam (n = 4)	156 ± 14	160 ± 13	180 ± 9*	157 ± 10
	Placebo (n = 4)	150 ± 35	157 ± 26	175 ± 15	160 ± 4
MAP, mm Hg	Fenoldopam (n = 4)	113 ± 9	108 ± 9	90 ± 10*	105 ± 7
	Placebo (n = 4)	108 ± 6	103 ± 5	89 ± 11*	101 ± 5
CI, ml·min^{-1}·kg^{-1}	Fenoldopam (n = 4)	113 ± 17	105 ± 13	57 ± 5*	98 ± 9
	Placebo (n = 4)	110 ± 14	109 ± 15	63 ± 8*	94 ± 12
SVR, dynes/cm^{-5}	Fenoldopam (n = 4)	7469 ± 835	7608 ± 549	11743 ± 1460*	7949 ± 448
	Placebo (n = 4)	7806 ± 632	7558 ± 972	11192 ± 572*	8477 ± 1168
RVR, mm Hg·mL^{-1}·min^{-1}	Fenoldopam (n = 4)	1.5 ± 0.2	1.3 ± 0.2	1.3 ± 0.2	1.9 ± 0.7
	Placebo (n = 4)	1.6 ± 0.5	1.6 ± 0.3	1.9 ± 0.4	2.1 ± 0.6
Urine output, mL/min	Fenoldopam (n = 4)	0.3 ± 0.19	0.34 ± 0.27	0.14 ± 0.05	0.36 ± 0.24
	Placebo (n = 4)	0.26 ± 0.15	0.18 ± 0.08	0.08 ± 0.05*	0.25 ± 0.07
Creatinine, μmol/L	Fenoldopam (n = 4)	48 ± 5.1	45 ± 4.8	43 ± 8.0	46 ± 7.9
	Placebo (n = 4)	53 ± 4.4	51 ± 3.1	52 ± 6.0	53 ± 6.1

CrCl mL·min⁻¹·kg⁻¹	Fenoldopam (n = 4)	3.0 ± 1.0	3.9 ± 0.6	2.9 ± 0.5	3.9 ± 0.8
	Placebo (n = 4)	3.0 ± 0.4	2.9 ± 0.4	1.8 ± 0.8*	2.9 ± 0.8
RBF, mL/min⁻¹	Fenoldopam (n = 4)	75 ± 14	90 ± 18	73 ± 17	63 ± 24
	Placebo (n = 4)	72 ± 20	67 ± 11	47 ± 6*	52 ± 12†
FENa, %	Fenoldopam (n = 4)	1.9 ± 1.1	1.3 ± 0.9	1.7 ± 2.7	0.7 ± 0.4
	Placebo (n = 4)	1.7 ± 0.9	1.4 ± 0.65	0.4 ± 0.2*	0.6 ± 0.2†
LiCl mL·min⁻¹·kg⁻¹	Fenoldopam (n = 4)	1.1 ± 0.9	1.7 ± 1.1	0.7 ± 0.5	1.2 ± 0.8
	Placebo (n = 4)	1.3 ± 0.5	1.3 ± 0.6	0.6 ± 0.5*	1.2 ± 0.6
P Osmo, mOsm⁻¹	Fenoldopam (n = 4)	309 ± 7	307 ± 8	308 ± 7	308 ± 7
	Placebo (n = 4)	306 ± 4	306 ± 5	304 ± 7	306 ± 6
U Osmo, mOsm⁻¹	Fenoldopam (n = 4)	1125 ± 342	1262 ± 309	1209 ± 197	1006 ± 190
	Placebo (n = 4)	1123 ± 322	1244 ± 338	1219 ± 303	865 ± 62
Arterial pH	Fenoldopam (n = 4)	7.4 ± 0.04	7.4 ± 0.03	7.4 ± 0.03	7.4 ± 0.04
	Placebo (n = 4)	7.4 ± 0.05	7.4 ± 0.06	7.4 ± 0.05	7.4 ± 0.03
FF	Fenoldopam (n = 4)	0.45 ± 0.1	0.5 ± 0.1	0.5 ± 0.2	0.8 ± 0.4
	Placebo (n = 4)	0.45 ± 0.1	0.4 ± 0.1	0.4 ± 0.1	0.6 ± 0.1

Data are mean ± SD.
*P < .01 compared with control period.
†P < .05 compared with control period.
(Courtesy of Halpenny M, Markos F, Snow HM, et al: Effects of prophylactic fenoldopam infusion on renal blood flow and renal tubular function during acute hypovolemia in anesthetized dogs. *Crit Care Med* 29:855-860, 2001.)

output, creatinine clearance, and fractional excretion of sodium at 4 different time points: (1) before infusion of fenoldopam or normal saline; (2) during infusion of fenoldopam or normal saline (1 hour); (3) during a 90-minute period of hypovolemia (induced by acute partial exsanguination), with current infusion of fenoldopam or normal saline; and (4) during a 1-hour period after retransfusing the dogs.

Results.—Administration of fenoldopam was not correlated with hemodynamic instability. Renal blood flow and urine output dropped significantly from baseline ($P < .01$) during the hypovolemic period in the placebo group (mean, 72 to 47 mL/min and 0.26 to 0.08 mL/min, respectively) but not in the fenoldopam group (mean, 75 to 73 mL/min and 0.3 to 0.14 mL/min, respectively). Creatinine clearance and fractional excretion of sodium dropped significantly from baseline ($P < .01$) in the placebo group during the hypovolemic period (mean, 3.0 to 1.8 mL·kg^{-1}·min^{-1} and 1.7% to 0.4%, respectively); this did not occur in animals that received fenoldopam (mean, 3.0 to 2.9 mL·kg^{-1}·min^{-1} and 1.9% to 1.7%, respectively) (Table 1).

Conclusion.—Fenoldopam eradicated the tubular prerenal response to profound hypovolemia and maintained renal blood flow, glomerular filtration rate, and natriuresis without causing hypotension. This indicates that fenoldopam may have a renoprotective effect in acute ischemic injury.

▶ An agent with pharmacodynamic purity; other animal trials and a few human trials have at least indirectly supported these findings as well. We have a positive anectodel experience of our own in patients with hepatorenal syndrome before liver transplantation. Other applications include attenuating mesenteric ischemia (that is early unpublished data from our laboratory) and augmenting alveolar fluid clearance in the injured lung. Currently, it is approved for hypertensive urgency, and hospital pharmacy and therapeutics committees monitor its use pretty closely because of the costs. I expect future evidence to shine a positive light on fenoldopam, and that it will supplant ineffective agents such as dopamine.

J. D. Lang, Jr, MD

Impact of a Rotating Empiric Antibiotic Schedule on Infectious Mortality in an Intensive Care Unit
Raymond DP, Pelletier SJ, Crabtree TD, et al (Univ of Virginia, Charlottesville)
Crit Care Med 29:1101-1108, 2001   8–18

Background.—In critically ill patients, the development of antibiotic-resistant bacteria leads to significant morbidity and death. Quarterly rotation of empirical antibiotics may reduce infectious complications from resistant organisms in the ICU.

Methods.—Data on 540 epidsodes of infection occurring in an ICU during 2 years were obtained prospectively. The study period included 1 year of nonprotocol-driven antibiotic use and 1 year of rotating empirical antibiotics. More than 100 variables were recorded for each infectious episode, including patient, infection, treatment, and outcome characteristics.

Findings.—Between the 2 study years, there were no differences in age, APACHE II score, race, overall antibiotic use, or treatment duration. During the year of rotation, significant reductions were noted in the incidence of antibiotic-resistant gram-positive coccal infections, antibiotic-resistant gram-negative bacillary infections, and deaths associated with infection. In a logistic regression analysis, variables independently predicting death included age, APACHE II score, solid organ transplantation, and malignant disease. Antibiotic rotation independently predicted survival.

Conclusions.—Implementation of a quarterly, empirical antibiotic rotation schedule in an ICU is feasible and effective in reducing the incidence of infection, antibiotic-resistant organism infection, and death due to infection. This practice does not increase the cost of antibiotic treatment. Further research is warranted.

▶ A superb study reinforcing the concept of "rotating" antibiotic regimens to inhibit microbial resistance. Quarterly rotation of antibiotic therapy reduced a number of key outcomes, including number of infections per 100 admissions. Both crude mortality and attributable mortality rates were decreased in the rotating group. It is important that the percentages of infections caused by resistant bacteria (both gram-negative rods and gram-positive cocci) were significantly decreased. There were no demonstrable increases in side effects from rotating antibiotics. Also, in the rotating group there was a trend toward a reduction in antibiotic costs per patient. Protocol violations were insignificant. Limitations included the evolution of additional infection control measures during the study period, which included antibiotic substitutions, the distribution of alcohol handwash dispensers, and the initiation of an antibiotic surveillance program.

J. D. Lang, Jr, MD

Assessment of Two Hand Hygiene Regimens for Intensive Care Unit Personnel
Larson EL, Aiello AE, Bastyr J, et al (Columbia Univ, New York; 3M Health Care, St Paul, Minn; Columbia Presbyterian Med Ctr, New York)
Crit Care Med 29:944-951, 2001 8–19

Background.—Hand hygiene can significantly reduce the transmission of potentially infectious agents, but health care personnel must practice it consistently and effectively. Skin damage and dermatologic problems may also occur among personnel who practice hand hygiene too vigorously. A balance must be maintained between maximizing antimicrobial effectiveness and minimizing changes in skin health and microflora that could lead to nosocomial infection. Two hand-care regimens were compared for

TABLE 4.—Microbial Counts on Hands of Participants ($\log_{10}$ CFU)

A. Differences Between ALC and CHG Groups

Time Interval	ALC Group (+/− SE)	CHG Group (+/− SE)	p Value
Baseline	5.03 (0.15)	4.41 (0.19)	0.02
Mid-day 1	4.64 (0.17)	4.47 (0.17)	0.56*
Wk 2	4.59 (0.19)	4.50 (0.16)	0.20*
Wk 4	4.72 (0.19)	4.64 (0.17)	0.40*

B. Differences Between Baseline and Subsequent Cultures for ALC and CHG Groups

$\log_{10}$ CFU Difference From Baseline

Group	Mid-Day 1	p Value†	Wk 2	p Value†	Wk 4	p Value†
ALC	−0.43 log	0.03	−0.46 log	0.04	−0.31 log	0.18
CHG	+0.07 log	0.69	+0.09 log	0.59	+0.24 log	0.12

*Analysis of covariance.
†Paired t test.
Abbreviations: CFU, colony-forming units.
(Courtesy of Larson EL, Aiello AE, Bastyr J, et al: Assessment of two hand hygiene regimens for intensive care unit personnel. *Crit Care Med* 29:944-951, 2001.)

effectiveness in impact on skin microbiology and skin condition among health care workers in an intensive care environment.

Methods.—All 50 subjects worked full time (more than 30 h/wk), were aged 18 to 65 years, were free of known allergy to the study products, were not using topical or systemic steroids or antibiotics, and had no current dermatologic conditions. Over the course of this 4-week prospective, randomized, clinical trial, all participants' skin condition was assessed; diaries were completed outlining potential confounding effects of gloving and use of lotion, frequency of hand washing and numbers of patient contacts; and hands were sampled for microbiologic status and skin condition. One group used a 2% chlorhexidine gluconate (CHG)-containing traditional antiseptic wash; the other group used a waterless handrub that contained 61% ethanol with emollients (ALC).

Results.—An average of 116.9 hours of time was reported in the hand hygiene diaries, with a mean reported hand washing total for a 12-hour shift being 11.7 and a mean application of ALC of 17.7. The mean number of lotion applications was 5.5 times. An average of 3.96 patients were contacted per shift. On average, 15.7 glovings per shift were reported, with gloves worn an average of 2.6 hours per shift. The number of applications of lotion correlated significantly with the amount of lotion used. The CHG group had significantly more hand washings per shift than the ALC group, per study design. Nurses and other staff put on gloves approximately 3 times as often as physicians did; they also touched patients more often. Physicians and nurses used significantly less lotion than did other staff. The ALC group showed improved skin condition, whereas the CHG group showed worsening at all points except week 2. By the fourth week, the ALC group had significantly better moisture scores than did the CHG group, even though the CHG group applied lotion 50% more often than the ALC group. All participants had coagulase-negative staphylococci isolated from hands; 13 isolates had methicillin-sensitive *Staphylococcus aureus*, and 40 isolates had gram-negative bacteria. Only at baseline did either group have a significantly different colony-forming unit count (Table 4). Significantly less time was required for the ALC regimen than for the CHG process (12.7 seconds vs 21.1 seconds). In addition, the ALC regimen was associated with a 50% reduction in material costs.

Conclusions.—The use of a waterless lotion that contained alcohol and emollient and the use of a detergent-based antiseptic agent were essentially equal in microbiologic effectiveness, but the lotion improved the skin condition of these critical care personnel and required significantly less time to use.

▶ Fundamental infection control measures can easily be undermined if undesirable side effects are encountered. This study demonstrates that being in tune with the latest formulations available for hygiene could pay dividends. We know from previous studies that health care personnel, particularly physicians, are prone to wash their hands less than other personnel and for a shorter duration. Physicians are also more apt not to change their behavior. Although not a conclusion of this study, an inference could be made that early education coupled with hygiene agents that have few side effects could increase compliance, thus contributing to a decrease in nosocomial infections rates. Our ICU currently has available both chlorhexidine and ethanol-based antiseptic washes.

J. D. Lang, Jr, MD

Inhibitory Effects of S-(−) and R-(+) Bupivacaine on Neutrophil Function

Welters ID, Menzebach A, Langefeld TW, et al (Justus-Liebig Universität, Giessen, Germany)
Acta Anaesthesiol Scand 45:570-575, 2001   8–20

Introduction.—Local anesthetics constrain migration, enzyme release, and superoxide anion generation of polymorphonuclear leukocytes. The ability of polymorphonuclear leukocytes to phagocytose and kill bacteria makes them a major defense mechanism in the circulating blood. The influence of racemic bupivacaine and its enantiomers [S-(−) and R-(+)] on neutrophil phagocytic activity, oxidative burst, and surface expression of complement and Fcγ receptors was examined.

Methods.—Venous blood was preincubated with different concentrations of racemic bupivacaine, R-(+) bupivacaine, or S-(−) bupivacaine. Fluoresceine isothiocyanate (FITC)-labeled antibodies against Fcγ receptor 3 (CD11b) were used to ascertain surface receptor expression. Phagocytic activity was determined by ingestion of FITC-labeled vital *Staphylococcus aureus*. Oxidative burst was gauged by conversion of nonfluorescent dihydrorhodamine 123 into fluorescent rhodamine 123. Flow cytometry was used to assess the fluorescent intensity of each sample.

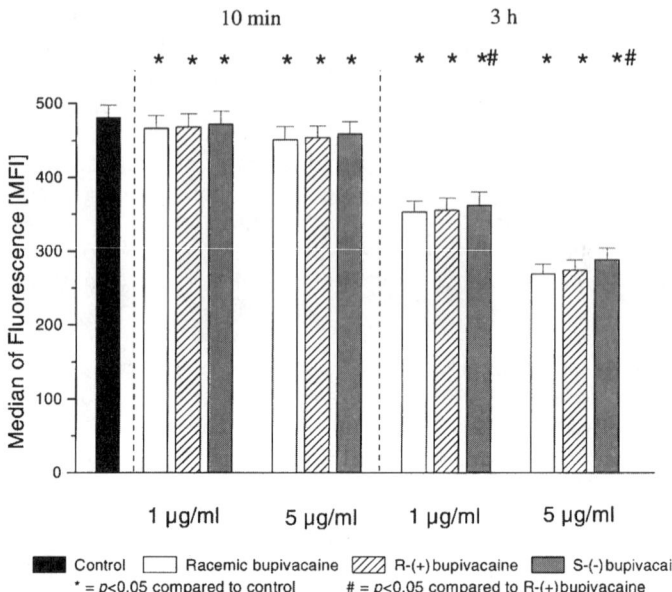

FIGURE 5.—Influence of racemic bupivacaine and bupivacaine enantiomers on neutrophil oxidative burst. Different time intervals and concentrations were tested. Mean and standard deviation of 10 different experiments are shown. (Courtesy of Welters ID, Menzebach A, Langefeld TW, et al: Inhibitory effects of S-(−) and R-(+) bupivacaine on neutrophil function. *Acta Anaesthesiol Scand* 45:570-575, 2001.)

Results.—Racemic bupivacaine restricted surface receptor expression, phagocytosis, and oxidative burst in a time- and concentration-dependent manner (Fig 5). The S-(−) enantiomer applied significantly less inhibitory action on neutrophil function, compared with R-(+) and racemic bupivacaine; these effects were small when compared with overall changes.

Conclusion.—Bupivacaine may inhibit surface receptor expression and thus contribute to decreased phagocyte activity and oxidative burst. The enantiomer-specific effects of bupivacaine may have a small role in the inhibition of these leukocyte functions.

▶ This study provides additional evidence bolstering the positive influences of analgesia on inflammatory processes. Regardless of the enantiomer studied, decreased neutrophil surface receptor expression, phagocytic activity, and neutrophil superoxide radical formation were demonstrated at concentrations routinely achieved with the clinical use of bupivacaine. No, the methodology was not in vivo, but it adds to the accumulating database supporting antinociceptive therapies and their anti-inflammatory effects. To what extent will it contribute to the patient's outcome? At this time that is unquantifiable, but analgesia and inhibition of thrombus formation as demonstrated in other studies, coupled with attenuation of inflammation, are solid reasons to incorporate local anesthetics into a "multimodal" pain management plan for the critically ill patient.

J. D. Lang, Jr, MD

The Effect of Vancomycin and Third-Generation Cephalosporins on Prevalence of Vancomycin-Resistant Enterococci in 126 US Adult Intensive Care Units

Fridkin SK, for the Intensive Care Antimicrobial Resistance Epidemiology (ICARE) Project and the National Nosocomial Infections Surveillance (NNIS) System Hospitals (Natl Ctr for Infectious Diseases, US Ctrs for Disease Control and Prevention, Atlanta, Ga; Emory Univ, Atlanta, Ga)
Ann Intern Med 135:175-183, 2001   8–21

Introduction.—Most hospitals in the United States during the past decade have observed the epidemic rise in vancomycin-resistant enterococci (VRE) isolates from hospitalized patients. Few investigations have reported data on the institutional risk factors of VRE, including rates of antimicrobial use that predict rates of VRE. Determining modifiable institutional factors can be useful in quality improvement efforts to minimize hospital-acquired infections with VRE. Data were used from hospitals participating in the 1996 Project Intensive Care Antimicrobial Resistance Epidemiology (ICARE) to examine the relationship between institutional characteristics (including rates of nosocomial infection or antimicrobial use) and the prevalence of VRE in adult ICUs.

Methods.—All patients admitted to the 126 participating adult ICUs from 60 US hospitals from January 1996 through July 1999 were evaluated in this prospective ecologic investigation. The monthly use of antimicrobial agents (defined as daily doses per 1000 patient-days), nosocomial infection rates, and susceptibilities of all tested enterococci isolated from clinical cultures were recorded.

Results.—The prevalence of VRE (median, 10%; range, 0%-59%) did not vary significantly by type of ICU. The rate of VRE was significantly higher among teaching centers (12.6% vs 5.6% overall) and larger hospitals (those with more than 500 beds 12.5% vs 6.5% for smaller hospitals). The prevalence of VRE was strongly correlated with VRE prevalence among inpatient non-ICU areas ($r = 0.63$; confidence interval [CI], 0.52-0.73) and outpatient areas in the hospital ($r = 0.53$; CI, 0.39-0.66). Ventilator use was weakly correlated with VRE ($r = 0.20$; CI, 0.01-0.38). The rate of VRE in an ICU was significantly associated with ICU-specific use of vancomycin ($r = 0.44$; CI, 0.29-0.57). Rates of other antimicrobial agents were not significantly associated with VRE rates. In a weighted linear regression model controlling for type of ICU and rates of VRE among non-ICU inpatient areas, rates of vancomycin use ($P < .001$) and third-generation cephalosporin use ($P = .02$) were independently correlated with VRE prevalence.

Conclusion.—Higher rates of vancomycin or third-generation cephalosporin use were correlated with an increased prevalence of VRE, independent of other ICU characteristics and the endemic VRE prevalence elsewhere in the hospital. Reducing the rates of use of these antimicrobial agents could decrease the rates of VRE in ICUs.

▶ VRE remains a problem at most institutions. However, we have seen dramatic reductions in isolates both inside and outside our surgical ICU with restrictions on the use of third-generation cephalosporins and on the use of cephalosporins in general. These protocols were initiated after VRE was essentially eradicated in our trauma-burn ICU.[1] Strategies such as more control over vancomycin use, better education of perioperative antibiotic use, improved antimicrobial education for residents (especially for those in anesthesiology), cycling of antibiotics, and basics such as the strict enforcement of hand washing are all essential steps in reducing isolate rates. These strategies coupled with very frequent surveillance of your own ICU and institutional isolates and antibiograms can assist in greatly affecting VRE rates.

J. D. Lang, Jr, MD

Reference

1. May A, Melton S, McGwin G, et al: Reduction of vancomycin-resistant enterococcal infections by limitation of broad-spectrum cephalosporin use in a trauma and burn intensive care unit. *Shock* 14:259-264, 2000.

Motivating Factors in Futile Clinical Interventions
Rivera S, Kim D, Garone S, et al (Cedars-Sinai Med Ctr, Los Angeles)
Chest 119:1944-1947, 2001   8–22

Background.—Remarkable advances in medical technology have made possible the significant prolongation of life. The extension of life by medical intervention may result in meaningful attainment of goals, but there are situations in which these technological interventions will never achieve the patient's desired level of function. Interventions that prolong life despite outcomes that are both ethically and medically unacceptable are considered to be futile and medically inappropriate. Therapies that have even a low probability of clinical benefit or a slight chance of achieving a patient's goal may not be absolutely futile. Serious ethical, medical, and societal dilemmas have resulted from those patients for whom outcomes are such that their hospital stay is lengthened without hope of achieving any realistic goal. Many articles have been written on the subject of futile care, and some have addressed medically inappropriate care, but there has previously been no attempt to rigorously define the persons and factors that lead to these interventions. The parties who are primarily responsible for these interventions and the factors that motivate them were determined. In addition, the role of a timely bioethical consultation in curtailing such interventions was analyzed.

Methods.—In a retrospective review, 100 patients of 331 bioethical consultations were identified who had either futile or medically inappropriate therapy.

Results.—The average patient age was 73.5 ± 32 years, and 57% were men. Fifty-seven percent of the patients had been admitted with a degenerative disorder, 21% had an inflammatory disorder, and 16% had a neoplastic disorder. In 62% of cases, the family was responsible for the futile treatment, and the physician was responsible for futile treatment in 37% of cases. In one case, a conservator was responsible for the futile treatment. In 7 of the 62 cases in which the family was responsible for the futile treatment, family dissent was also involved. However, there was no family dissent in the cases in which the physician was primarily responsible for the futile treatment. In 12 of 37 cases involving physician responsibility, liability issues were a key motivation; however, physician liability was a motivation in only 1 of 62 cases in which the family was responsible for the futile treatment. When therapy was discontinued as a result of the bioethics consultation, patients died in a median of 2 days. When therapy was continued, patients died in a median of 16 days.

Conclusions.—It is believed that these findings are indicative of the benefits of a timely bioethical consultation in the ameliorating of needless patient suffering and in the reduction of unnecessary costs.

▶ A very interesting study addressing futility of care and the potential contributors driving this type of care. The study lacked good design, being retrospective, and subjectively determining what cases were classified as futile care. However, it probably keeps in the ballpark the contributing factors and consequences of futile clinical interventions. Families were the responsible parties in nearly two thirds of the cases. Of interest, was that physicians continued futile in approximately a third of the cases because they feared medicolegal consequences. Ethics consultations allowed resolution in approximately 75% of the physician-driven cases and approximately 50% of the patient family-driven cases. It was calculated that cost savings resulting from the prevention of futile care could approach $11,000 per patient, emphasizing the importance of realizing futile care is being delivered and that using the appropriate resources available to assist in addressing these complicated and emotional issues, such as a bioethics consultation.

J. D. Lang, Jr, MD

Conflict Associated With Decisions to Limit Life-Sustaining Treatment in Intensive Care Units

Breen CM, Abernethy AP, Abbott KH, et al (VA Med Ctr, Durham, NC; Duke Univ, Durham, NC)
J Gen Intern Med 16:283-289, 2001   8–23

Introduction.—Most conflicts associated with end-of-life decision making do not involve the legal system. Little is known about the prevalence

TABLE 2.—Prevalence and Characteristics of Conflict

Code	Cases (%) N = 102
Conflict	80 (78)
No conflict	22 (22)
Participants	
Family-family	24 (24)*
Staff-family	49 (48)*
Staff-staff	49 (48)*
Issue	
Treatment decision	64 (63)*
Other task	46 (45)*
Social	19 (19)*

*Totals more than 78% because more than 1 conflict was possible per case.
(Courtesy of Breen CM, Abernethy AP, Abbott KH, et al: Conflict associated with decisions to limit life-sustaining treatment in intensive care units. *J Gen Intern Med* 16:283-289, 2001. Reprinted by permission of Blackwell Science, Inc.)

of interpersonal conflicts or their causes or effects when patients in the ICU are considered for limitation of life-sustaining treatment. These factors were examined by qualitatively analyzing prospectively gathered data from interviews in 6 ICUs at a university medical center.

Methods.—Semistructured interviews were conducted among 406 physicians and nurses involved in the care of 102 patients. The interviews addressed disagreement during life-sustaining treatment decision making. Two raters coded the transcripts of the interviews, which were audiotaped.

Results.—At least 1 health care provider in 78% of the cases described a situation that was coded as conflict (Table 2). The conflict was between the staff and family members in 48% of the cases, among staff members in 48%, and among family members in 24%. In 63% of the cases, conflict arose over the decision concerning life-sustaining treatment itself. In 45% of the cases, the conflict was over other tasks, including communication and pain control. The conflict concerned social issues in 19% of the cases.

Conclusion.—Conflict is more prevalent in the setting of ICU decision making than previously reported. Treatment decisions may not be the only or even the most important issue causing conflict.

▶ A very revealing study that thoroughly exposes the "real world" dynamic of conflict that exists between patients, family, and staff. Not only was there conflict between the patient or patient's family and the health care delivery team, more profound was the conflict among the health care delivery team members, whether that was between faculty physicians, a faculty physician and a resident physician, or a nurse and a resident. The study findings reemphasize the need for further education at all levels of the health care hierarchy regarding the spectrum of events entailed in the critical care setting (do not resuscitate [DNR], withdrawing or withholding life-sustaining treatments, pain control, and ethics). Conflict arose between primary care physicians and intensivists regarding treatment plans, which is common in "semiopen" critical care units where many physicians are involved in decision making (another legitimate reason for "closed" critical care units). Other issues that commonly surfaced were an inability to discriminate between DNR status and the treatment plan of the patient, and what is deemed as appropriate pain management (not enough vs too much). This is a great study for all to read.

J. D. Lang, Jr, MD

The Impact of Organisational Change on Outcome in an Intensive Care Unit in the United Kingdom
Baldock G, Foley P, Brett S (Hammersmith Hosp, London)
Intensive Care Med 27:865-872, 2001   8–24

Background.—Three factors that have been deemed important in the quality delivery of care for ICUs are the presence of a consultant who has administrative responsibility for the unit, 24-hour availability of an intensive care medicine specialist, and the continuous presence of resident staff on the unit who have few or no commitments elsewhere. In an open ICU environment, either the admitting medical or surgical team, with the ICU consultants in an advisory role, make ongoing management decisions. In a closed ICU, ongoing care is managed by ICU consultants who are in close contact with the admitting team. Variations between these 2 extremes also work. An open ICU that became a closed ICU and sought to detect the impact of organizational changes on patient survival rate was studied.

Methods.—Data were prospectively collected from an ICU in a postgraduate teaching hospital. A total of 476 of 1134 admissions to the ICU had elective surgery. Risk of death was calculated for each admission. Hospital mortality rate corrected for the severity of illness was determined.

Results.—Before becoming a closed unit, the crude hospital mortality rate was 28%. This fell to 20% ($P = .01$). In addition, a reduction of nearly half was noted in probability of death. After making adjustments for other risk factors, risk of death, transfers, and hematologic status all had an impact on mortality rate. The risk of death was increased 5-fold among patients who were referred from another ICU; the risk of death for patients with hematologic disorders was almost 3 times as high as for patients without these disorders.

Conclusions.—The hospital mortality rate fell substantially after changing the ICU organization from open to closed. This is consistent with other studies of closed versus open ICU models.

▶ This is another credible study supporting the concept of a closed ICU. The reduction in mortality rate was statistically significant. All patients benefited except the ICU admissions for care after elective surgery, which had the same mortality rate when compared with previous data. Certainly, one major design flaw was that 2 organizational changes were implemented: more house staff were added and the unit was closed. Other studies have been published, and the data have generally supported the closed concept because of decreased mortality rate, decreased ICU days, decreased ventilator days, or a reduction in resource utilization. The data are accruing; we must embrace the concept. Organizations such as the Leapfrog Group (www.leap-froggroup.org) have made issues such as the staffing of ICUs with critical care trained physicians a central component of their mission to improve patient safety. Although they have made no reference to ICU design, the closed concept offers many more advantages to patients, physicians, and other health care personnel.

J. D. Lang, Jr, MD

Comparison of Premortem Clinical Diagnoses in Critically Ill Patients and Subsequent Autopsy Findings
Roosen J, Frans E, Wilmer A, et al (Univ Hosps Gasthuisberg, Leuven, Belgium)
Mayo Clin Proc 75:562-567, 2000   8–25

Introduction.—Although there is compelling scientific evidence in favor of autopsy, the rate of autopsies in general hospitals and in university hospitals in particular seems to be declining from levels as high as 50% in the 1940s, to 22% to 35% in the 1970s, and to 10% to 25% in the 1980s. One hundred patients who died in a medical ICU of a university hospital were evaluated retrospectively to determine whether the practice of re-questing an autopsy continues to be a valid approach to obtain clinically and educationally relevant information.

Methods.—Medical records were compared for clinical diagnoses and postmortem major diagnoses of 100 patients who died in 1996 (autopsy rate, 93%).

Results.—Of 100 patients evaluated, 40% were female, 98% were medical patients, 14% were immunosuppressed, 40% were admitted from hospital wards, 10% were admitted from critical care units from other hospitals, and 2% were admitted from the operating room. The mean patient age was 63.6 years (range, 17-90 years). The mean Acute Physiology and Chronic Health Evaluation (APACHE) II score was 25, and the average length of stay in the medical ICU was 11.8 days. Clinical diagnoses were confirmed at autopsy in 81% of patients. In 16% of patients, autopsy findings showed a major diagnosis that, if known before death, may have led to a change in therapy and prolonged survival (class I missed major diagnosis). The most common class I missed major diagnoses were fungal infection, cardiac tamponade, abdominal hemorrhage, and myocardial infarction. An additional 10% of autopsies showed a diagnosis that, if known before death, probably would not have resulted in a change in therapy (class II error).

Conclusion.—Autopsy continues to be an important tool for both education and quality control. In the ICU setting, the number of missed major diagnoses continues to be high. There has been a clear shift during the past 20 to 30 years in the types of missed diagnoses. Nosocomial and opportunistic infections are currently the diagnoses most likely to be missed in the ICU. Bedside applicable techniques including ECG recordings with supplemental posterior chest leads, echocardiography, and meticulous abdominal ultrasonography may improve the outcome in selected ICU patients.

▶ No doubt autopsy rates are decreasing. Today's house staff and physicians in general seem more reluctant to inquire or "push" for an autopsy. This study revealed that the rate of class I missed diagnoses can be fairly high (the literature ranges between 10% and 27%). The autopsy can serve multiple purposes including (1) exposing diagnostic weaknesses within a particular unit; (2) lending insight into newly emerging diseases; (3) serving as a great teaching tool; and (4) assisting in providing closure to a patient's family and physicians. This study has reminded me yet again of the importance of an autopsy.

J. D. Lang, Jr, MD

Twenty-four Hour Presence of Physicians in the ICU
Burchardi H, Moerer O (Univ Hosp Göttingen, Germany)
J Crit Care 5:131-137, 2001   8–26

Background.—High-quality, cost-effective intensive care medicine (ICM) is best achieved when the responsibility and management are given to those who have the expertise. The 24-hour presence of physicians in the ICU was discussed.

Discussion.—Increasing evidence shows that the responsible involvement of intensivists results in better patient outcomes and a more efficient use of resources. The team model involves an on-site team of dedicated nurses and physicians who are directly responsible for treatment but who also draw on the expertise of various consultants from different disciplines. This team runs the ICU under the direct supervision of a full-time intensivist who is fully trained in the spectrum of ICM and who is able to handle all emergency procedures. Twenty-four-hour coverage by on-site physicians is necessary. These physicians do not need the same level of specialized expertise as an intensivist as long as an experienced specialist is available on call.

▶ In a comprehensive review of the ICU concept, the authors discuss the differences between the concept in Europe versus the USA. Other aspects discussed are 24-hour coverage, challenges of the future, and the role of telemedicine for the practicing intensivist. A quality review that I recommend to all.

J. D. Lang, Jr, MD

Protocol-Driven Care in the Intensive Care Unit: A Tool for Quality

Wall RJ, Dittus RS, Ely EW (Vanderbilt Univ, Nashville, Tenn)
J Crit Care 5:283-285, 2001   8–27

Background.—Advances in ICU organization and patient management have resulted in decreased morbidity and mortality rates. Protocol-driven care in the ICU was discussed.

Discussion.—Two important advances in ICU management are the use of multidisciplinary teams (MDTs) and the development of clinical protocols. Although some authorities have worried that protocols will replace clinical judgment, many randomized controlled trials have shown that outcomes are improved when such protocols are used in critical care decision making. A well-designed ICU protocol does not restrict clinician decision making but focuses the clinician's attention on the common features of patients with a well-described illness. Protocol-driven care does not remove the need for clinical judgment. Rather, it requires attention to the subtleties of each case and possible deviation from the protocol. Although the use of protocol-driven care and MDTs does not guarantee high-quality care, it does offer tools for achieving this objective. Protocols must be applied with clinical acumen, attention to individual subtleties, and an understanding of the basic theories of quality improvement.

▶ A concise review of the evidence and future potential of protocols in the ICU setting. No doubt they ensure a certain level of care, and data exist to support their role. The authors also discuss that lack of systems analysis by physicians and point out that "change-process illiteracy" that exists among many intensivists will have to be overcome to achieve success (consistent high-quality critical care).

J. D. Lang, Jr, MD

Who Bounces Back? Physiologic and Other Predictors of Intensive Care Unit Readmission

Rosenberg AL, Hofer TP, Hayward RA, et al (Univ of Michigan, Ann Arbor)
Crit Care Med 29:511-518, 2001   8–28

Background.—Patients who are readmitted to the ICU have significantly higher mortality rates and hospital costs than patients who do not require ICU readmission. Whether severity of illness measures can help identify which patients are at risk of ICU readmission was examined prospectively in a 4-year, single-center study.

Methods.—The subjects were 3310 patients with a first medical ICU admission who survived to ICU discharge. The diagnosis was recorded at admission, and the Acute Physiology Score (APS) and treatment status were determined daily throughout the ICU stay. For patients who were readmitted, the cause of the readmission (recurrence of initial disease or development of a new problem), its timing, and the location from which they were readmitted were also noted. Logistic regression analysis was used to identify significant predictors of in-hospital mortality in the readmitted patients.

Results.—Of the 3310 patients at risk for ICU readmission, 317 (9.6%) were readmitted. Almost half (47%) were readmitted within 72 hours of their initial ICU discharge. Patients readmitted to the ICU were significantly more likely than patients who were not readmitted to have sepsis (13% vs 8%) and hepatic failure (7% vs 4%) at admission. Patients who were readmitted also had a significantly higher APS score at ICU discharge (mean, 42 vs 34). The length of hospitalization was twice as long in the readmitted patients (mean, 32 vs 16 days; $P < .001$), and mortality rates were 5 times higher (43% vs 8%; $P < .0001$). Three independent predictors of ICU readmission were identified: an APS score of > 40 at ICU discharge (odds ratio [OR], 2.1), admission to the ICU from a general medical ward (OR, 1.9), and admission to the ICU after transfer from another hospital (OR, 1.7).

Conclusion.—Patients readmitted to the ICU had twice the length of hospital stay and 5 times the risk of mortality as did patients who were not readmitted. The findings of logistic regression analyses (higher APS score at ICU discharge and previous unsuccessful therapy on a general medical unit or at another hospital) suggest that a poor response to treatment is associated with an increased risk of ICU readmission. These findings have implications for tertiary care ICUs in that referral centers treating substantial numbers of transfer patients may have higher-than-expected ICU readmission rates and higher costs because of these patients' poor response to treatment.

▶ These are data that continue to bolster the importance of the need for improved predictive indexes to detect those patients who are at "high-risk" for readmission so that additional care, either within the ICU setting or perhaps in a specialized area for such patients, may be administered. An APACHE III score of more than 40 on discharge was found to be an independent predictor of ICU readmission, which should probably warrant prospective study. A striking discovery is the near 50% mortality rate of patients transferred to the ICU from other hospitals. This is particularly problematic for tertiary care medical centers because of the aging patient population, increasingly more critically ill patient population, and economically stressed medical community.

While most ICU readmission rates still remain below 10%, the trend is for increases in readmission rates. A comparison between the impact of intensivists versus nonintensivists and open versus closed ICUs would be a very important endeavor, especially with issues such as the Leapfrog Group (which I support) impacting on how we practice critical care medicine and staff our ICUs.

J. D. Lang, Jr, MD

Doctors' Perceptions of the Effects of Interventions Tested in Prospective, Randomised, Controlled, Clinical Trials: Results of a Survey of ICU Physicians

Ferreira F, Vincent J-L, Brun-Buisson C, et al (Erasme Univ, Brussels, Belgium; Henri Mondor Hosp, Paris; Hadassah-Hebrew Univ, Jerusalem, Israel; et al)
Intensive Care Med 27:548-554, 2001   8–29

Background.—Medical professionals are under increasing pressure to demonstrate the efficacy of treatment interventions, especially in the ICU. The current study surveyed ICU physicians as to which interventions they believed have been tested by prospective, randomized, controlled clinical trials (RCTs) in critically ill patients.

Methods.—A survey was distributed to 3250 registrants at an international symposium on intensive care and emergency medicine in Belgium. Respondents were asked to list the ICU interventions they believed have been shown by RCTs to improve survival. Respondents were then to rate their assessment of the efficacy of each intervention on a 5-point Likert scale and to indicate their level of confidence in their own assessments on a 3-point scale. Of the 527 questionnaires completed, 446 were suitable for analysis.

Findings.—Five hundred twelve interventions were identified as having been tested by RCTs. Forty-two were named more than 12 times. Of that subset, 31 were believed to be beneficial, and 11 were believed to have harmful effects. Many of the interventions named have, in fact, not been studied in RCTs, and some interventions tested in RCTs were not mentioned.

Conclusions.—Many ICU interventions thought to have been shown effective in RCTs by the current survey respondents have not been studied in such trials. Few interventions used in ICUs have actually been demonstrated by RCTs to positively influence outcomes.

▶ A rather revealing study demonstrating the confusion among intensivists, and probably all other groups of practitioners, regarding the evolution of clinical evidence used in our day-to-day decision making in critically ill patients and the paucity of RCTs that lead to these decisions. Cardiologists have been ahead of the curve, and the rest are now poised to get into the competition to form study groups powered to prospectively answer crucial clinical questions. The last 1 to 2 years may have been the most pivotal with respect to the importance of RCTs in the area of critical care medicine. Significant findings were that low tidal ventilation strategies in patients with acute lung injury/acute respiratory distress syndrome and the administration of activated protein C in patients with septic shock demonstrated reductions in patient mortality rates. However, judging from this study, however flawed it may be, there are significant strides to be made in the perception of the physician's mind.

J. D. Lang, Jr, MD

Outcome of Long-Stay Intensive Care Patients

Hughes M, MacKirdy FN, Norrie J, et al (Glasgow, Scotland; Victoria Infirmary, Glasgow, Scotland; Univ of Glasgow, Scotland; et al)
Intensive Care Med 27:779-782, 2001   8–30

Background.—Efforts to control ICU costs must address the issue of continued care for long-term patients. The outcomes of patients requiring long-term intensive care were investigated in a study conducted in the United Kingdom.

Method.—Data were obtained in 23 Scottish ICUs during a 3-year period. Three hundred twenty-three patients staying in the ICU for 30 days or longer were included in the study.

Findings.—These long-term ICU patients represented only 1.6% of the patients but used 15.7% of bed-days. However, 60% of these long-term ICU patients survived to hospital discharge. Survivors could not be discriminated from nonsurvivors on the basis of data collected in this study.

Conclusions.—Because long-term ICU patients have a relatively high hospital survival rate, resources should not be withheld on the basis of prolonged ICU stay alone. Clinical, economic, or political pressure to withdraw treatment at an earlier stage of ICU care should be resisted.

▶ A study such as this re-energizes me, because it reinforces the notion of "hard work pays dividends." In this case, the dividend is a pretty robust survival rate, even in patients whose hospital stay is more than 30 days. The patient population comprised both medical and surgical disciplines and, therefore, was pretty heterogeneous in make-up. Survivors were significantly younger, as would be expected. If patients were over 70 years of age, the mortality rate was 50%. Surgical patients fare better than nonsurgical patients. There was no subgroup analysis comparing surgical subspecialties, medical conditions requiring admission, or emergent versus nonemergent surgical cases. There was also no discussion regarding the costs the hospital stay or the physiologic and neurologic status of these patients on hospital discharge. Were intensivists in charge of the delivery of care? Were the patients functional? Did they pose a financial or psychological burden to their families and society? These questions are unanswerable in this study; however, extrapolating from a study presented in this section (Abstract 8–31), one might think (and hope) that these patients would enjoy an acceptable quality of life. Again, these issues will continue to be discussed with an increasing elderly patient population coupled with financial stress on the world's health care systems.

J. D. Lang, Jr, MD

Quality of Life and Functional Level in Elderly Patients Surviving Surgical Intensive Care

Udekwu P, Gurkin B, Oller D, et al (Univ of North Carolina, Chapel Hill; Wake Med Education Inst, Raleigh, NC)
J Am Coll Surg 193:245-249, 2001   8–31

Introduction.—The elderly use up to one third of all health care resources and represent between 26% and 51% of all ICU admissions. This age group is a target for cost reduction efforts. Elderly survival of surgical critical illness was examined by using perceived quality of life (PQOL) and activities of daily living (ADL) as indicators of value of care.

Methods.—A total of 672 patients aged 70 years or older who were admitted to a surgical ICU between October 1, 1992 and March 31, 1995 were evaluated. The following data were obtained from a computerized ICU database: age, gender, ICU and hospital length of stay, admission type and service, severity of illness as indicated by the Acute Physiology and Chronic Health Evaluation (APACHE) II scoring system, and admission diagnosis codes. Patients who survived hospitalization were interviewed with a standardized format, using a previously published PQOL index to acquire postillness subjective quality-of-life information. For noncommunicative or incompetent patients, family members or long-term care personnel were interviewed.

Results.—For ADL and PQOL measures, data were obtainable for 342 (50.9%) and 240 (35.7%) patients, respectively. The median duration from admission date to assessment was 21 months. The ADL scores diminished significantly overall, from a mean of 4.75 to 4.22. The proportion of completely independent patients decreased from 84.9% to 72.0%. The number of completely dependent patients increased from 0% to 3.8%. The PQOL scores were not significantly different from the scores of healthy patients living in the community. Regression models showed no relationship changes between ADL and age, service, APACHE II score, and emergent operation or admission.

Conclusion.—Although overall functional levels decreased, rates of full dependency increased only slightly. The PQOL was high among elderly patients who survived surgical intensive care. High hospital and postdischarge mortality rates should not prompt restriction of care in elderly patients who need surgical ICU services.

▶ The findings of this study were in some respects surprising. In the patients that survived (227 of 672 died during ICU stay or after discharge prior study completion), the ADL index was quantitatively different, but the patient's perception via the PQOL index was not markedly different. Much of these data were gathered from surrogates, so accuracy could be questioned in a number of cases. I am given a perspective that I did not expect, since intensivists generally are not involved in longitudinal care outside of the ICU setting. Our surgery colleagues keep us updated on certain patients or send us reports on the odd patient periodically. I think there will be bias towards somewhat positive conclusions versus, say, the medical intensive care patients. These patients will have severe chronic disease and have much less reserve to survive or, if that should occur, to return home after discharge and resume near-normal life activities or have the perception that their quality of life is acceptable. On the other hand, internal medicine–based specialities may also make decisions before an intensive care admission that may select out for a comparable result, as seen in this study (admit to an intermediate care unit for care or offer comfort care measures only). No doubt, an enormous amount of health care dollars is spent on end-of-life care issues. And with the octogenarian patient population being one of the fastest growing segments, issues such as these will need to be continually addressed. Should care be rationed?

J. D. Lang, Jr, MD

A Preliminary Analysis of Psychophysiological Variables and Nursing Performance in Situations of Increasing Criticality
Smith AM, Ortiguera SA, Laskowski ER, et al (Mayo Clinic, Rochester, Minn)
Mayo Clin Proc 76:275-284, 2001   8–32

Introduction.—ICU nursing is not more stressful overall than non-ICU nursing, yet it is likely that some ICU nurses experience high levels of stress. Although the technology to understand the effects of stress on nurses is available, no trials have addressed the relationship between psychophysiologic variables, situations of criticality, and nursing performance. The influence of psychologic variables and physiologic response on endotracheal tube (ET) suctioning was prospectively examined in novice ICU nurses in situations of increasing criticality.

Methods.—Psychophysiologic variables and ET suctioning performance were evaluated in a classroom, a skills laboratory, and an ICU. Situation-specific anxiety (state anxiety) and the predisposition to view situations as threatening (trait anxiety), cognitive appraisal, and heart rate were determined and compared with self-appraisal measures and a nurse instructor's rating of successful performance. Baseline data were gathered during a class for 45 novice ICU nurses.

Results.—Complete data were available on 26 ICU nurses. This included nurses being videotaped and monitored in the classroom, skills laboratory, and in the ICU during suctioning. High-state anxiety was significantly predictive of poor ICU suctioning performance ($P < .04$). Nurses who were high in state and trait anxiety, worry, and heart rate had poor performance, compared with nurses with less anxiety. The nurses with the best performance had a mean heart rate of 94 beats/min.

Conclusion.—The ICU nurses who were in a high state of anxiety, were high-trait anxious, and worried had a faster heart rate and performed less well than nurses who were more relaxed. Nurses who were high-state anxious may be at risk for attrition, burnout, medical errors, and poor performance in other ICU nursing tasks.

▶ An intriguing study that provides behavioral insight of our critical care nursing colleagues and can probably in some way be extrapolated to ourselves. High anxiety trait predisposed to a high anxiety state, leading to a negative performance (ET suctioning) in this particular cohort. Physicians of various specialities have undergone physiologic testing while performing their craft. These data revealed anesthesiologists to have the lowest heart rates, followed by cardiologists and lastly surgeons. These data are derived from different trials and did not prospectively evaluate differences between specialities. Nor did these data correlate a physiologic parameter to a psychologic one, such as an anxiety score. This is an area that is ripe for research. Psychophysiologic profiling may allow for more individualized training that can positively affect patient care and professional careers at all levels of the health care delivery system. No doubt, the specialty of anesthesiology has a higher-than-average rate of work-related stress disorders. Although this study has significant design flaws, it may serve as an impetus for prospective work to emerge, allowing more insights (maybe allowing physicians to be more sensitive to their work environment) and interventions for productive, gratifying, and sustained careers.

J. D. Lang, Jr, MD

Comparison of Performance 2 Years After the Old and New (Interactive) ATLS Courses
Ali J, Adam R, Pierre I, et al (Univ of West Indies; Univ of Toronto)
J Surg Res 97:71-75, 2001   8–33

Background.—Beginning in 1997, changes were made in the delivery of the Advanced Trauma Life Support (ATLS) course to emphasize an interactive format. A study performed soon after introduction of the new course showed significant improvement in clinical performance compared with the old course, but no change in cognitive performance. A 2-year follow-up study was performed to see how well these changes were maintained.

Methods.—Of the 32 physicians participating in the first study, 26 were available for the follow-up study: 13 from the "interactive" group and 13 from the "old" group. The physicians were evaluated on a 40-item MCQ test on trauma topics and on 4 trauma objective structured clinical examinations (OSCE) using simulated trauma patients. Comparisons included overall OSCE scores, adherence to priority scores, and overall approach scores.

Results.—Cognitive scores had deteriorated significantly from the previous study—none of the physicians in either group achieved a passing score of 80%. However, OCSE scores suggested no significant deterioration in clinical assessment and management skills. As in the previous study, clinical performance scores remained higher in the interactive group.

Conclusions.—The superior clinical performance documented after introduction of the interactive ATLS course is well maintained at 2 years' follow-up. The interactive program appears to be associated with a persistently high confidence level in applying clinical trauma management skills. However, with both the old and new formats, cognitive scores show significant deterioration after 2 years.

▶ The study seems to confirm what has been observed but has gone unpublished. Retention of facts not used frequently and brought up in the context of a clinical approach are very difficult to retain. This may simply have to do with traditional memorization techniques versus open dialogue and discussion of how facts integrate with a certain clinical concept or approach. An interactive design, as this study demonstrates, allows for better clinical examination and priority scores over time, supporting the notion of better retention. Judging from the study design, it is doubtful that more intelligent or motivated individuals were selected out. This gives credence to the integration of problem-based learning, simulators, and on-line interactive forms of instruction within a given curriculum.

J. D. Lang, Jr, MD

Complications of Femoral and Subclavian Venous Catheterization in Critically Ill Patients: A Randomized Controlled Trial
Merrer J, for the French Catheter Study Group in Intensive Care (Hôpital de Poissy, France; et al)
JAMA 286:700-707, 2001   8–34

Introduction.—Major femoral or retroperitoneal hematoma is the most common major mechanical complication of femoral venous catheterization. It occurs in up to 1.3% of cases. Pneumothorax is the most common major complication of subclavian venous catheterization (incidence, 1.5%-2.3%). Catheter-related thrombosis ranges from 6.6% to 25% with femoral catheterization and from 10% to 50% with subclavian catheterization. Subclavian catheterization has been linked to a lower rate of infection, compared with femoral catheterization. The rates of mechanical, infectious, and thrombotic complications associated with femoral and subclavian venous catheterization were examined in a multicenter, prospective, concealed, randomized, controlled trial in ICU patients between December 1997 and July 2000.

Methods.—Two hundred eighty-nine adult patients from 8 ICUs in France receiving a first central venous catheter were randomly assigned to undergo central venous catheterization at either the femoral or subclavian site. Patients were followed up for rates and severity of mechanical, infectious, and thrombotic complications (289, 270, and 223 patients, respectively).

Results.—Femoral catheterization was linked to a higher incidence rate of overall infectious complications (19.8% vs 4.5%, $P < .001$; incidence density of 20 vs 3.7 per 1000 catheter-days), major infectious complications (clinical sepsis with or without bloodstream infection, 4.4% vs 1.5%, $P = .07$; incidence density of 4.5 vs 1.2 per 1000 catheter-days), overall thrombotic complications (21.5% vs 1.9%, $P < .001$), and complete thrombosis of the vessel (6% vs 0%, $P = .01$). Rates of overall and major mechanical complications were similar between the femoral and subclavian groups (17.3% vs 18.8%, $P = .74$; and 1.4% vs 2.8%, $P = .44$, respectively). Risk factors for mechanical complications included duration of insertion ($P < .001$), insertion in 2 of the centers ($P = .001$), and insertion during the night ($P = .03$). The only factor associated with infectious complications was femoral catheterization ($P < .001$). Antibiotic administration via the catheter reduced the risk of infectious complications ($P = .03$). The only risk factor for thrombotic complications was femoral catheterization ($P < .001$).

Conclusion.—Catheterization of the femoral vein was associated with a significantly higher risk of overall complications, compared with catheterization of the subclavian vein. Femoral catheterization increased the risk of catheter-related infection and thrombosis. The rates of mechanical complications were similar for both femoral and subclavian catheterization.

▶ The results of this trial were pretty dramatic and should not fall on deaf ears. If a third arm including internal jugular catheters had been included, the impact would be even more exciting. In our unit, internal jugular cannulations (although the reported rate of infectious complications is greater than that for subclavian catheters) occur with the greatest frequency, followed by subclavian cannulations; the femoral route generally is used as a last resort or for continuous renal replacement. The most commonly encountered mechanical complications were arterial punctures, in a few cases requiring surgical intervention and blood transfusion therapy. Several independent risk factors were observed, but the insertion at night got my attention. This was possibly caused by operator fatigue or because lower-level, inexperienced personnel were responsible for catheter placement. There were no differences between the 2 groups, with both near 20%. The divergence in results was caused by infectious and thrombotic-related complications, which were significant. Often, femoral catheters are placed under urgent or emergent situations, but because of the study design, they were placed under "elective" circumstances in patients receiving their first catheter. A very informative study.

J. D. Lang, Jr, MD

Growth Hormone Together With Glutamine-Containing Total Parenteral Nutrition Maintains Muscle Glutamine Levels and Results in a Less Negative Nitrogen Balance After Surgical Trauma

Hammarqvist F, Sandgren A, Andersson K, et al (Huddinge Univ Hosp, Stockholm; Södertälje Hosp, Stockholm; State Univ of New York, Stony Brook)

Surgery 129:576-586, 2001   8–35

Background.—Muscle protein catabolism, reflected by a decrease in glutamine (GLN), a decrease in muscle protein synthesis, and a negative nitrogen balance can be reduced by either administration of GLN or growth hormone (GH). In this study, the effects of a combination of GH and GLN were studied.

Methods.—Patients (n = 16) undergoing abdominal operation were given total parenteral nutrition (TPN) containing either GLN alone or GLN together with GH (GH/GLN) during 3 postoperative days. The amino acid concentration and protein synthesis in muscle tissue and the nitrogen balance were measured.

Results.—GH/GLN reduced nitrogen losses compared with GLN alone (-5.8 ± 1.4 g nitrogen versus -10.6 ± 1.1 g nitrogen, $P < .05$). GH/GLN maintained muscle GLN at preoperative levels compared with a 47.5% ± 6.3% decline in the GLN group. A similar decrease was seen in the fractional synthesis rate of muscle protein postoperatively in both groups.

Conclusions.—GH has an additive effect given together with GLN on muscle amino acid metabolism, preventing the decrease in the GLN concentration in skeletal muscle and diminishing the loss of whole body nitrogen. However, the improvements in muscle amino acid concentrations and nitrogen loss were not associated with differences between the groups in muscle protein synthesis postoperatively.

▶ This study comes on the heels of a recent study demonstrating an increased mortality rate in critically ill patients receiving GH.[1] The authors sought to decrease the cellular efflux of GLN by the nitrogen-sparing effects of GH. The addition of GH to the glutamine/TPN formulation did just that at 3 days after lower abdominal surgery. Nitrogen balance improved with the addition of GH, but without evidence of an increase in protein synthesis. Since GH is known to deplete peripheral GLN stores, stress on vital organ systems may have been caused by GH monotherapy. Perhaps prospective randomized studies can be performed on critically ill patients using TPN versus total enteral nutrition and the concomitant use of GH/GLN.

J. D. Lang, Jr, MD

Reference

1. Takala J, Ruokonen E, Webster NR, et al: Increased mortality associated with growth hormone treatment in critically ill adults. *N Engl J Med* 341:785-792, 1999.

Evaluation of Delirium in Critically ill Patients: Validation of the Confusion Assessment Method for the Intensive Care Unit (CAM-ICU)
Ely EW, Margolin R, Francis J, et al (Vanderbilt Univ, Nashville, Tenn; Yale Univ, New Haven, Conn)
Crit Care Med 29:1370-1379, 2001   8–36

Background.—ICU patients are at very high risk of the development of delirium. An instrument to accurately diagnose delirium in critically ill patients in the ICU was developed and validated.

Methods.—The Confusion Assessment Method was modified for use in the ICU (CAM-ICU) and tested. Thirty-eight patients admitted to adult medical and coronary ICUs at 1 center were included in the prospective cohort study. Daily CAM-ICU ratings by 2 nurses and an intensivist were compared with the reference standard, delirium criteria from the *Diagnostic and Statistical Manual of Mental Disorders* as assessed by a delirium expert. A total of 293 daily, paired evaluations were completed and analyzed.

Findings.—The reference standard diagnoses were delirium in 42% of all observations and coma in 27% of all observations. Delirium developed in 87% of the patients during their ICU stay, the mean duration of which was 4.2 days. When assessments of comatose patients were excluded (because of a lack of characteristic delirium features), the nurses and the intensivist showed high interrater reliability for their CAM-ICU ratings, with kappa statistics of 0.84, 0.79, and 0.95, respectively. Compared with the reference standard, the sensitivities of CAM-ICU as applied by the 2 nurses and the intensivist were 95%, 96%, and 100%, respectively. Specificities were 93%, 93%, and 89%, respectively.

Conclusions.—The CAM-ICU applied by ICU nurses and physicians is highly valid and reliable for diagnosing delirium in ICU patients. This may be a useful tool in both clinical settings and research studies.

▶ Delirium in the critical care setting is commonplace, as this study indicates (87% during the ICU stay). Tools that assist in diagnosing and following the course of delirium are badly needed and will alter the care plan if significant findings are revealed. Like many things in the ICU, the primary problem that results in the admission gets most of the attention, and sequelae such as delirium go unnoticed or at least unattended. In my opinion, this study will serve 2 purposes in the many ICUs: (1) allow for more focused attention and interventions as needed and (2) serve as a springboard for more education and emphasis on this disorder. Validation of the CAM-ICU should be undertaken with a larger number of patients and with other critically ill patient populations, such as the surgical, trauma, and burn patients.

J. D. Lang, Jr, MD

Postoperative Fibrinolysis Diagnosed by Thrombelastography

Liu G, Bowkett J, Przybylowski G, et al (Univ of Melbourne, Heidelberg, Victoria)
Anaesth Intensive Care 28:77-81, 2000   8–37

Background.—Thrombelastrography (TEG) is useful for monitoring bedside coagulation, especially in patients with fibrinolysis. A case in which TEG enabled early detection of fibrinolysis with significant clinical bleeding immediately after hip replacement surgery was presented.

> *Case Report.*—Man, 79, was undergoing a left total hip replacement. His history included non–insulin-dependent diabetes, hypertension, and chronic renal insufficiency. Routine medications included nifedipine, salbutamol, resonium, and paracetamol and codeine. A transfusion of packed red blood cells for anemia and subcutaneous heparin were given prophylactically. The preoperative coagulation profile and other test results were normal. Spinal anesthesia was achieved with bupivacaine. Sedation during surgery included intermittent bolus doses of midazolam and propofol. Intravenous cefazolin was administered intraoperatively. At the end of the procedure, which lasted 110 minutes, the patient's hemodynamics were stable. Considerable oozing of blood was noted at the wound closure site. Postoperatively, 600 mL drained in the first hour. The patient was being monitored perioperatively with TEG as part of a research project. A blood sample obtained in the middle of the surgical procedure showed a hypocoagulable state, as evidenced by prolonged r and k values and a decreased angle. A fibrinolytic pattern was seen on postoperative TEG. Subsequent coagulation tests demonstrated a normal clotting profile, except for a greatly increased D-dimer. A bolus injection of epsilon aminocaproic acid resulted in a marked reduction in blood drainage. Three hours later, the TEG demonstrated some hypocoagulability but no fibrinolysis. At 5 hours, the TEG was normal and the D-dimer level had declined. On postoperative days 1, 3, and 5, TEG tracings were normal. On day 7, unilateral venography showed no evidence of deep venous thrombosis on the surgically treated limb.

Conclusions.—Early diagnosis of fibrinolysis by TEG made possible the initiation of appropriate therapy. Monitoring with TEG probably resulted in less blood product transfusion and may have prevented unnecessary surgical re-exploration.

▶ This article featured a case report demonstrating the efficacy of TEG in a patient with intraoperative fibrinolysis. Use of the TEG assisted in the diagnosis and was used as a tool to follow the effects of antifibrinolytic therapy. With coagulation becoming much more of a "mainstream" topic because of therapies such as Xigris, the value of TEG should become more appreciated by intensivists. A critical mass of TEG research has been published recently, allowing for descriptive and mechanistic insights into coagulation disturbances caused by a number of pathophysiologic states.

J. D. Lang, Jr, MD

Efficacy and Safety of Recombinant Human Activated Protein C for Severe Sepsis
Bernard GR, for the Recombinant Human Activated Protein C Worldwide Evaluation in Severe Sepsis (PROWESS) Study Group (Vanderbilt Univ, Nashville, Tenn; et al)
N Engl J Med 344:699-709, 2001   8–38

Background.—A generalized inflammatory and procoagulant infection response can lead to severe sepsis, which is associated with a very high mortality rate. Treatment with activated protein C may improve the outcome of severe sepsis. Phase 2 clinical trials demonstrated that treatment of patients with severe sepsis with recombinant activated protein C (drotrecogin alfa activated) resulted in dose-dependent reductions in markers of coagulopathy and inflammation. The effect of treatment with drotrecogin alfa activated on the mortality rate of patients with severe sepsis was examined in a phase 3 clinical trial.

Study Design.—A study group of 1690 patients with systemic inflammation and organ failure participated in the randomized, double-blind, placebo-controlled, multicenter trial from July 1998 to June 2000. The primary end point was all-cause mortality, which was evaluated 28 days after the beginning of treatment. Adverse effects were also monitored.

Results.—The mortality rate among patients with severe sepsis was 30.8% in the placebo group and 24.7% in the treatment group. Treatment with drotrecogin alfa activated was associated with a reduction in the relative risk of mortality of 19.4% and an absolute reduction in the risk of mortality of 6.1%. Levels of plasma D-dimer, a marker of coagulopathy, were significantly lower in patients receiving drotrecogin alfa activated than in those receiving placebo on days 1 through 7 after the beginning of the infusion. The incidence of serious bleeding was higher in the treatment group than in the placebo group, as would be expected with a protein with antithrombotic properties.

Conclusions.—The administration of drotrecogin alfa activated to patients with severe sepsis reduced all-cause mortality. The results of this phase 3 trial indicate that 1 additional life could be saved for every 16 patients with severe sepsis treated. Treatment is associated with a higher incidence of serious bleeding.

▶ This is an important study. Recombinant human activated protein C reduced mortality in patients with severe sepsis; the mortality rate was 30.8% in the placebo group and 24.7% in the treatment group. This may appear to be a small difference, but given the frequency and seriousness of severe sepsis in the ICU setting in the United States, it may be an important advance. The incidence of bleeding was higher in the activated protein C group, an adverse event that might be expected when a drug with such pharmacologic activity is administered.

M. Wood, MD, FRCA

Intensive Insulin Therapy in Critically Ill Patients
Van den Berghe G, Wouters P, Weekers F, et al (Catholic Univ of Leuven, Belgium)
N Engl J Med 345:1359-1367, 2001   8–39

Background.—Hyperglycemia and insulin resistance will develop in many ICU patients, even if they have no previous history of diabetes. Insulin therapy can return blood glucose levels to normal, although the prognostic impact of this treatment is uncertain. The effects of intensive insulin therapy to correct blood glucose levels on the outcomes of ICU patients were studied.

Methods.—Participants were 1548 patients in a surgical ICU who were receiving mechanical ventilation. They were randomly assigned to receive intensive insulin therapy or conventional treatment. In the intervention group, insulin was given to maintain blood glucose levels within a target range of 80 to 110 mg/dL; in the control group, insulin infusion was given

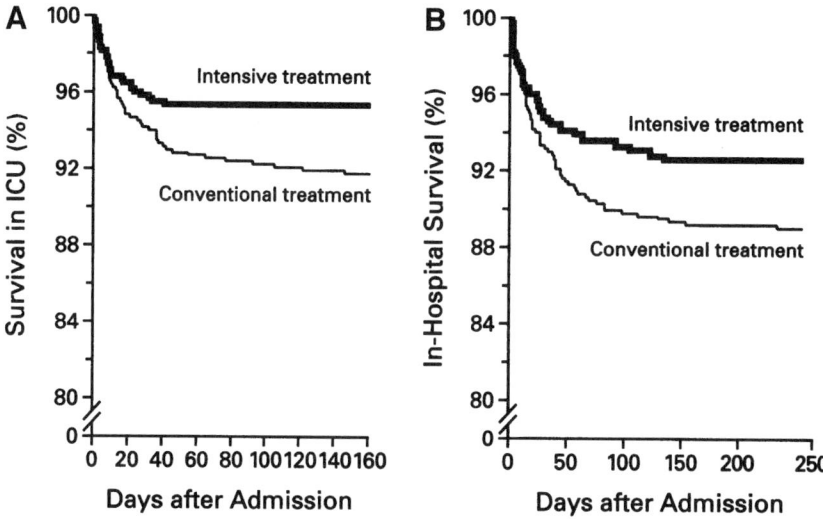

FIGURE 1.—Kaplan-Meier curves showing cumulative survival of patients who received intensive insulin treatment or conventional treatment in the ICU. Patients discharged alive from the ICU (**A**) and from the hospital (**B**) were considered to have survived. In both cases, the differences between the treatment groups were significant (survival in ICU, nominal $P = .005$ and adjusted $P < .04$; in-hospital survival, nominal $P = .01$). P values were determined with the use of the Mantel-Cox log-rank test. (Reprinted by permission of *The New England Journal of Medicine*, courtesy of Van den Berghe G, Wouters P, Weekers F, et al: Intensive insulin therapy in critically ill patients. *N Engl J Med* 345:1359-1367, 2001. Copyright 2001, Massachusetts Medical Society. All rights reserved.)

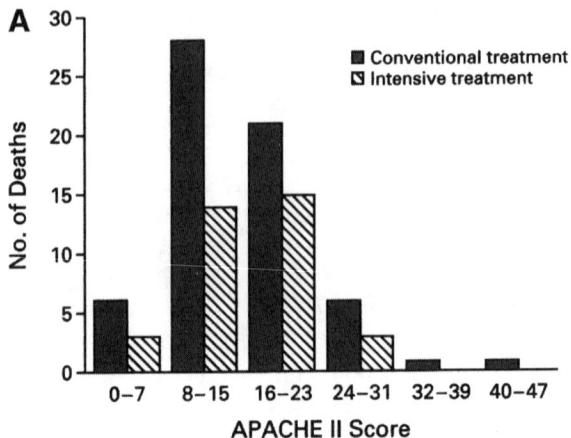

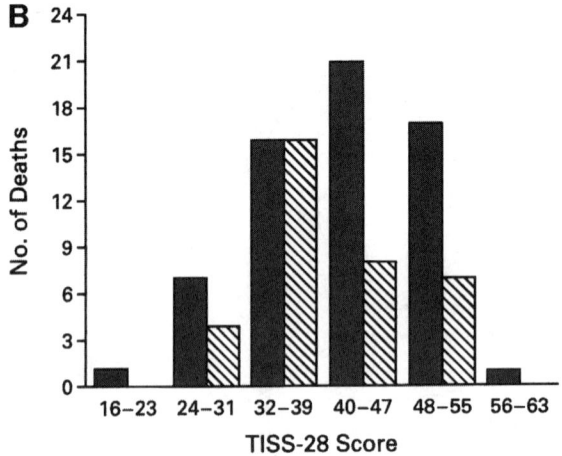

FIGURE 2.—Number of deaths in the intensive care unit according to the Acute Physiology and Chronic Health Evaluation (*APACHE II*) score (**A**) and the Simplified Therapeutic Intervention Scoring System (*TISS-28*) score (**B**) in the first 24 hours. Higher APACHE II scores indicate more severe illness, and higher TISS-28 scores indicate a higher number of therapeutic interventions. (Reprinted by permission of *The New England Journal of Medicine*, courtesy of Van den Berghe G, Wouters P, Weekers F, et al: Intensive insulin therapy in critically ill patients. *N Engl J Med* 345:1359-1367, 2001. Copyright 2001, Massachusetts Medical Society. All rights reserved.)

only if blood glucose levels rose above 215 mg/dL, with a target range of 180 to 200 mg/dL. Morbidity and mortality rates were compared between groups.

Results.—The mortality rate in the ICU was 4.6% in the intensive insulin group, compared with 8.0% in the conventional therapy group (Fig 1). Much of the prognostic impact of intensive insulin therapy came in the reduction of deaths from multiple organ failure with a confirmed septic focus. Intensive insulin therapy was effective in almost all subgroups of patients defined according to the Acute Physiology and Chronic Health

Evaluation (APACHE II) score and the Simplifed Therapeutic Intervention Scoring System (TISS-28) score during the first 24 hours after admission (Fig 2). Patients receiving intensive insulin therapy also had a 34% reduction in in-hospital mortality. Significant reductions in morbidity were noted as well, including a 46% reduction in bloodstream infections, a 41% decrease in acute renal failure requiring dialysis or hemofiltration, a 50% reduction in red blood cell transfusion, and a 44% reduction in critical illness polyneuropathy.

Conclusion.—For surgical ICU patients, intensive insulin therapy to maintain good control of blood glucose levels is associated with significant improvement in measures of morbidity and mortality. Blood glucose levels should be maintained at 110 mg/dL or below, whether or not the patient has a history of diabetes.

▶ This is a landmark study for anesthesiologists and intensivists, and highlights the importance of rigorous control of blood glucose levels in critically ill patients.

M. Wood, MD, FRCA

The Protective Effect of Acadesine on Lung Ischemia-Reperfusion Injury
Matot I, Jurim O (Hebrew Univ of Jerusalem, Israel)
Anesth Analg 92:590-595, 2001   8–40

Background.—Injury to the lung occurs when it is exposed to periods of ischemia and reperfusion (I-R), but the mechanism involved in producing the injury is unknown. Acadesine, a nucleoside of the class of adenosine-regulating drugs, increases the concentration of extracellular tissue adenosine when net adenosine triphosphate breakdown is occurring. Its effect is localized to the ischemic tissues only and the substance is both safe and tolerated well when given intravenously. The agent has cardioprotective properties, attenuates mucosal lesions, and reduces the pulmonary dysfunction of posttraumatic endotoxemia in pigs. Its effectiveness in managing I-R lung injury when given intravenously before or after reperfusion was assessed.

Methods.—One group of intact-chest spontaneously breathing cats underwent occlusion of the lobar artery of the left lower lung lobe for 2 hours (ischemia), and a second group was reperfused for 3 hours (I-R). Three protocols were then performed randomly on the animals: animals were given acadesine intravenously 15 minutes before ischemia, animals received acadesine intravenously 15 minutes before reperfusion, or animals received acadesine 30 minutes after reperfusion. The dosage of acadesine was initial dose, 2.5 mg/kg/min for 5 minutes, then 0.5 mg/kg/min until reperfusion was completed. Histologic examination was performed to evaluate injury, with comparisons made with the animals' right lobes.

Results.—All of the left lower lung lobes of the ischemic animals were pale. Those of the I-R group had hemorrhagic lesions throughout the lobe.

TABLE 1.—Quantitative Assessment of Lung Injury

Groups	Injured Alveoli (%)*		Alveoli With Exudate (%)		Average Number of Leukocytes†		Average Number of Erythrocytes‡		Wet/Dry Weight Ratio	
	LLL	RLL	LLL	RLL	LLL	RLL	LLL	RLL	LLL	RLL
1: Ischemia (I)	3 ± 1	4 ± 1	2 ± 1	1 ± 1	2 ± 2	2 ± 1	0.3 ± 0.2	0.2 ± 0.1	4 ± 1	4 ± 0.5
2: I-reperfusion (R)	63 ± 9§	3 ± 2	34 ± 13§	1 ± 1	8 ± 2§	3 ± 1	1.9 ± 0.4§	0.3 ± 0.2	9 ± 2§	4 ± 1
3: I-R + acadesine before I	4 ± 1	4 ± 2	1 ± 1	2 ± 1	3 ± 2	3 ± 1	0.3 ± 0.3	0.4 ± 0.2	5 ± 1	5 ± 0.5
4: I-R + acadesine before R	6 ± 2‖	2 ± 1	4 ± 1‖	1 ± 1	4 ± 2	2 ± 2	0.5 ± 0.2	0.3 ± 0.1	6 ± 1	4 ± 1
5: I-R + acadesine after R	62 ± 8§	2 ± 1	28 ± 10§	1 ± 1	11 ± 3§	2 ± 1	1.7 ± 0.6§	0.3 ± 0.2	10 ± 2§	5 ± 1
6: Nonischemic control	3 ± 1	4 ± 2	1 ± 1	2 ± 1	3 ± 1	3 ± 1	0.2 ± 0.2	0.2 ± 0.1	5 ± 0.5	4 ± 1

Note: Values are mean ± SD.

* Alveoli containing exudate, more than two leukocytes, or more than two erythrocytes.
† Average number of leukocytes in a single injured alveolus.
‡ Average number of erythrocytes in a single injured alveolus.
§ Groups 2 and 5 (LLL) were significantly different from the other groups and from their corresponding RLL in all parameters with the use of one-way analysis of variance with Newman-Keuls multiple comparison test as the *post hoc* test ($P < 0.01$). There was no difference among the six groups in the control (RLL) lobes.
‖ LLL of Group 4 was significantly different from its control lobe in the percentage of injured alveoli and alveoli with exudate ($P < 0.05$).

Abbreviations: LLL, left lower lobe; *RLL*, right lower lobe.

(Courtesy of Mattot I, Jurim O: The protective effect of acadesine on lung ischemia-reperfusion injury. *Anesth Analg* 92:590-595, 2001.)

The lungs undergoing I-R that had received acadesine before the ischemia or the reperfusion showed no abnormal findings macroscopically. Those receiving acadesine after reperfusion had gross hemorrhagic foci. The left lower lung lobe of the I-R animals had disrupted alveolar structure and 63% injured alveoli. Ischemia without reperfusion did not produce injury. The number of injured alveoli was significantly reduced when acadesine was given before the ischemia or the reperfusion (Table 1).

Conclusions.—It appears that reperfusion after ischemia causes injury to the lungs, but this injury can be managed with the intravenous administration of acadesine before ischemia and/or reperfusion. This protective effect was not present when acadesine was given after reperfusion.

▶ Acadesine has cardioprotective properties; this study shows, in an animal model, that acadesine has protective effects on lung ischemia-reperfusion injury. The long-term use of such a drug is unknown but may be of value in lung transplantation.

M. Wood, MD, FRCA

Pediatric Critical Care Medicine

Reversal of Catabolism by Beta-Blockade After Severe Burns
Herndon DN, Hart DW, Wolf SE, et al (Univ of Texas, Galveston)
N Engl J Med 345:1223-1229, 2001   8–41

Objective.—Severely burned patients have a hypermetabolic response mediated by endogenous catecholamines and leading to increased energy expenditure and catabolism of muscle protein. Previous studies have shown decreased energy expenditure with β-blockade after burns. The effects of long-term β-blockade with propranolol on energy expenditure and muscle protein catabolism in children with severe burns were examined.

Methods.—The randomized trial included 25 children with burns involving more than 40% of the total body surface area. One group received β-blockade with oral propranolol for 2 weeks or longer, and children in the other group were left untreated as control subjects. The propranolol dosage was adjusted as necessary to maintain resting heart rate at a level 20% lower than baseline.

Results.—With propranolol therapy, heart rate and resting energy expenditure decreased significantly. This was so within the β-blockade group, compared with baseline, and for the propranolol group versus the control group (Fig 2). Compared with baseline, net muscle-protein balance increased by 82% in the propranolol group and decreased by 27% in the control group, although the difference was nonsignificant. Whole-body potassium scanning showed no change in fat-free mass in patients receiving propranolol, compared with a mean 9% decrease in untreated control subjects.

Conclusion.—β-Blockade with propranolol significantly reduces hypermetabolism in children with burns. Propranolol therapy also reverses the

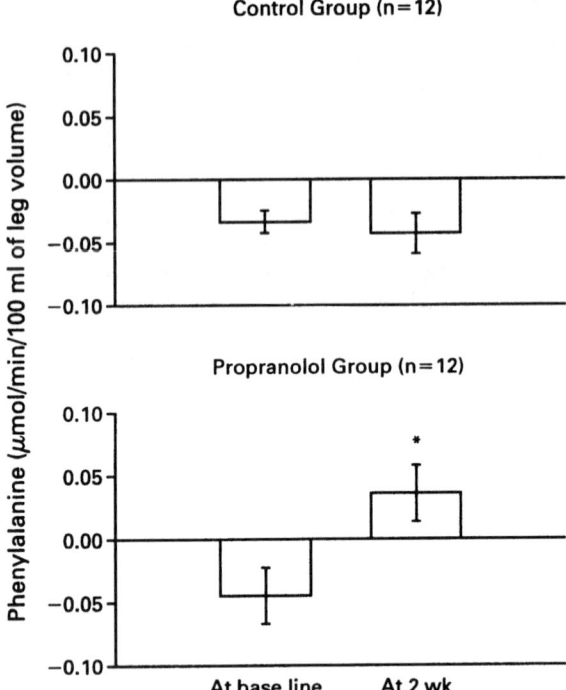

FIGURE 2.—Mean (±SE) change from baseline in the net balance of muscle-protein synthesis and breakdown during 2 weeks of treatment. Values were obtained with use of a 5-hour kinetic study that used isotopically labeled phenylalanine. The *asterisk* indicates a significant difference between the 2 groups (P = .001 by t test) and a significant difference between the baseline value and the value at 2 weeks (P = .002 by paired t test). (Reprinted by permission of *The New England Journal of Medicine* from Herndon DN, Hart DW, Wolf SE, et al: Reversal of catabolism by beta-blockade after severe burns. N Engl J Med 345:1223-1229. Copyright 2001, Massachusetts Medical Society. All rights reserved.)

post-burn muscle protein catabolic state. Propranolol is a safe, simple, and effective therapy that may improve patients' ability to recuperate.

▶ A sophisticated analysis of protein utilization that demonstrates promising application for these unfortunate children. The method is extremely rigorous and has pitfalls, but all 3 techniques were consistent in their message of enhanced muscle protein synthesis. β-Blockade was very well tolerated. On a few occasions, propranolol was withheld because of a decrease in MAP to 60 to 65 mm Hg, but there were no cases of bronchospasm. The net dose required was 6.3 mg/kg/d orally, which is substantial. An obvious question is, will benefit be gained. Only larger trials powered to make these determinations will answer that, but they should be undertaken. Because the treatment cost is low, immediate implementation of such a strategy is not problematic. Extrapolation to the older burn patient population may be more difficult because of differences in protein muscle metabolism and potential intolerance of higher dose of propranolol.

J. D. Lang, Jr, MD

Low-Dose Nitric Oxide Therapy for Persistent Pulmonary Hypertension of the Newborn

Clark RH, for the Clinical Inhaled Nitric Oxide Research Group (Duke Univ, Durham, NC; et al)
N Engl J Med 342:469-474, 2000   8–42

Background.—Inhaled nitric oxide (NO) is known to improve gas exchange in neonates. However, the efficacy of low-dose inhaled NO in decreasing the need for extracorporeal membrane oxygenation (ECMO) has not been determined.

Methods.—Two hundred forty-eight neonates were enrolled in a clinical study to see whether low-dose inhaled NO reduces the use of ECMO in newborns with pulmonary hypertension. All infants were born after 34 weeks' gestation, were 4 days old or younger, needed assisted ventilation, and had hypoxemic respiratory failure as defined by an oxygenation index of 25 or greater. One hundred twenty-six neonates were assigned to NO, 20 ppm for a maximum of 24 hours, followed by 6 ppm for no more than 96 hours. One hundred twenty-two infants were assigned to the control group.

Findings.—Thirty-eight percent of the NO group and 64% of the control group needed ECMO. The mortality rate at 30 days was comparable in the 2 groups, at 8% and 7%, respectively. Chronic lung disease developed less frequently in the NO recipients than in the control group infants.

Conclusions.—Inhaled NO decreases the need for ECMO in neonates with hypoxemic respiratory failure and pulmonary hypertension. The current study differs from previous research in its use of a low dose of NO for a shorter duration.

▶ An excellent example of a properly designed trial. This study definitively demonstrated that inhaled NO decreases the need for ECMO in neonates who have pulmonary hypertension diagnosed via echocardiography. These data are very important because compared with ECMO, the costs are significantly different (NO being much cheaper). Morever, ECMO is not available in many regions and it has a certain complication profile associated with it. Because NO was FDA approved in December of 1999, its use in this patient population should almost become "routine." The concentrations used were low (20 ppm for 24 hours and the 5 ppm not exceeding 96 hours), thus the complications were low. The only patient population that did not benefit were neonates born with congenital diaphragmatic hernias. In addition to reductions in ECMO, neonates who received inhaled NO also demonstrated significant reductions in pulmonary outcome. While mechanism was not part of the study design, one may speculate that attenuation of the inflammatory response may have been responsible.

J. D. Lang, Jr, MD

Adverse Effects of Early Dexamethasone Treatment in Extremely-Low-Birth-Weight Infants

Stark AR, for the National Institute of Child Health and Human Development Neonatal Research Network (Brigham and Women's Hosp, Boston; Univ of Alabama, Birmingham; Univ of Texas, Houston; et al)

N Engl J Med 344:95-101, 2001   8–43

Introduction.—The early administration of high doses of dexamethasone may decrease the risk of chronic lung disease in premature infants. Infants in trials with high-dose dexamethasone experienced adverse effects, including hypertension and hyperglycemia. Treatment with a moderate dose of dexamethasone was evaluated to determine whether it could reduce the risk of chronic lung disease and have minimal adverse effects in infants with birth weights ranging from 501 to 1000 g who were treated with mechanical ventilation within 12 hours after birth.

Methods.—The study included 220 very low birth weight infants who were randomly assigned to treatment with either dexamethasone or placebo with either routine ventilatory support or permissive hypercapnia. Dexamethasone was administered within 24 hours after birth at 0.15 mg/kg of body weight per day for 3 days, then tapered over 7 days. The main outcome measures were death or chronic lung disease at 36 weeks' postmenstrual age.

Results.—Compared with placebo, the relative risk of death or chronic lung disease was 0.9 in the dexamethasone group. The effect of dexamethasone did not differ with respect to ventilatory approach, so the dexamethasone and placebo groups were combined. In comparison with the placebo group, infants in the dexamethasone group were less likely to require oxygen supplementation at 28 days after birth ($P = .004$), were less likely to receive open-label glucocorticoid treatment during hospitalization (34% vs 51%; $P = .01$), were more likely to have hypertension (P

TABLE 4.—Complications Attributable to the Study Drug

Complication	Dexamethasone (N = 111) no. (%)	Placebo (N = 109)	Relative Risk (95% CI)*	P Value
Systolic pressure				
>80 mm Hg	30 (27)	4 (4)	7.4 (2.7-20.2)	<0.001
>90 mm Hg	7 (13)	0	—	0.01
Treatment for hypertension	14 (13)	5 (5)	2.7 (1.0-7.4)	0.04
Blood glucose >180 mg/dl (10 mmol/liter)	52 (47)	44 (40)	1.2 (0.9-1.6)	0.30
Insulin treatment	26 (23)	13 (12)	2.0 (1.1-3.6)	0.02
Upper gastrointestinal bleeding	6 (5)	2 (2)	2.9 (0.6-14.3)	0.18

*Relative risks indicate the occurrence of the complication in the dexamethasone group as compared with the placebo group.

Abbreviation: CI, Confidence interval.

TABLE 5.—Gastrointestinal Perforation Within 14 Days After Birth, According to Whether Indomethacin Was Administered With or Without Dexamethasone

Treatment	All Infants	Infants With Perforation
	no.	no. (%)
Dexamethasone and indomethacin	70	13 (19)
Dexamethasone alone	41	1 (2)
Placebo and indomethacin	82	4 (5)
Placebo alone	27	0
Total	220	18 (8)

< .001), and were more likely to receive insulin treatment for hyperglycemia ($P = .02$) (Table 4). During the first 14 days, infants in the dexamethasone group were also more likely than those in the placebo group to have spontaneous gastrointestinal perforation (13% vs 4%; $P = .02$). Perforation appeared to be correlated with indomethacin treatment during the first 24 hours, and the effect of dexamethasone on the perforation rate appeared to be greater when indomethacin was also being administered (Table 5). Dexamethasone-treated infants had lower body weight ($P = .02$) and a smaller head circumference ($P = .04$) at 36 weeks' postmenstrual age, compared with placebo-treated infants.

Conclusion.—The early administration of dexamethasone in moderate doses had no effect on death or chronic lung disease in very low birth weight preterm infants; it was associated with gastrointestinal perforation and diminished growth.

▶ This is the second article this year to conclude that dexamethasone administered in low birth weight infants (500-1000 g) is associated with significant complications and no reduction in mortality.[1] Because approximately 30% of these infants develop chronic lung disease and many have low baseline cortisol levels, supplementation would assist in attenuating lung injury and associated consequences. The gastrointestinal perforation rate was so high in the treatment limb that the study was terminated. The hypothesis as to the etiology was suppression of prostaglandin production, which is an integral component in maintaining gut integrity. Requirements for oxygen at 28 days were less versus placebo, but when compared with the other observed results, dexamethasone it was concluded could not be routinely recommended.

J. D. Lang, Jr, MD

Reference

1. The Vermont Oxford Network Steroid Study Group: Early postnatal dexamethasone therapy for the prevention of chronic lung disease. *Pediatrics* 108:741-748, 2001.

Routine Chest Radiographs in Pediatric Intensive Care Units
Quasney MW, Goodman DM, Billow M, et al (Univ of Tennessee, Memphis; Northwestern Univ, Evanston, Ill; Children's Hosp Med Ctr of Akron, Ohio; et al)
Pediatrics 107:241-248, 2001   8–44

Introduction.—Most trials evaluating the efficacy and value of routine chest radiographs have been performed in adult ICUs and have shown a high incidence of unsuspected or abnormal findings that frequently lead to changes in patient management. The usefulness of routine chest radiographs in critically ill children may be different than in adults for various anatomic and physiologic reasons. The usefulness of routine morning chest radiographs was prospectively assessed in 15 pediatric ICUs by examining the frequency of interventions performed based on the results of the routine chest radiograph.

Methods.—The following data were recorded from patients in the pediatric ICU who had a routine morning chest radiograph: weight, diagnosis, presence of active cardiopulmonary problems, length of stay, and number and type of devices. The number and type of interventions based on the interpretation of the chest radiographs were noted.

Results.—There were 512 routine chest radiographs evaluated, most of which were obtained from patients admitted because of cardiovascular disease (195/512; 38%) or respiratory failure (186/512; 36%). Ninety-one percent (465/512) of the routine chest radiographs were obtained in patients with 1 or more devices. Of the 512 routine chest radiographs, 231 (45%) resulted in 1 or more interventions. One hundred fifty-five of the 284 routine chest radiographs (55%) obtained in patients who weighed 10 kg or less resulted in 1 or more interventions, compared with 61 of the 152 (40%) and 15 of the 76 (20%) routine chest radiographs obtained in patients who weighed 10 to 40 kg and 40 kg or more, respectively. The frequency of interventions increased from 19% in patients with no devices to more than 50% in children with 2 or more devices. Of patients with no active cardiopulmonary problems, 27% required 1 or more interventions as a result of findings on chest radiographs, compared with 51% of patients with active cardiopulmonary problems. Diagnosis and length of ICU stay at the time routine chest radiographs were obtained did not affect the percentage of chest radiographs that resulted in interventions.

Conclusion.—Interventions were most likely to occur as a result of findings on routine chest radiographs in the smaller, critically ill child with 1 or more devices and if active cardiopulmonary problems were present.

▶ The conclusion of this study is consistent with most intensivists' practice and most of the peer-reviewed literature. Amazingly, in children weighing 10 kg or less, daily chest x-rays (CXRs) result in an intervention 55% of the time. The most common intervention was adjustment of the endotracheal tube followed by changes in physiotherapy and then changes in diuretic therapy. In an era of cost-containment, the routine daily CXRs is undergoing scrutiny. However information gained by this procedure probably lessens cost by allowing conditions, some potentially devastating, from advancing to a greater degree of seriousness, thus worsening clinical outcome and re-sources being used. The risk of performing a CXR in the critically ill must be considered but has been at an acceptable level up to now (less than 1% in this study). A prospective randomized study evaluating daily CXRs versus CXRs ordered because of a clinical change would be informative.

J. D. Lang, Jr, MD

**Energy Metabolism of Infants and Children With Systemic Inflamma-
tory Response Syndrome and Sepsis**
Turi RA, Petros AJ, Eaton S, et al (Univ College London)
Ann Surg 233:581-587, 2001   8–45

Introduction.—Investigations in adults with sepsis have demonstrated increased energy expenditure and mobilization of endogenous fat. Energy metabolism and substrate utilization during sepsis have never been characterized in infants or children. Critically ill children with systemic inflammatory response syndrome (SIRS) or sepsis were evaluated to determine whether they experience altered resting energy expenditure (REE) or substrate utilization.

Methods.—Twenty-one critically ill children with SIRS or sepsis underwent metabolic evaluations and were matched for weight with 21 stable control children. Seven patients needed inotropic support and 17 underwent mechanical ventilation. Fifteen patients with SIRS had evidence of bacterial, fungal, or viral infection and were considered to have sepsis. Respiratory gas exchange was measured with the use of computerized indirect calorimetry for 1 to 2 hours continuously.

Results.—The REE of patients with SIRS or sepsis was similar to that of controls. There were no differences in carbon dioxide production and oxygen consumption. Resting energy metabolism was similar in patients with SIRS and those with sepsis. In addition, the presence of a low platelet count or the need for inotropic support did not affect resting energy metabolism. The median respiratory quotient of patients with SIRS or sepsis was 0.88 (range, 0.75-1.12), suggesting mixed utilization of fat and carbohydrates; this did not differ significantly from controls (Fig 1). The Pediatric Risk of Mortality Score was not significantly associated with REE or the respiratory quotient.

Conclusion.—Children with SIRS or sepsis do not have increased energy requirements. The resting metabolism for children is based on both car-

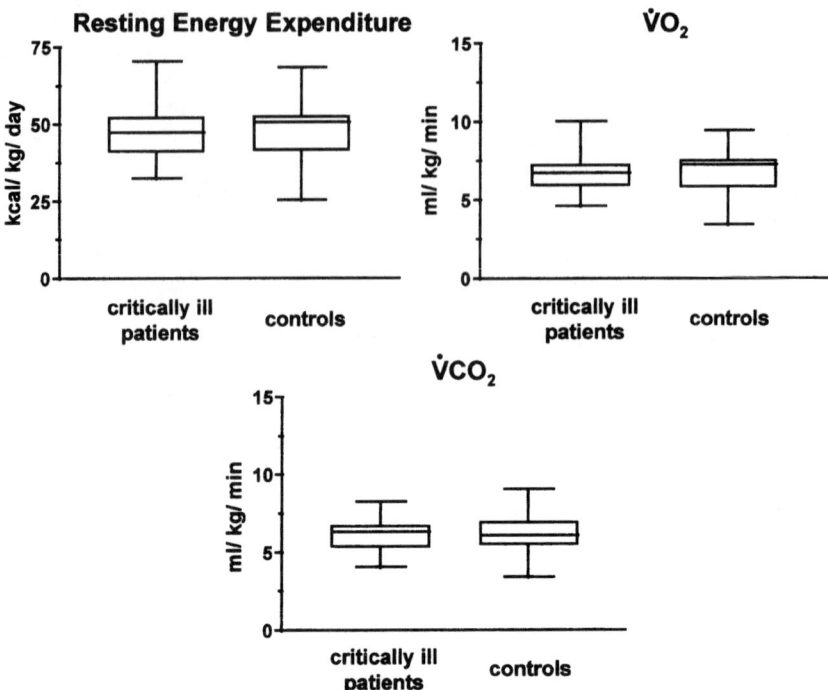

FIGURE 1.—Respiratory gas exchange in critically ill patients and controls. Indirect calorimetry was performed on critically ill patients (n = 21) and control patients matched for weight (n = 21). Resting energy expenditure, oxygen consumption (VO_2), and carbon dioxide production (VCO_2) were calculated. There were no significant differences between critically ill patients and controls for resting energy expenditure (P = .828), VO_2 (P = .828), or VCO_2 (P = .993). Results are expressed as median, range, and interquartile range (Wilcoxon matched pairs test). (Courtesy of Turi RA, Petros AJ, Eaton S, et al: Energy metabolism of infants and children with systemic inflammatory response syndrome and sepsis. *Ann Surg* 233:581-587, 2001.)

bohydrate and fat utilization. It may be that these children divert the energy for growth into recovery processes.

▶ The overall net effect of nutrition in critically ill patients is still unknown. One circumstance that does appear deleterious is the effect of overfeeding on pulmonary dynamics, especially during the period of ventilator weaning. In addition, other vital organ systems such as the liver, especially if dysfunctional, can incur an additional insult from nutritional supplementation. Deriving the appropriate caloric requirements for adult patients with SIRS, sepsis, severe sepsis, and septic shock is extremely challenging and if using indirect calorimetery can be extremely variable; however, the derived caloric requirement is generally higher than that for the nonstressed adult. In this study, the authors have demonstrated that children's energy requirements differ significantly from those of their parents but not from those of their non-stressed playmates, and must therefore be supplemented accordingly.

J. D. Lang, Jr, MD

9 Other Perioperative Patient Care Issues

Effects of Preoperative Warming on the Incidence of Wound Infection After Clean Surgery: A Randomised Controlled Trial
Melling AC, Ali B, Scott EM, et al (Univ Hosp of North Tees, Stockton-on-Tees, England)
Lancet 358:876-880, 2001

9–1

Purpose.—Wound infection after "clean" surgery is an expensive problem that may be more common than generally thought. Among patients undergoing colorectal surgery, patient warming reduces the risk of infection. The effects of warming on infection rates in patients undergoing brief, clean surgical procedures were investigated.

Methods.—The randomized trial included 421 patients undergoing various short-duration, clean surgical procedures, including breast, varicose vein, and hernia surgery. Patients were assigned to undergo either local or systemic warming instituted at least 30 minutes before the operation or no preoperative warming. Infection rates and wound scores were assessed at 2 and 6 weeks' follow-up.

Results.—The wound infection rate was 5% in the warmed groups versus 14% in the nonwarmed group (Table 3). Warming was also associated with lower wound scores. Rates of hematoma and seroma were similar with and without warming. Patients in the nonwarmed group were significantly more likely to receive postoperative antibiotics. Breast surgery

TABLE 3.—The Effects of Warming Therapies Compared With Standard Treatment

	Systemic Warming	Local Warming
Absolute risk reduction (95% CI)	7·9% (1·0-14·8)	10·1% (3·6-16·6)
Relative risk reduction	57·7%	73·7%
Numbers needed to treat relative to the standard treatment	15 patients	10 patients

TABLE 4.—Characteristics of Patient by Wound Infection

	Wound Infection (n=32)	Non-wound Infection (n=384)
Age (years)*	48·06 (13·47)	49·96 (14·48)
Body mass index (kg)*	28·04 (5·44)	25·51 (3·98)
Male/female	12/20	162/222
Smokers	11 (34%)	118 (31%)
Type of surgery		
Breast	18 (56%)	157 (41%)
Hernia	10 (31%)	145 (38%)
Varicose veins	4 (13%)	82 (21%)
Previous surgery	3 (9%)	29 (8%)
(in the last 3 months)		
Cancer diagnosis	11 (34%)	106 (28%)
Shaving times†		
Didn't shave	9 (28%)	101 (27%)
Within 7 h	6 (19%)	110 (30%)
7 h or more	17 (53%)	166 (44%)
Fasting times‡		
8 h or less	23 (72%)	250 (67%)
More than 8 h	9 (28%)	125 (33%)
Theatre		
Day case unit	30 (94%)	330 (86%)
Main theatre	2 (6%)	54 (14%)
Initial core temperature (°C)*	36·7 (0·55)	36·6 (0·53)
Postwarming temperature (°C)*	36·9 (0·28)	36·9 (0·58)
Postoperative temperature (°C)*	36·6 (0·66)	36·4 (0·59)
Prophylactic antibiotics	6 (19%)	115 (30%)
Operation time*	51·3 (18·5)	48·69 (17·4)
Seniority of surgeon§		
Senior house officer	12 (38%)	175 (51%)
Registrar	17 (53%)	136 (40%)
Consultant	3 (9%)	31 (9%)

*Values are mean (SD).
†Data missing for 7 patients.
‡Data missing for 9 patients.
§Data missing for 42 patients.
(Courtesy of Melling AC, Ali B, Scott EM, et al: Effects of preoperative warming on the incidence of wound infection after clean surgery: A randomized controlled trial. *Lancet* 358:876-880, 2001. Copyright by The Lancet Ltd, 2001.)

had a higher rate of wound infection than did hernia surgery or varicose vein surgery (Table 4).

Conclusion.—Among patients undergoing brief, clean surgical procedures, preoperative warming is associated with a lower postoperative infection rate. With further study, preoperative warming could become a safe and effective alternative to prophylactic antibiotics in this group of patients.

▶ Relatively simple treatments can have profound effects. Further studies are needed—but as the authors say, preoperative warming might provide an alternative to prophylactic antibiotics for specific types of surgery.

M. Wood, MD, FRCA

Vasopressin Versus Epinephrine for Inhospital Cardiac Arrest: A Randomised Controlled Trial

Stiell IG, Hébert PC, Wells GA, et al (Univ of Ottawa, Ontario, Canada; Univ of Western Ontario, London, Canada; Univ of Alberta, Edmonton, Canada)
Lancet 358:105-109, 2001   9–2

Background.—High doses of epinephrine and other adrenergic agents do little to improve survival rates after cardiac arrest. Some evidence suggests that vasopressin may improve survival rates when used in the out-of-hospital setting. Whether vasopressin is an effective and safe alternative to epinephrine for the treatment of in-hospital cardiac arrest was studied in a prospective trial.

Methods.—The research subjects were 200 patients with in-hospital cardiac arrest who were treated according to the American Heart Association Advanced Cardiac Life Support protocols. None of the research subjects had cardiac arrest secondary to obvious exsanguination or had cardiac arrest before arrival at the hospital or in the operating, recovery, or delivery rooms. Patients were randomly assigned to receive either one 40-U dose of IV vasopressin (n = 104; 63% men; mean age, 70 years) or one 1-mg dose of IV epinephrine (n = 96; 64% men; mean age, 70 years) at the point during the Advanced Cardiac Life Support protocol when epinephrine is first indicated. Patients who did not respond with a return of pulse after the initial dose of vasopressin or epinephrine were then given 1-mg doses of epinephrine every 3 to 5 minutes. Differences in survival to hospital discharge, in survival to 1 hour after discontinuation of resuscitation, and in neurologic function between the vasopressin and epinephrine groups were examined. Differences in survival were also examined according to age (≤70 or >70 years old), cause of cardiac arrest, and initial cardiac rhythm.

Results.—The mean time from collapse to administration of the study drug was 6.1 minutes and was similar in both groups. Baseline clinical and

TABLE 3.—Survival and Adverse Outcomes

Outcome Measure	Vasopressin (n=104)	Epinephrine (n=96)	p	Percentage Absolute Difference (95% CI)
Primary survival measures				
1 h	40 (39%)	34 (35%)	0·66	3·1 (−10·5 to 17·3)
Hospital discharge	12 (12%)	13 (14%)	0·67	−2·0 (−11·6 to 7·8)
Other survival measures				
Any return of pulse	62 (60%)	57 (59%)	0·97	0·2 (−14·0 to 14·5)
Pulse >20 min	45 (43%)	38 (40%)	0·60	3·7 (−10·6 to 17·9)
24 h	27 (26%)	23 (24%)	0·74	2·0 (−10·6 to 14·6)
30 days	13 (13%)	13 (14%)	0·83	−1·0 (−11·0 to 8·9)
Adverse outcomes				
Tachyarrhythmias	10 (10%)	8 (8%)	0·75	1·3 (−7·2 to 9·8)
Uncontrolled hypertension	0	0		
Mesenteric infarction	0	0		

(Courtesy of Stiell IG, Hébert PC, Wells GA, et al: Vasopressin versus epinephrine for inhospital cardiac arrest: A randomized controlled trial. *Lancet* 358:105-109, 2001. Copyright by the Lancet Ltd, 2001.)

demographic variables were also similar between the vasopressin and epinephrine groups. Primary and secondary survival measures did not differ significantly between the 2 groups (Table 3). Subgroup analyses could identify no significant differences in survival based on age, cause of cardiac arrest, or initial rhythm. No differences were found in adverse events or in neurologic function between the vasopressin and epinephrine groups, as determined by Mini-Mental State Examination (median scores, 36 vs 35, respectively) and cerebral performance category (median score, 1 vs 1).

Conclusions.—Vasopressin administration did not provide a survival advantage over epinephrine in these patients with cardiac arrest, neither for the group as a whole nor for subgroups based on cause of arrest, initial rhythm, or age. Thus, these findings do not support the use of vasopressin as an alternative to epinephrine for patients with in-hospital cardiac arrest.

▶ A tremendous interest exists in the use of vasopressin as a vasopressor in the management of cardiac arrest. Recently, the American Heart Association added vasopressin to their guidelines for treatment of cardiac arrest. This randomized, controlled trial fails to provide support for their recommendation.

M. Wood, MD, FRCA

Ischemic Optic Neuropathy After Liver Transplantation
Janicki PK, Pai R, Wright JK, et al (Vanderbilt Univ, Nashville, Tenn)
Anesthesiology 94:361-363, 2001   9–3

Background.—The most commonly reported cause of sudden, devastating postoperative visual loss is anterior ischemic optic neuropathy (ION), which occurs as a result of decreased delivery of oxygen to the optic nerves. Previous reports have described postoperative blindness in association with pressure-induced eye injury, arterial hypotension, low hematocrit concentration, and obstruction of venous outflow. Superior vena cava syndrome (SVCS), one reported cause of venous obstruction, is an uncommon complication of liver transplantation in patients with a history of central venous thrombosis, indwelling catheters, or peritoneovenous shunts. A case of ION after liver transplantation was described.

> *Case Report.*—Man, 43, with hepatitis C cirrhosis and intractable ascites, and a history of repeated placement of peritoneojugular shunts and placement of a transjugular intrahepatic portosystemic shunt underwent liver transplantation. Insertion of peripheral, larger bore catheters was unsuccessful because of poor peripheral venous access. Central lines were placed after several attempts. Large-bore intravenous catheters ultimately were inserted into both internal jugular veins and the subclavian veins. An oximetric pulmonary artery catheter was placed through the right

internal jugular catheter. The procedure was uneventful until the third hour, when it was terminated because malignancy within the donor organ was identified on postmortem examination. During closure, the previously placed, nonfunctional peritoneojugular shunt was removed by sliding the venous end from the subcostal incision. Swelling and cyanosis were subsequently noted on the patient's face and neck. In the ICU, the patient's face became significantly edematous and cyanotic, and a diagnosis of acute SVCS was made. Three of 4 larger bore catheters were removed. Doppler studies revealed total occlusion of both subclavian veins and the left and right internal jugular veins, as well as a clot in the superior vena cava. A second liver transplant procedure was performed uneventfully, during which the blood loss was estimated to be about 6 L. The patient received 12 L of crystalloids, 1 L of albumin 5%, 13 units of packed erythrocytes, 10 units of fresh-frozen plasma, and 20 units of platelets. The postoperative course was initially uneventful, but on the fourth postoperative day the patient indicated that he could not see. The patient subsequently received a diagosis of bilateral anterior ION. He was discharged on postoperative day 21 with resolving SVCS and complete bilateral blindness.

Conclusions.—Postoperative anterior ION results from decreased oxygen delivery from multiple causes. Usually, postoperative anterior ION is associated with hypotension and blood loss, but often other variables, such as venous obstruction or vascular abnormalities, are contributing factors. In a recent study of 350 patients who experienced massive trauma, anterior ION developed in 2.6% of patients, with a significant association of ION with massive fluid resuscitation and prolonged ventilatory support. Most of these patients were placed in the supine position.

▶ ION and postoperative blindness are rarely reported, but there is a recognition that it is perhaps more common than we once realized. Although we can identify what we think are precipitating factors, the etiology is really not known.

M. Wood, MD, FRCA

Volume Standards for High-Risk Surgical Procedures: Potential Benefits of the Leapforg Initiative
Birkmeyer JD, Finlayson EVA, Birkmeyer CM, et al (Dartmouth-Hitchcock Med Ctr, Lebanon, NH; Univ of California, San Francisco)
Surgery 130:415-422, 2001   9–4

Background.—As part of a broader effort aimed at improving hospital safety, a large coalition of employers, the Leapfrog Group, will soon require hospitals caring for their employees to meet volume standards for

TABLE 2.—Projected In-hospital Mortality Rates With 5 Procedures at Low-Volume (LVHs) and High-Volume (HVHs) Hospitals

Procedure	Overall Mortality	Relative Risk of Mortality (LVH vs HVH)	Projected In-Hospital Mortality HVH	LVH
CABG	2.9%	1.38	2.4%*	3.3%*
Coronary angioplasty	1.0%	1.33	0.9%*	1.2%*
Elective AAA repair	4.9%	1.60	4.2%	6.7%
CEA	0.6%	1.28	0.5%*	0.7%*
Esophagectomy	14%	3.01	5.9%	15.8%

*"Back-calculated" from estimates of overall mortality rate (above), relative risks of mortality at LVHs and HVHs, and estimated distribution of patients at LVHs and HVHs.
(Courtesy of Birkmeyer JD, Finlayson EVA, Birkmeyer CM: Volume Standards for high-risk surgical procedures: Potential benefits of the Leapfrog initiative. *Surgery* 130:415-422, 2001.)

5 high-risk surgical procedures. We estimated the potential benefits of full nationwide implementation of these volume standards.

Methods.—Using data from Nationwide Inpatient Sample and other sources, we first estimated the total number of each of the 5 procedures— coronary-artery bypass graft, abdominal aortic aneurysm repair, coronary angioplasty, esophagectomy, and carotid endarterectomy—performed each year in hospitals in US metropolitan areas. (Leapfrog exempts hospitals in rural areas to avoid issues.) We then projected the effectiveness of volume standards (in terms of relative risks of mortality) for each procedure using data from a published structured literature review (Table 2).

Results.—With full implementation nationwide, the Leapfrog volume standards would save 2581 lives. Of the procedures, volume standards would save the most lives with coronary-artery bypass graft (1486), followed by abdominal aortic-aneurysm repair (464), coronary angioplasty (345), esophagectomy (168), and carotid endarterectomy (118) (Fig 2). In our estimates of the number of lives saved, we considered assumptions about how many patients would be affected and the effectiveness of volume standards (ie, strength of underlying volume-outcome relationships with each procedure).

Conclusios.—If the Leapfrog volume standards are successfully implemented, employers and health-care purchasers could prevent many surgical deaths by requiring hospital volume standards for high-risk procedures (Table 4).

▶ The Leapfrog Group safety initiative will have impact on anesthesiologists more than they expect! To care for leapfrog employees, hospitals will be required to meet 3 safety standards: (1) computerized order entry, (2) intensive care units staffed by full-time intensivists, and (3) volume standards as outlined in this manuscript.

M. Wood, MD, FRCA

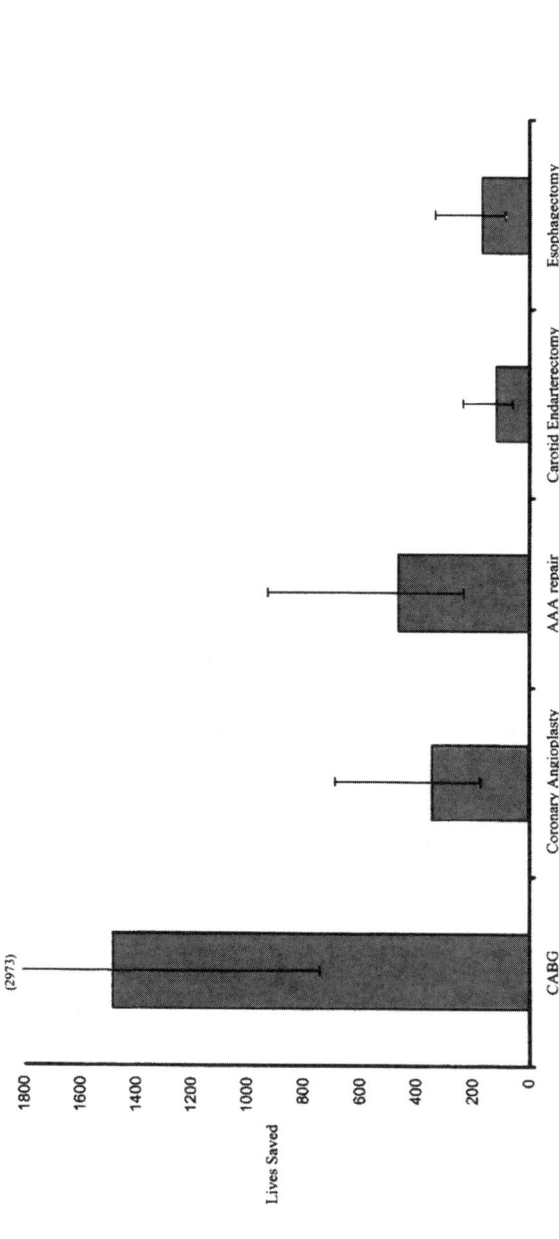

FIGURE 2.—Number of lives saved by Leapfrog volume standards for 5 procedures according to excess mortality at low-volume hospitals. *Shaded columns* indicate projected lives saved from baseline estimates. *Error bars* indicate projected lives saved in sensitivity analysis when excess mortality estimate is varied from 50% to 200% of our baseline estimate. (Courtesy of Birkmeyer JD, Finlayson EVA, Birkmeyer CM: Volume standards for high-risk surgical procedures: Potential benefits of the Leapfrog Initiative. *Surgery* 130:415-422, 2001.)

TABLE 4.—Summary of Volume-Outcome Studies of Procedures Selected for Inclusion by Leapfrog Group, as Summarized by Dudley et al

Procedure	Total	Number of Studies			
		High Volume SS* Better	NS† Trend Toward High Volume Better	NS† Trend Toward High Volume Worse	High Volume SS* Worse
CABG	11	9	2	0	0
Coronary angioplasty	6	6	0	0	0
Elective AAA repair	9	9	0	0	0
CEA	9	6	3	0	0
Esophagectomy	2	2	0	0	0

*Statistically significant.
†Not significant.
(Courtesy of Birkmeyer JD, Finlayson EVA, Birkmeyer CM: Volume standards for high-risk surgical procedures: Potential benefits of the Leapfrog initiative. *Surgery* 130:415-422, 2001.)

How Much Are Patients Willing to Pay to Avoid Postoperative Nausea and Vomiting?

Gan TJ, Sloan F, de L Dear G, et al (Duke Univ, Durham, NC)
Anesth Analg 92:393-400, 2001   9–5

Background.—Much has been written about the benefits of newer drugs introduced in anesthesia in terms of the physiologic and pharmacologic responses in patients. However, much less is known regarding the value that patients put on the benefits of these new drugs. Postoperative nausea and vomiting are frequent occurrences after surgery, and no drug used in anesthesia is completely effective in preventing postoperative nausea and vomiting. But how important is the absence of postoperative nausea and vomiting to patients? Several studies have indicated that beyond ranking the absence of postoperative nausea and vomiting as important, patients rate it as more important than earlier discharge from an ambulatory surgical unit. Cost-benefit analysis was used to evaluate the hypothesis that patients are willing to pay for an antiemetic agent that would prevent postoperative nausea and vomiting, and that the willingness to pay is related to the demographic characteristics of the patient.

Methods.—Participants included 80 elective day surgical patients. After recovery in the postanesthesia care unit, the patients completed an interactive computer questionnaire regarding demographic data, the value they placed on avoiding postoperative nausea and vomiting, and their willingness to pay for an antiemetic.

Results.—Patients indicated an overall willingness to pay an average of $56 (range, $26-$97) for an antiemetic agent that would completely prevent postoperative nausea and vomiting. Patients who had developed nausea and vomiting postoperatively were willing to pay a higher price ($73 and $100, respectively). Avoidance of nausea and vomiting was ranked as important by 76% and 78% of patients, respectively. Several independent covariates were found to increase the willingness to pay, including the experience of nausea or vomiting in the postanesthetic care unit, a higher patient income, a history of postoperative nausea or vomiting, increasing age, and being married.

Conclusions.—Postoperative nausea and vomiting are unpleasant experiences that patients are willing to pay to avoid. Patients are willing to pay from $56 to $100 for an antiemetic that is completely effective.

▶ In the days when hospitals are cost cutting, and administrators prefer the use of droperidol to a more expensive 5-hydroxytryptamine receptor antagonist, this is a small but interesting study that attempts to put a cost on the prevention of postoperative nausea and vomiting from the patient's perspective.

M. Wood, MD, FRCA

Meta-Analysis of Low Molecular Weight Heparin in the Prevention of Venous Thromboembolism in General Surgery

Mismetti P, Laporte S, Darmon J-Y, et al (Univ Hosp, Saint-Etienne, France; Medibridge Clinical Research, Velizy, France)
Br J Surg 88:913-930, 2001   9–6

Background.—The use of low molecular weight heparins (LMWHs) has been justified by their ability to reduce the incidence of deep vein thrombosis (DVT), which may provide prophylaxis against venous thromboembolism (VTE). However, this is not certain; therefore, reevaluation of the role of LMWH was indicated. This assessment focused on the actual clinical effect of LMWHs, the magnitude of their effect in comparison to that of unfractionated heparin (UFH), and the optimal dose to achieve prophylactic importance.

Methods.—Data were obtained through an exhaustive literature search that identified all open-label, single- or double-blind randomized studies of LMWH that used a control group. The incidence of DVT detected systematically at the end of treatment using ultrasonography, fibrinogen uptake testing, impedance plethysmography, thermography, or venography was the primary end point, with a secondary emphasis on the incidence of symptomatic pulmonary embolism (PE), symptomatic VTE, death, major hemorrhage, wound hematoma or other hemorrhage, and percent of patients who needed transfusions postoperatively. Two meta-analyses and two sensitivity analyses were performed.

Results.—From 1984 to 1999, 82 studies were identified that dealt with the effect of LMWH prophylaxis; 59 met the study criteria. In comparing LMWHs to placebo or no treatment, systematically detected DVT carried an adjusted incidence of 14.5%, the incidence of PE was 0.5%, clinical VTE was 0.9%, and death was 0.0%. The risk of DVT was reduced 72% in those receiving LMWHs compared to the placebo or no treatment group, with a reduction of 75% for PE, 71% for VTE, and 46% for overall mortality. Hemorrhage occurred more frequently in patients on LMWHs. The comparison of LMWHs and UFH showed that the incidence of systematically detected DVT was 5.0%, clinical PE was 0.4%, clinical VTE was 1.3%, and death was 1.7%. The reduction in risk of DVT achieved with LMWHs was only 10% and that for PE, 12%. Clinical VTE was significantly reduced; death remained the same. The incidence of major hemorrhage in the UFH patients was 3.2% and that of wound hematoma, 6.1%; the reduction achieved with LMWHs did not reach significance. In double-blind studies, LMWHs had an advantage over UFH in both efficacy and safety. In cancer surgery the safety and efficacy of LMWHs and UFH were similar. Comparing low and high prophylactic dose regimens of LMWHs and UFH showed no significant increase in risk reduction with low doses of LMWHs, although risk of hemorrhage, particularly major hemorrhage, was reduced over the use of UFH. High-dose LMWHs had greater effectiveness than UFH, especially in the prophylaxis of PE. However, the risk of hemorrhage increased with the higher dose, especially the risk of major hemorrhage.

Conclusions.—The use of LMWHs was at least as effective and safe as the use of UFH in prophylaxis for venous thromboembolism. The optimal dose to be used is yet to be determined.

▶ LMWHs are frequently used to prevent venous thromboembolism in general surgery—but are they effective? This metaanalysis shows that they are as effective and as safe as unfractionated heparin. The discussion in this article is informative and outlines the adverse effects of LMWHS.

M. Wood, MD, FRCA

10 Complications and Mishaps in Anesthesia

Perioperative Complications After Living Donor Lobectomy
Battafarano RJ, Anderson RC, Meyers BF, et al (Washington Univ, St Louis)
J Thorac Cardiovasc Surg 120:909-915, 2000   10–1

Background.—The availability of suitable cadaveric donor lungs has not kept pace with the increasing need for donor lungs in the management of patients with end-stage pulmonary disease requiring lung transplantation. In 1998, 498 patients died while awaiting cadaveric lung transplants. Most of these patients had inflammatory lung diseases such as cystic fibrosis and pulmonary fibrosis. The technique of living donor lobectomy has been developed to meet this need for donor lungs. In living donor lobectomy, right and left lower lobes are obtained from a pair of living donors. An experience with living donor lobectomy from July 1994 to February 2000 was reviewed.

Methods.—A total of 62 donor lobectomies were performed during this period. Hospital and outpatient records from these donors were retrospectively analyzed for the incidence of perioperative complications.

Results.—No perioperative complications occurred in 24 of 62 donors (38.7%). These 24 had a median hospital stay of 5.0 days. Postoperative complications occurred in 38 of 62 donors (61.3%). Ten patients had 12 major complications, including pleural effusions necessitating drainage (4 patients); bronchial stump fistulas (3 patients); bilobectomy (1 patient); and hemorrhaging requiring red cell transfusion, phrenic nerve injury, and bronchial stricture requiring dilatation (1 patient each). Among the 38 donors with postoperative complications, 9 donors each had persistent air leaks and pericarditis; 8 donors had pneumonia; 7 donors had arrhythmia; 3 donors each had atelectasis, ileus, and subcutaneous emphysema; 2 donors each had urinary tract infections, loculated pleural effusions, and transfusion; and 1 donor each had colitis as a result of *Clostridium difficile* infection, puncture of a saline breast implant, and severe contact dermatitis secondary to adhesive tape. No postoperative deaths occurred, and only 1 donor required reoperation.

Conclusion.—Living donor lobectomy will continue to be a significant alternative for potential recipients of lung transplants who cannot wait for cadaveric lung allografts. The procedure can be performed with low mortality; however, the morbidity rate is high, and this must be taken into consideration during counseling of potential living donors.

▶ I knew that if living donor lobectomy were ever done, it would be done at Washington University in St Louis by the Cooper group. However, I was surprised to find that living donor lobectomy was being performed. Clearly, the currently available numbers of suitable cadaveric donors for lungs are not great enough to meet the increased needs of patients with end-stage pulmonary disease requiring lung transplantation. The authors state that more than 498 patients died while awaiting lung transplants in 1998. In this operation, a pair of donor lobes was transplanted into pediatric recipients. These lung lobes are usually taken from family members. The pediatric recipients have cystic fibrosis in the vast majority of cases. Those interested in learning about how this operation is done, in terms of removing the lobes—also note, the significant rate of complications—can read this article. That pericarditis and pneumonia are listed as minor complications says something about the risk of serious complications. On the other hand, if you were a parent and your child was going to die and this operation was available to you, these risks may seem minimal.

M. F. Roizen, MD

Breakage of Epidural Catheters: A Comparison of an Arrow Reinforced Catheter and Other Nonreinforced Catheters

Asai T, Yamamoto K, Hirose T, et al (Kansai Med Univ, Osaka, Japan)
Anesth Analg 92:246-248, 2001   10–2

Introduction.—Advantages of the Arrow reinforced epidural catheter over conventional nonreinforced catheters include ease of insertion and an infrequent incidence of associated paresthesias and epidural vein cannulation. In this case, an Arrow catheter broke during removal.

> *Case Report.*—A woman, 57, was scheduled for total knee arthroplasty. A 19-gauge undamaged Arrow catheter was passed easily through a 17-gauge Arrow Tuohy needle into the L3-4 epidural space. The catheter was used successfully for anesthesia and for postoperative analgesia. On the fourth day after surgery, removal of the catheter proved difficult. Although the catheter was removed with additional traction, its distal part was missing. The inner metal coil, however, remained attached to the withdrawn catheter segment. The metal coil was easily pulled from the patient's body and the catheter tip surgically removed with local anesthesia.

Methods.—The problem encountered in this case prompted an ex vivo examination of the strength of the Arrow reinforced epidural catheter, particularly of the segment between the 7- and 8-cm marks where the density of the inner stainless steel coil changes and where an intact catheter makes a natural curve. The Arrow catheter and 3 types of 19-gauge non-reinforced catheters were evaluated using a weight and a scale for degree of stretching, force required to snap the catheter, and site of breakage.

Results and Discussion.—Compared with the other 3 catheters, the Arrow catheter stretched significantly more and snapped at a significantly lower weight. All catheters snapped at the fixed site or pulling site, never between. The incidence of breakage of epidural catheters during removal is not known. During several years of use, the authors reported 1 case of breakage and 3 other cases of difficult removal of the Arrow catheter. Because the patient's body movements may relieve a trapped catheter, one should reattempt removal 30 to 60 minutes later and avoid pulling the catheter forcefully.

▶ This study study, is an excellent technology assessment study. These authors use the Arrow catheter routinely in their practice, but in an analysis of their data clearly found that the Arrow catheter had a higher breakage rate and broke at a lower tension that did other non-reinforced catheters. The authors also give us a take-home message: they suggest that if there is difficultly in removing the catheter, one should avoid pulling the catheter forcefully and should reattempt removal 30 to 60 minutes later. They postulate that success with this technique occurred because the patient's body movements during those 30 to 60 minutes fortuitously relieved trapped catheters. While that postulate is supported by their case reports, there is no other support for it.

M. F. Roizen, MD

Medication Errors in Anesthetic Practice: A Survey of 687 Practitioners
Orser BA, Chen RJB, Yee DA (Univ of Toronto)
Can J Anesth 48:139-146, 2001   10–3

Background.—It is estimated that 180,000 hospitalized patients in the United States die each year as a result of adverse medical events, and the major contributing factor is medication error. Deaths from medical errors in this country are thus higher annually than the mortality from automobile collisions (45,000). Beyond the human cost, these adverse drug events place a significant financial burden on health care systems. At one institution, the annual cost of medication-related problems was estimated at $1.5 million. Effective strategies are needed to reduce medication error and enhance patient safety and lower costs. The incidence of medication error associated with anesthetic practice is not known, but there is a potential for disastrous errors, given the potency, variety, and frequency of the drugs administered to patients undergoing anesthesia. Anesthesiologists in Canada were surveyed to determine how many had experienced a medication error and to identify the causal factors. In addition, the perceived value of a Canadian reporting agency for medication errors and improved standards for labels on drug ampules was investigated.

Methods.—A survey was mailed to 2266 members of the Canadian Anesthesiologists' Society. Respondents answered fixed-response questions and described medication errors.

Results.—The response rate was 30% (687 anesthesiologists). Responses indicated that 85% of the participants had experienced at least one drug error or "near miss." Most errors (98%) had minor consequences, but 4 deaths were reported. The error most commonly reported involved the administration of muscle relaxants instead of a reversal agent. Common contributing factors were syringe swaps (70.4%) and label misidentification (46.8%). Most of the respondents (97.9%) indicated that they read the ampule label "most of the time," but the color of the label was an important secondary cue. About half of the respondents indicated that they would report the error if a reporting program existed, and most of the respondents (84%) indicated agreement that improved standards for drug labels would help to reduce the incidence of medication errors.

Conclusions.—Most of the anesthesiologists responding to this survey experienced at least 1 drug error. The most common error involved a syringe swap in which a muscle relaxant was administered instead of a reversal agent. These findings are supportive of the need for the improvement of standards for drug labels and the establishment of reporting agencies for medication errors.

▶ One wonders when bar-coding will be common and techniques to prevent drug errors and wrong drug administration will gain acceptance. But clearly "syringe swaps" and the misidentification of the label are the most common causes of problems now.

M. F. Roizen, MD

Anterior Spinal Artery Syndrome Following Total Hip Arthroplasty Under Epidural Anaesthesia
Hong DK, Lawrence HM (Canberra Hosp, Australia)
Anaesth Intensive Care 29:62-66, 2001   10–4

Background.—Anterior spinal artery syndrome is a rare, devastating condition caused by inadequate blood supply to the spinal cord through the spinal artery. The syndrome is characterized by paralysis and loss of bowel and bladder function, with intact or impaired sensory function. Anterior spinal artery syndrome has been reported to occur spontaneously and after both general and regional anesthesia. A case of anterior spinal artery syndrome after lumbar epidural anesthesia for total hip arthroplasty was reported. The possible etiologies of anterior spinal artery syndrome in patients undergoing regional anesthesia were discussed.

Case Report.—Man, 57, with osteoarthritis was to undergo left total hip arthroplasty. His weight at presentation was 100 kg. The patient's medical history was negative for ischemic heart disease, peripheral vascular disease, hypertension, and diabetes. He wore a brace for scoliosis for 4 years as an adolescent. On examination his lumbar spine was straight, but preoperative lumbar radiography showed osteophyte formation, generalized disk space narrowing, mild scoliosis, and evidence of old Scheuermann's disease. The patient was taking no medications and had no known allergies. His preoperative blood pressure was 150/80 mm Hg, and his preoperative hemoglobin, electrolytes, and creatinine levels and chest radiography and ECG findings were normal. Epidural anesthesia was initiated, and the patient was positioned on his right side with padding under the chest, head, and neck. Oxygen was delivered via Hudson mask at 5 L/min, and the patient was lightly sedated with a total dose of midazolam of 5 mg during the operation. An additional 5 mL of lignocaine with adrenaline was administered after movement of the operative leg early in the procedure. The surgery was uneventful and concluded about 1 hour after placement of the epidural anesthesia. Blood loss was less than 300 mL. The patient's systolic blood pressure remained greater than 100 mm Hg throughout the procedure, but there were 2 brief periods of hypertension lasting less than 5 minutes. In each instance, the hypotension responded to boluses of intravenous fluid. Two liters of crystalloid solution and 500 mL of gelatin-based colloid were administered intraoperatively. The patient was moved to the recovery room free of pain and with slight movement of his right leg. The patient had good analgesia 7 hours after surgery. All movement in both lower limbs was absent with the exception of weak flexion and extension in the right ankle. The patient had normal touch sensation, and the prolonged motor block was attributed to the initial dose of local anesthetic. The infusion of bupivacaine 0.125% with 5 μg/mL fentanyl, which had commenced postoperatively at 10 mL/h, was continued. The epidural infusion was discontinued at 24 hours because the patient's neurologic status was unchanged. An MRI at that time showed no sign of epidural hematoma or abscess. No other anatomic cause for his paralysis was evident. Motor responses were bilaterally absent below T12, except for profound weakness of ankle flexion and extension on the right, and there was loss of bowel and bladder sphincter function. A second MRI at 48 hours postoperatively indicated an abnormal signal within the spinal cord from the level of T8 to the conus, a sign that was consistent with infarction. A diagnosis of anterior spinal artery syndrome was made. The patient had no recovery of motor function and remained paralyzed 9 months after surgery.

Conclusions.—Paraplegia after epidural anesthesia is a rare complication. It is easy to incriminate regional anesthesia in such a case, but complications attributed to epidural anesthesia may result from preexisting neurologic or vascular disease that was not detected before surgery.

► I chose this devastating case report to highlight the fact that this syndrome does still occur after general and regional anesthesia. Many times the distinguishing etiology cannot be identified—and this is a major cause for concern.

M. Wood, MD, FRCA

North American Malignant Hyperthermia Population: Screening of the Ryanodine Receptor Gene and Identification of Novel Mutations
Sambuughin N, Sei Y, Gallagher KL, et al (Barrow Neurological Inst, Phoenix, Ariz; Wake Forest Univ, Winston-Salem, NC; Trinity Communications Inc, Conshohocken, Pa; et al)
Anesthesiology 95:594-599, 2001   10–5

Background.—Malignant hyperthermia (MH) occurs in susceptible individuals after they are exposed to inhalational anesthetics and succinylcholine and is noted in 1 of 15,000 anesthetic administrations in children and in 1 of 50,000 anesthetic administrations in adults. Inheritance is as an autosomal dominant trait with reduced penetrance; typically the patient does not appear abnormal until the exposure occurs, so the diagnosis of MH before surgical problems occur is difficult. A common cause of MH involves mutations of the gene that encodes for the skeletal muscle ryanodine receptor, and more than 20 of these mutations have been identified, plus some are expressed as central core disease. The main targets for mutation screening of patients with MH are the N-terminal and the central regions of the ryanodine receptor. A systematic screening of the ryanodine receptor gene was carried out among a population of MH patients in North America.

Methods.—Samples of skeletal muscle were obtained from 73 persons susceptible to MH as determined by the North American MH caffeine-halothane contracture test. Mutational analysis was carried out, screening the genomic DNA using polymerase chain reaction-based restriction fragment length polymorphism, single-strand conformation polymorphism, and sequencing analysis. The restriction fragment length polymorphism method was used to analyze most of the known ryanodine receptor gene mutations; new mutations underwent analysis using the single-strand conformation polymorphism in exons 12, 15, 39, 40, 44, 45, and 46 of the gene.

Results.—Seven previously reported mutations were detected (Arg163Cys, Gly248Arg, Arg614Cys, Val2168Met, Thr2206Met, Gly2434Arg, and Arg2454His). The frequencies with which these mutations were found were 2.7%, 1.4%, 1.4%, 1.4%, 1.4%, 5.5%, and 4.1%.

The frequency with which the 3 novel amino acid substitutions (Val2214Ile, Ala2367Thr, and Asp2431Asn) occurred was 1.4% each. Thus 10 different mutations of the ryanodine receptor gene were found in 16 unrelated individuals screened because they were MH susceptible. This corresponds to 21.9% of the screened population in North America.

Conclusions.—The MH-susceptible patients screened revealed 7 known and 3 novel candidate mutations in the ryanodine receptor gene. These mutations accounted for 21.9% of the North American population. These results resemble those obtained in recent studies of German and Italian individuals who are MH susceptible.

▶ Genotyping patients who are at risk for malignant hyperthermia is a relatively unexplored area; at present, our tests for malignant hyperthermia are not easy and we do not really understand the relationship between the genotype and phenotype, that is, how the abnormal genotype is expressed in a clinical setting. This is not easy to explore, because the disorder is rare and life-threatening. This does not make for easy testing in a clinical research center.

M. Wood, MD, FRCA

Transient Neurologic Symptom (TNS) Following Intrathecal Ropivacaine

Ganapathy S, Sandhu HB, Stockall CA, et al (Univ of Western Ontario, London, Canada)
Anesthesiology 93:1537-1539, 2000   10–6

Background.—Transient neurologic symptom (TNS) occurs in 0% to 37% of cases following hyperbaric spinal anesthesia, with the incidence varying with the surgical position and the drug used. The highest incidence occurs with hyperbaric 5% lidocaine, lithotomy position, and flexion of the knee. Ropivacaine has been associated with less motor blockade than the other agents. Low-dose ropivacaine (10 mg) intrathecally has not been previously noted to produce TNS, but this case report documents a patient receiving this dose in whom the syndrome developed.

Case Report.—Woman, age 38 years, had spinal anesthesia in the right lateral decubitus position with 10 mg 1% ropivacaine and was made hyperbaric with 0.5 mL 10% dextrose. On spinal puncture the cerebrospinal fluid was clear and no paresthesia was present. She turned supine after sensory block to pinprick reached the T12 level and soon reported severe low backache in the sacral area before surgery commenced. She received no sedation or other analgesics but suffered discomfort for the duration of the procedure (41 minutes). No pain or nausea occurred in the postanesthesia care unit. The supine position relieved the backache. The morning after surgery, she had moderate-to-severe headache and nausea that improved when she lay down. Neck pain was present, but no auditory symptoms occurred. The severe backache grew worse with coughing but she denied sciatica pain. Her wound pain was 30 to 40 on a 100-point scale. The next day her wound pain had increased to 50 to 60, headache was moderate, and backache was again worsened with coughing. Headache and surgical pain showed improvement on the third day, but her backache now radiated to the buttocks, back of both thighs, and calves. At 5 days postoperatively, she noted significant pain radiating to the thighs, severe calf ache, and numbness on the inner aspect of her soles. On detailed examination, straight leg-raising was limited to 45 degrees by pain, but other aspects were normal, except for slightly reduced sensation on the inner aspect of the soles. Based on the absence of other findings, a diagnosis of TNS was tentatively made, but no interventions were performed. After 20 days, only a mild ache in her sacrum remained that resolved over 6 weeks, along with a return of sensation to her foot.

Conclusions.—TNS had not been associated with the use of ropivacaine for ambulatory anesthesia, although a higher incidence of backache with its use had been noted. The TNS symptoms noted in this case were bilateral and of the same degree on each side. The backache developed as soon as the drug was administered. Further evaluation is required to determine the true incidence of this complication following the intrathecal administration of ropivacaine.

Is Transient Lumbar Pain After Spinal Anaesthesia With Lidocaine Influenced by Early Mobilisation?

Lindh A, Andersson A-S, Westman L (Ersta Hosp, Stockholm; Astrazeneca R&D, Södertälje, Sweden)
Acta Anaesthesiol Scand 45:290-293, 2001   10–7

Background.—Transient radicular irritation was identified as postoperative pain that radiated to the buttocks and thighs and below the knees, lasting 72 hours. The reported incidence is 10% to 30% and treatment with paracetamol or dextropropoxyphene or nonsteroidal antiinflammatory drugs or other analgesics has proved successful. Renamed transient lumbar pain (TLP), a link may be noted with lidocaine or other local anesthetics. Early ambulation after spinal anesthesia has been postulated to be a risk factor for the development of TLP, a theory tested in patients undergoing inguinal hernial repair.

Methods.—A total of 107 patients were randomly assigned to be ambulated early or late, with early defined as beginning as early as possible after total regression of spinal block and late defined as remaining in bed for at least 12 hours. Assessments were done 4, 8, and 12 hours after the anesthesia to measure wound pain, nausea, tiredness, and symptoms of TLP, plus patients completed a diary detailing symptoms once a day for the first 3 days at home postoperatively. On the fifth through the seventh day postoperatively, patients were contacted by telephone.

Results.—Symptoms of TLP occurred in 25 patients (23%): 12 who ambulated early, and 13 who ambulated late, so no significant difference was found for this parameter. Symptoms were noted the first day after surgery and occurred in the buttocks, thighs, and lower limbs. In two patients, TLP lasted more than 3 days. Fourteen patients who ambulated early had a visual analogue scale (VAS) pain score more than 50 on 1 of the first 3 days or over several days. Of those who ambulated late, 14 had a score greater than 50 during the postoperative period. Among the TLP patients, 4 had a VAS score exceeding 50 in the early group and 1 had a score exceeding 50 in the late group. The pain score exceeded 50 in 20% of the patients in whom TLP developed. Twenty-eight percent of the patients in whom TLP did not develop had a pain score greater than 50.

Conclusions.—No difference was seen in the incidence of TLP between those ambulating early and those ambulating late in the surgical course. In addition, no correlation with severe pain was found. Thus other factors must be associated with TLP, possibly pain caused by overstretching of the ligaments, fascies, and muscles.

▶ The first study (Abstract 10–6) suggests that TNS can occur following administration of the new local anesthetic, ropivacaine, while the second study (Abstract 10–7) indicates early mobilization in ambulatory surgery has no effect on the incidence of translumbar pain.

M. Wood, MD, FRCA

A Multiple-Hospital Anaesthetic Problem Register: Establishment of a Regionally Organized System for Facilitated Reporting of Potentially Recurring Anaesthetic-Related Problems
Kerridge RK, Crittenden MB, Vutukuri VLSP (John Hunter Hosp, Newcastle, New South Wales)
Anaesth Intensive Care 29:106-112, 2001   10–8

Background.—When problems occur in association with anesthesia and have the potential to recur, patients should be warned, documentation should be carried out, and all parties should be informed to help with any future management problems. However, current systems do not always work effectively. A system was developed to facilitate the reporting and retrieval of information on patients such as this, covering 20 separate hospitals.

Methods.—The components included in the system are a reporting package to make it easy for anesthetists in busy clinical practices to make appropriate reports, centralized clerical support, supervision by anesthetists, provision of the reports and laminated cards to the patient, and a database that remains accessible indefinitely. The system also developed a new classification system for use in identifying airway management difficulties.

Results.—The project began with 16 patients, and 26 were added over the course of development. Reports are submitted 3 times each week, covering 50,000 surgical anesthetics each year. Most reports concern dif-

TABLE 2.—Reporting Doctor

Reporting Doctor	Number
Staff Specialist	88
Visiting Specialist	155
Fellow/Senior Registrar	20
Registrar	72
GP Anaesthetist	15

(Courtesy of Kerridge RK, Crittenden MB, Vutukuri VLSP: A multiple-hospital anaesthetic problem register: establishment of a regionally organized system for facilitated reporting of potentially recurring anaesthetic-related problems, *Anaesth Intensive Care* 29:106-112, 2001.)

ficulties in airway management, although anaphylaxis, malignant hyperthermia, suxamethonium apnea, and atypical reactions to anesthetic are also represented. The new classification system relates to difficulty of intubation and has 5 grades. Among the physicians reporting are salaried specialists, specialists in private practice, anesthetists in training, and general practitioner anesthetists (Table 2). Indications are that the frequency of reporting from the various anesthetic locations is reasonably consistent with the workload and complexity noted at the various locations. No medicolegal actions have been related to the cases on the database, but it appears that the duty of care is fulfilled by this system. Anesthetists in the area generally agree that the system meets a public relations concern, impressing patients with the concern of professionals for their welfare, and fulfills the need for professional satisfaction.

Conclusions.—The system works well in the current environment and improves on previous systems for handling the future needs of patients in whom anesthesia-related problems develop with the potential for recurrence.

▶ The airline industry has long had a process for the confidential reporting of near misses or critical incidents. With the increased interest in medical errors, anesthesiologists are now starting to recognize the value of such a system.

M. Wood, MD, FRCA

11 Obstetric Anesthesia

Analgesia for Labor

Lateral Recumbent Head-Down Posture for Epidural Catheter Insertion Reduces Intravascular Injection

Bahar M, Chanimov M, Cohen ML, et al (Tel-Aviv Univ, Israel)
Can J Anaesth 48:48-53, 2001
11–1

Objective.—Accidental and unrecognized cannulation of an epidural vein can result in serious complications. The incidence of puncturing of a blood vessel in laboring women was tested during epidural catheter insertion in the sitting, lateral recumbent horizontal, and lateral recumbent head-down positions.

Methods.—Between 1996 and 1999, 900 healthy laboring women were randomly allocated to receive an epidural puncture and catheter insertion in the sitting position (n = 300), in the left lateral horizontal position (n = 300), or in the left lateral head-down position (n = 300). Outcome measures included the presence of blood in the epidural catheter, blood on needle puncture, subarachnoid puncture, and more than 1 attempt at epidural cannulation.

Results.—The fewest complications occurred when the patient was in the lateral recumbent head-down position (Table).

Conclusion.—A lumbar epidural blockade, performed with the patient in the lateral recumbent head-down position, reduces the incidence of a vein being punctured.

▶ This study has confirmed a long-held bias of mine. I believe that the results can be explained by the likelihood that the lateral position results in less aortocaval compression, improved venous return, and decreased epidural venous congestion than does the sitting position. However, I acknowledge that others have concluded otherwise.

D. H. Chestnut, MD

TABLE.—Complications in Performance of Epidural Analgesia: The Effect of 3 Different Positions

Patients	Position	Blood in Epidural Catheter	Blood on Needle Puncture	Inadvertent Subarachnoid Puncture	More Than 1 Attempt at Epidural Cannulation
300	Sitting (S)	32 (10.7%)	6 (2%)	2 (0.7%)	40 (13.3%)
300	Lateral recumbent horizontal (LH)	18 (6.0%)	4 (1.3%)	3 (1.0%)	24 (8.0%)
300	Lateral recumbent head-down (LHD)	6 (2.0%)	1 (0.3%)	1 (0.3%)	21 (7.0%)
900	Total	56 (6.2%)	11 (1.2%)	6 (0.7%)	85 (9.4%)
Pairwise	S v LH	3.68	0.10	0.00	3.94
Tests*	S v LHD	17.56†	2.31	0.00	5.91†
(Chi-square)	LH v LHD	5.25	0.81	0.25	0.1

*The chi-square test is not strictly suitable for the comparisons in the second and third columns where the numbers of complications are small. However, apart from the first column, the comparisons are informal, and the test results provide a rough guide only.
†Exceeds the critical level 5.48 derived from the Tukey-Kramer pairwise comparison procedure.
(Courtesy of Bahar M, Chanimov M, Cohen ML, et al: Lateral recumbent head-down posture for epidural catheter insertion reduces intravascular injection. *Can J Anaesth* 48:48-53, 2001.)

The Limitations of Ropivacaine With Epinephrine as an Epidural Test Dose in Parturients

Kee WDN, Khaw KS, Lee BB, et al (Chinese Univ of Hong Kong, China)
Anesth Analg 92:1529-1531, 2001   11–2

Background.—The best composition of epidural test doses has not been established. A randomized, double-blind study was performed to determine whether ropivacaine-epinephrine is an effective test dose in parturients undergoing elective cesarean delivery.

Methods.—Thirty-six women undergoing elective cesarean section at term were enrolled in the study. Twelve women (group E) received 2 mL ropivacaine 0.75% and epinephrine 15 µg epidurally, with 2 mL saline intrathecally and 2 mL saline IV. Another 12 women (group IV) received 2 mL ropivacaine 0.75% and epinephrine 15 µg IV, with 2 mL saline epidurally and 2 mL saline intrathecally. The remaining 12 women (group S) received 2 mL ropivacaine 0.75% and epinephrine 15 µg intrathecally, plus 2 mL saline epidurally and 2 mL saline IV.

Findings.—Eight group S patients had adequate block for surgery after the test dose. Epidural anesthesia was established uneventfully through the epidural catheter in the rest of the patients. All group IV patients had positive heart rate changes. One group S patient could not cooperate with sensory assessments. The remainder in this group had sensory changes with upper level of T11 or greater after 10 minutes. Three group E patients and 2 group IV patients also had sensory changes. All group S patients had Bromage scores of 1 or more, compared with none in the other groups. All infants were born in good condition.

Conclusion.—This combination of ropivacaine and epinephrine used as a test dose had serious limitations. It should not be used to replace lidocaine-epinephrine for this purpose.

▶ In my judgment, 3 mL of 1.5% lidocaine with 1:200,000 epinephrine is the preferred epidural test dose for most obstetric patients receiving epidural anesthesia.

D. H. Chestnut, MD

Quality of Analgesia When Air Versus Saline Is Used for Identification of the Epidural Space in the Parturient

Beilin Y, Arnold I, Telfeyan C, et al (Mount Sinai School of Medicine, New York)
Reg Anesth Pain Med 25:596-599, 2000   11–3

Objective.—Air or saline is typically used for identification of the epidural space. Whether there is a difference in the frequency of unacceptable analgesia when air or saline is used as part of the loss-of-resistance (LOR) technique was investigated during epidural analgesia in women in labor.

The incidence of side effects and complications was compared between the 2 groups in a randomized, prospective study.

Methods.—Women requesting epidural analgesia were randomly allocated to receive 2 mL of air (n = 80) or 2 mL of saline (n = 80) as part of the LOR technique. Before catheter placement, each woman was asked to rate her pain. Analgesia was administered, and the adequacy of pain relief was assessed after 15 minutes.

Results.—Catheters could not be threaded or were improperly threaded in 6 patients in the air group and in 8 patients in the saline group. Significantly more patients in the air group (n = 27, 36%) than in the saline group (n = 14, 19%) had incomplete analgesia at 15 minutes and required additional medication. The L-1 dermatome was the most common location of pain in both groups. Pain scores were higher in the air group than in the saline group.

Conclusion.—Laboring women receiving saline as part of the LOR technique had a higher frequency of adequate epidural analgesia than women receiving air as part of the LOR technique.

▶ The authors observed a modest increase in the number of patients who required additional medication in the air group when compared to the saline group. I have used the loss-of-resistance-to-air technique for most of my career. However, during the last several years, my residents have persuaded me that it is preferable to use the loss-of resistance-to-saline technique. This is proof that a middle-aged anesthesiologist—who is set in his ways—can change!

D. H. Chestnut, MD

Improved Epidural Analgesia in the Parturient in the 30° Tilt Position
Beilin Y, Abramovitz SE, Zahn J, et al (Mount Sinai School of Medicine, New York)
Can J Anaesth 47:1176-1181, 2000   11–4

Objective.—Studies of the effect of patient position on quality of epidural analgesia have been inconclusive. Whether there is a difference in the incidence of incomplete analgesia when a local epidural anesthetic is administered during labor while the woman is in the left lateral decubitus position versus the supine position and the incidence of complications were assessed.

Methods.—After catheter placement, laboring women were randomly placed in the left lateral decubitus position (n = 149) or in the supine position (n = 144) with a 30° left tilt. Thirteen milliliters of 0.25% bupivacaine was administered, and pain relief was assessed 15 minutes after the last dose of local anesthetic or 25 minutes after the test dose. Fetal heart rate slowing, hypotension, and the ephedrine requirement were recorded.

Results.—Three patients were excluded from the analysis because of changes in fetal heart rate, and 6 patients were excluded because they required catheter replacement. There were 145 patients in the lateral group and 139 in the tilt group who completed the study. At 15 minutes, significantly more women in the lateral group than in the tilt group required additional analgesia (38% vs 24%). Pain scores were also significantly higher in the lateral group than in the tilt group. Those who required more analgesia most commonly complained of pain on the right side at the T12 or L1 dermatome. The highest median dermatomic level of analgesia in the lateral group was T9 on the right side and T10 on the left side; in the tilt group, it was T9 on the right side and T8 on the left side. Although the incidence of hypotension was the same in both groups (5%), significantly more women in the lateral group than in the tilt group required ephedrine (10% vs 4%). The fetal heart rate slowed in 4% of the lateral group and in 5% of the tilt group. Catheter replacement was required in 3% of the lateral group and in 1% of the tilt group.

Conclusion.—Laboring women receiving epidural analgesia in the supine position with a 30° left tilt have better analgesia without an increase in complications than women placed in the lateral decubitus position.

▶ Most studies have noted that posture has little effect on the efficacy of epidural analgesia. Thus, I am unable to explain the results observed in the present study. The modest difference between groups in this study is not especially compelling. A 30° leftward tilt is probably safe—provided that it is really 30°! In my experience, there is a slippery slope between the leftward tilt position and the supine position, with its attendant risks of aortocaval compression.

D. H. Chestnut, MD

A Comparison of 0.0625% Bupivacaine With Fentanyl and 0.1% Ropivacaine With Fentanyl for Continuous Epidural Labor Analgesia
Fernández-Guisasola J, Serrano ML, Cobo B, et al (Fundación Hosp Alcorcón, Madrid)
Anesth Analg 92:1261-1265, 2001   11–5

Objective.—The analgesic efficacy and degree of motor block produced by epidural 0.0625% bupivacaine plus 2 μg/mL of fentanyl and 0.1% ropivacaine plus 2 μg/mL of fentanyl were prospectively compared in a double-blind study.

Methods.—After a test dose of lidocaine was administered, either 0.0625% bupivacaine plus fentanyl 2 μg/mL (group B = 52) or 0.1% ropivacaine plus fentanyl 2 μg/mL (group R = 48) were administered epidurally to laboring women. The infusion rate was 15 mL/h, with 5-mL boluses administered every 10 minutes when pain was perceived, until analgesia was affected. Pain intensity was measured on a verbal scale from 0 to 10 before and at 5, 10, 20, 30, 60, and 120 minutes after the first dose

TABLE 2.—Analgesia (Number of Boluses, Assessment, Level of Sensory Block) and Motor Block

	Bupivacaine (n = 51)	Ropivacaine (n = 47)
No. of boluses/patient		
First stage of labor	0.8 ± 1	0.5 ± 1
Second stage of labor	0.05 ± 0.3	0.1 ± 0.4
Patient satisfaction, no. (%)		
Excellent	42 (81.3)	37 (78.7)
Good	8 (15.7)	10 (21.3)
Fair	1 (1.9)	0 (0)
Level of sensory block	T8 (T7-T9)	T8 (T7-T9)
Motor block	4 (4-4)	4 (4-4)

Values are expressed as mean ± SD, incidence and percentage, or median (Q1-Q3 range). There were no significant differences between the groups.

(Courtesy of Fernández-Guisasola J, Serrano ML, Cobo B, et al: A comparison of 0.0625% bupivacaine with fentanyl and 0.1% ropivacaine with fentanyl for continuous epidural labor analgesia. *Anesth Analg* 92:1261-1265, 2001.)

of lidocaine and every 90 minutes thereafter. The Bromage scale was used to evaluate the degree of motor block. Levels of sensory block were assessed by temperature changes by using alcohol swabs. Arterial blood pressure was monitored for signs of hypotension. Maternal oxyhemoglobin and heart rate were measured for 10 minutes after the initial injection, and fetal heart rate and uterine activity were monitored. Incidents of nausea, vomiting, somnolence, and pruritus were recorded.

Results.—There were no differences between groups with respect to verbal pain scores, number of boluses administered, levels of sensory blocks obtained, degree of motor block, the number of spontaneous, forceps-assisted, and cesarean deliveries, or 1- and 5-minute Apgar scores or umbilical artery pH (Table 2). Three women in each group had nausea and vomiting.

Conclusion.—Both bupivacaine and ropivacaine are equally effective in producing analgesia with minimum motor block in laboring women.

▶ Other studies have suggested that ropivacaine is less potent than bupivacaine when administered epidurally for labor analgesia. When providing epidural analgesia for laboring women, anesthesiologists in contemporary practice typically give a relatively dilute solution of local anesthetic. When bupivacaine and ropivacaine are given epidurally in equipotent concentrations, it is unclear whether ropivacaine offers significant advantages over bupivacaine in laboring women.

D. H. Chestnut, MD

The Analgesic Effect of Sufentanil Combined With Ropivacaine 0.2% for Labor Analgesia: A Comparison of Three Sufentanil Doses

Debon R, Allaouchiche B, Duflo F, et al (Hôpel-Dieu Hosp, Lyon, France)
Anesth Analg 92:180-183, 2001   11–6

Objective.—Epidural analgesics and local anesthetics are often combined during labor to obtain a long-acting sensory block with minimal side effects. The effect on duration of labor analgesia of adding 1 of 3 sufentanil doses (5, 10, or 15 µg) to 0.2% ropivacaine was investigated in a prospective, randomized, double-blind study.

Methods.—One hundred parturients received 12 mL of 0.2% ropivacaine alone (20 patients) or with 5 (25 patients), 10 (20 patients), or 15 (17 patients) µg sufentanil injected over 1 minute. Motor block, heart rate, blood pressure, respiratory rate, oxygen saturation, nausea, and pruritus were recorded. Patients assessed pain on a visual linear analogue scale.

Results.—The average duration of anesthesia was 96 minutes for patients receiving ropivacaine only, 134 minutes for patients receiving 5 µg sufentanil, 135 minutes for patients receiving 10 µg sufentanil, and 130 minutes for patients receiving 15 µg sufentanil (Fig 1). Although visual

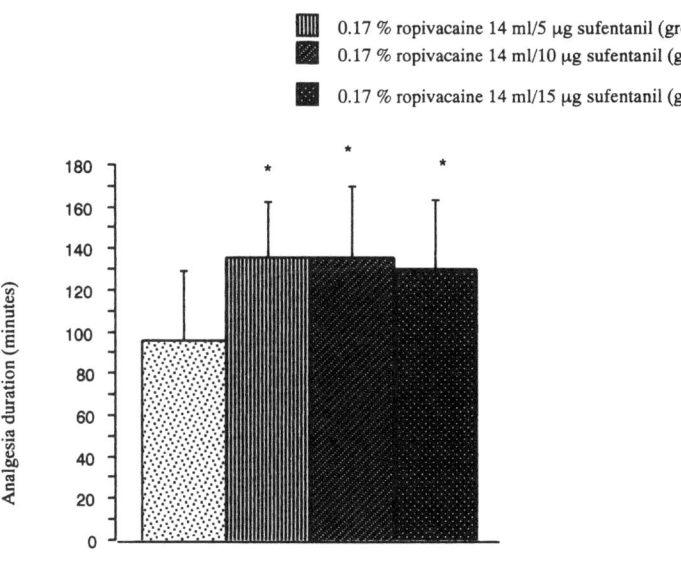

Analgesia duration in each group

FIGURE 1.—Mean analgesia duration in all groups. Analysis of variance showed a significant difference between all groups (P = .0002) and post hoc tests (Bonferroni adjustment comparisons) demonstrated a significantly longer analgesia duration in group 5, group 10, and group 15 (*asterisk* indicates P < .001) versus the control group. Mean and standard deviation are shown. (Courtesy of Debon R, Allaouchiche B, Duflo F, et al: The analgesic effect of sufentanil combined with ropivacaine 0.2% for labor analgesia: A comparison of three sufentanil doses. *Anesth Analg* 92:180-183, 2001.)

analogue scale scores were similar at baseline and 5 minutes after injection, they were significantly lower in the sufentanil groups, compared with the control group, 30 to 90 minutes after injection. All Bromage scores were 1 or less. There were no significant differences between groups with respect to any other maternal parameters measured.

Conclusion.—All doses of sufentanil, coupled with ropivacaine analgesia, significantly increased the duration of analgesia to a similar extent.

The Dose-Range Effects of Sufentanil Added to 0.125% Bupivacaine on the Quality of Patient-Controlled Epidural Analgesia During Labor

Bernard J-M, Le Roux D, Barthe A, et al (Polyclinique Jean-Villar, Bruges-Bordeaux, France)
Anesth Analg 92:184-188, 2001   11–7

Objective.—Sufentanil added to local anesthetics improves the quality and duration of epidural analgesia. The minimum sufentanil concentration that improves the quality of analgesia when it is controlled by women during labor was tested in a double-blind, randomized study.

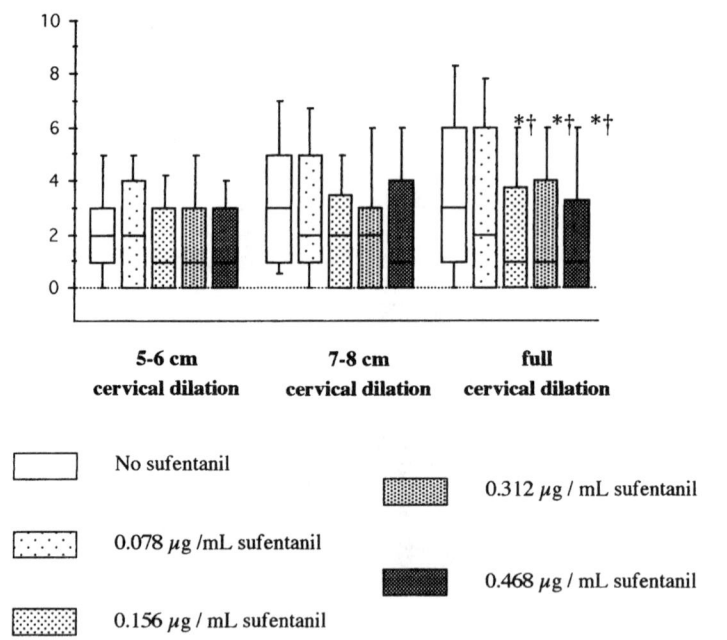

FIGURE 1.—Change in pain score during labor. The box plot displays 10th, 25th, median, 75th, and 90th percentiles of values. Analysis of variance followed by *t*-test with Bonferroni correction; F = 2.074, P = .084 at 5-6 cm cervical dilation; F = 2.694, P = .031 at 7-8 cm cervical dilation; and F = 5.541, P = .0003 at full cervical dilation. *Asterisk* indicates P < .05 versus no sufentanil, and *dagger* indicates P < .05 versus .078 μg/mL sufentanil. (Courtesy of Bernard J-M, Le Roux D, Barthe A, et al: The dose-range effects of sufentanil added to 0.125% bupivacaine on the quality of patient-controlled epidural analgesia during labor. *Anesth Analg* 92:184-188, 2001.)

Methods.—The efficacies of 0.125% bupivacaine with 1:800,000 epinephrine combined with 0 (66 patients), 0.078 (65 patients), 0.156 (65 patients), 0.312 (65 patients), or 0.468 (67 patients) µg/mL sufentanil were compared by means of the patient-controlled epidural analgesia technique.

Results.—During labor, 328 women used the patient-controlled epidural analgesia pump set to deliver a 12-mL bolus with a 25-minute lockout period. Six mL of 0.25% epidural bupivacaine was used as rescue analgesia. At full cervical dilation, pain was decreased for patients receiving at least 0.156 µg/mL sufentanil. Patients receiving 0 and 0.078 µg/mL sufentanil recorded similar pain (Fig 1). Women in all groups reported similar side effects. The incidence and severity of pruritus was dose related. Women receiving 0.312 and 0.468 µg/mL sufentanil recorded the highest degree of satisfaction with labor analgesia.

Conclusion.—Sufentanil added to 0.125% bupivacaine improved the quality of analgesia without increasing the requirement for rescue analgesia.

▶ In the first study (Abstract 11–6), the apparent lack of dose-response is somewhat surprising and prompts the following question: Is it possible that a dose of sufentanil smaller than 5 µg would have prolonged the duration of epidural ropivacaine analgesia? In my opinion, this study provides *indirect* evidence that epidural sufentanil augments epidural ropivacaine analgesia via an intraspinal effect.

The second study (Abstract 11–7) complements the first. The second study suggests that a dose of sufentanil as small as 0.156 µg/mL augments analgesia provided by epidural administration of 0.125% bupivacaine. When administered with a 12-mL bolus of 0.125% bupivacaine with 1:800,000 epinephrine, this represents only 1.872 µg of sufentanil. Together, these 2 studies suggest that there is little benefit to the epidural administration of a dose of sufentanil larger than 2 to 5 µg, when co-administered with either 0.2% ropivacaine or 0.125% bupivacaine. These results may not apply when sufentanil is co-administered with a more dilute solution of local anesthetic.

D. H. Chestnut, MD

Minimum Analgesic Dose of Epidural Sufentanil for First-Stage Labor Analgesia: A Comparison Between Spontaneous and Prostaglandin-Induced Labors in Nulliparous Women

Capogna G, Parpaglioni R, Lyons G, et al (AFaR-CRCCS Fatebenefratelli Gen Hosp, Rome; St James' Univ, Leeds, England; Withington Hosp, Manchester, England)
Anesthesiology 94:740-744, 2001   11–8

Objective.—The median effective dose (ED$_{50}$) for epidural sufentanil as the sole labor analgesic was determined by using the minimum local analgesic concentration model and defining this dose as the minimum analgesia dose of epidural sufentanil. The minimum analgesia dose was used to compare the analgesia requirement during spontaneous and prostaglandin-induced labors in a prospective, double-blind, sequential allocation study.

Methods.—A total of 70 healthy, nulliparous women, at more than 37 weeks' gestation, who had cervical dilatation of 2 to 4 cm, and who requested epidural analgesia during vertex presentation labor, were given sufentanil. The first woman in each group received 25 µg of sufentanil. Subsequent women in each group were given a higher or lower dose depending on the response of the previous patient in an up-down sequential allocation. Pain was assessed on a 100-mm visual analogue pain scale at 0, 15, and 30 minutes after administration of sufentanil. The women then progressed to spontaneous (n = 37) or induced (with dinoprostone, n = 33) labor.

Results.—Seven patients from the spontaneous group and 3 from the induced group were excluded from the study. The ED_{50} of sufentanil was significantly less for the spontaneous group than for the induced group (22.2 µg vs 27.3 µg).

Conclusion.—Women having labor induced with dinoprostone have a significantly higher analgesia requirement than do women having spontaneous labor.

▶ Obstetric anesthesiologists have long suspected that induction of labor results in greater dose requirements for effective analgesia than does spontaneous labor. This study suggests that induction of labor with prostaglandin significantly increases epidural sufentanil dose requirements. In contrast, a meta-analysis did not confirm that oxytocin administration increases the requirement for epidural bupivacaine in laboring women.[1]

D. H. Chestnut, MD

Reference

1. Columb MO, Lyons G, Polley LS, et al: Bupivacaine requirements for labor analgesia. *Anesthesiology* 90:A73, 1999.

Minimum Local Analgesic Dose of Intrathecal Bupivacaine in Labor and the Effect of Intrathecal Fentanyl
Stocks GM, Hallworth SP, Fernando R, et al (Royal Free Hosp, London; South Manchester Univ, Withington, England; St James's Univ, Leeds, England)
Anesthesiology 94:593-598, 2001   11–9

Introduction.—The combination of bupivacaine, 2.5 mg, with fentanyl, 25 µg, is a popular dosage for intrathecal analgesia in labor. Recent studies, however, suggest that effective analgesia can be achieved with lower doses. A study of women in the first stage of labor was designed to determine the median effective dose of intrathecal bupivacaine, defined as

TABLE 2.—Bupivacaine Requirements and Effect of Fentanyl

Group (n = 30)	MLAD (95% CI, mg)	Dunn *P* Value*
Bupivacaine-control	1.99 (1.71, 2.27)	
Bupivacaine-5 µg fentanyl	0.69 (0.35, 1.02)	< 0.001
Bupivacaine-15 µg fentanyl	0.71 (0.00, 1.53)	< 0.001
Bupivacaine-25 µg fentanyl	0.85 (0.58, 1.13)	< 0.001

*P value compared with bupivacaine control. Kruskal-Wallis, *P* <.0001.
Abbreviations: MLAD, Minimum local analgesic dose; *CI,* confidence interval.
(Courtesy of Stocks GM, Hallworth SP, Fernando R, et al: Minimum local analgesic dose of intrathecal bupivacaine in labor and the effect of intrathecal fentanyl. *Anesthesiology* 94:593-598, 2001. Copyright, American Society of Anesthesiologists, Inc. Used with permission of Lippincott-Raven Publishers.)

the minimum local analgesic dose (MLAD), when combined with various doses of fentanyl.

Methods.—Study participants were 124 parturients who requested labor analgesia. All were at more than 37 weeks' gestation and had between 2 cm and 6 cm of cervical dilatation when they were anesthetized by a combined spinal-epidural technique. The women were randomly assigned in a double-blind manner to receive bupivacaine alone or with 5, 15, or 25 µg fentanyl. Data recorded included analgesic effectiveness (assessed with 100-mm visual analogue pain scores), pruritus, and duration of spinal analgesia. The formula of Dixon and Massey was used to calculate MLAD.

Results.—Compared with the bupivacaine control group, there was a significant reduction in MLAD for all bupivacaine-fentanyl groups (Table 2). All bupivacaine-fentanyl groups had similar significant reductions in MLAD, so no dose-dependent effect of fentanyl on MLAD was observed. The addition of fentanyl significantly increased the duration of spinal analgesia, and this increase was dose-dependent. Nausea and vomiting occurred at a similar rate in all groups, but pruritus was significantly increased in the fentanyl groups.

Conclusion.—In this series of patients in the first stage of labor, the MLAD of intrathecal bupivacaine was estimated to be 1.99 mg. Bupivacaine dose-sparing was significant, even with the lowest dose (5 µg) of fentanyl, although lower doses reduced the duration of action of spinal analgesia.

▶ Years ago, one of my mentors, Dr Roy Pitkin, told me that the concluding paragraph of every clinical study should begin with the following phrase: "Under the conditions of the present study, we conclude. . ." Unfortunately, many clinical investigators do not follow this advice, and both investigators and readers inappropriately extrapolate results from 1 study—performed under 1 set of strictly controlled conditions—to all clinical settings. It is refreshing to see the authors of this study limit their conclusions to "the conditions of the (patient) study."

D. H. Chestnut, MD

The Addition of Morphine Prolongs Fentanyl–Bupivacaine Spinal Analgesia for the Relief of Labor Pain

Yeh H-M, Chen L-K, Shyu M-K, et al (Natl Taiwan Univ, Taipei; LAC-USC Med Ctr, Los Angeles)
Anesth Analg 92:665-668, 2001   11–10

Objective.—Combined spinal–epidural (CSE) analgesia lasts 2 to 3 hours. The addition of morphine to CSE may lengthen the duration of analgesia. Whether the addition of morphine (150 µg) to intrathecal fentanyl (25 µg) and bupivacaine (2.5 mg) would prolong labor analgesia was tested in a prospective, randomized, double-blind study.

Methods.—Laboring women requesting epidural analgesia were randomly assigned to receive fentanyl–bupivacaine (FB) (n = 50) or FB plus morphine (FBM) (n = 50) in the lateral position. The duration of analgesia and incidences of hypotension, nausea, pain, vomiting, pruritus, and operative delivery were recorded. Kaplan-Meier survival analysis was performed to compare the adequacy of analgesia between groups.

Results.—CSE was successful in 48 women in the FB group and in 47 women in the FBM group. The adequacy of analgesia and the duration of analgesia in the FBM group were significantly improved over that in the FB group (Fig 1). The incidence of complications was similar for both groups, including the incidence of pruritus.

Conclusion.—The addition of morphine to FB CSE prolongs the duration of labor analgesia and increases the adequacy of analgesia.

▶ Initial studies of intrathecal opioid administration for labor analgesia evaluated the use of intrathecal morphine. Troublesome pruritus, inadequate an-

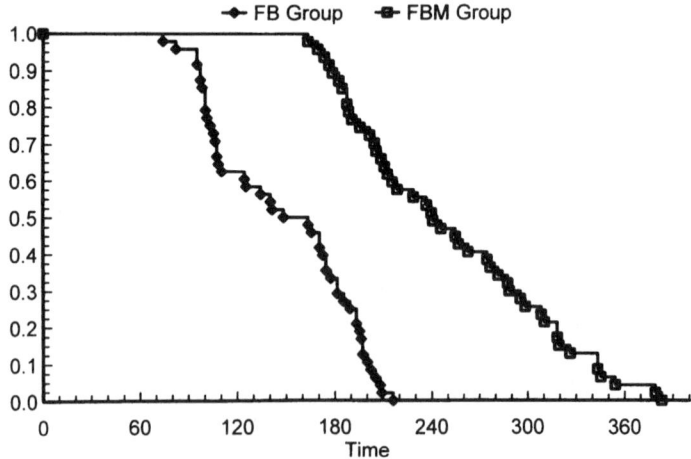

FIGURE 1.—Kaplan-Meier analysis of cumulative proportion of adequate intrathecal analgesia. The cumulative proportion of adequate analgesia was significantly different between the 2 groups (P < .05). (Courtesy of Yeh H-M, Chen L-K, Shyu M-K, et al: The addition of morphine prolongs fentanyl–bupivacaine spinal analgesia for the relief of labor pain. *Anesth Analg* 92(3):665-668, 2001.)

algesia during advanced labor, and the risk of maternal respiratory depression have limited the use of intrathecal morphine for labor analgesia. The results of this study are not surprising and are underwhelming. I reserve the use of intrathecal morphine in laboring women for special situations (eg, women with aortic stenosis).

D. H. Chestnut, MD

Maternal Satisfaction and Pain Control in Women Electing Natural Childbirth

Kannan S, Jamison RN, Datta S (Harvard Med School, Boston)
Reg Anesth Pain Med 26:468-472, 2001   11–11

Background and Objectives.—Many women who choose natural childbirth for labor ultimately request epidural analgesia to control labor pain. Unfortunately, parturients and family members may often be unprepared for epidural anesthesia, which can contribute to disappointment and dissatisfaction with their labor and delivery. This study examines how epidural analgesia for labor influences maternal satisfaction in women who initially choose natural childbirth.

Methods.—This study compared pain and maternal satisfaction in women who elected natural childbirth and successfully followed through (n = 23) with those who elected natural childbirth but requested epidural analgesia during their labor (24 women) (Fig 2). Subjects rated their pain throughout labor and completed pre- and postlabor questionnaires.

Results.—Women who requested epidural analgesia for pain during labor reported significantly lower pain scores than those women who had natural childbirth (*P* < .001). However, 88% of women who requested an

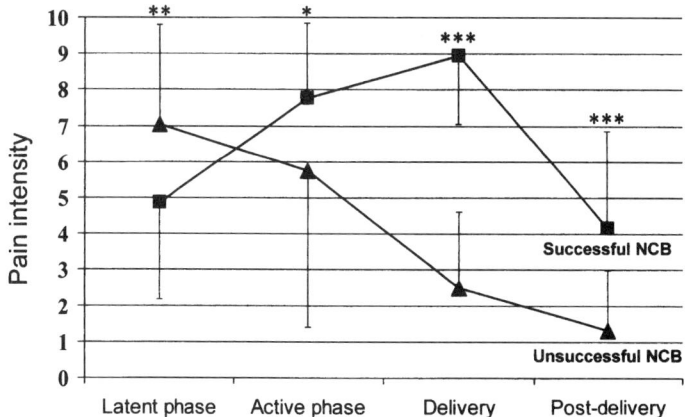

FIGURE 2.—Differences in patient mean pain intensity ratings during the stages of labor between women who succeeded with natural childbirth and those who did not succeed. *Single asterisk* indicates *P* < .05. *Double asterisk* indicates *P* < .01. *Triple asterisk* indicates *P* < .001. (Courtesy of Kannan S, Jamison RN, Datta S: Maternal satisfaction and pain control in women electing natural childbirth. *Reg Anesth Pain Med* 26:468-472, 2001.)

epidural for pain reported being less satisfied with their childbirth experience than those who did not, despite lower pain intensity. Antenatal survey results suggest that concerns about epidurals and their effect on the baby, greater than anticipated labor pain, perceived failure of requesting an epidural, and longer duration of labor may have accounted for these findings.

Conclusions.—This study examined the influence of epidural analgesia in parturients electing natural childbirth. Pain relief alone was not found to improve maternal satisfaction. This study highlights the importance of experience and prelabor expectations on maternal satisfaction with childbirth.

▶ Among pregnant women who plan natural childbirth, the provision of intrapartum pain relief via administration of epidural analgesia may not result in improved maternal satisfaction. An unplanned decision to receive epidural analgesia during labor may result in disappointment and feelings of failure in some of these patients.

D. H. Chestnut, MD

Patient-Controlled Analgesia for Labour Using Remifentanil: A Feasibility Study

Blair JM, Hill DA, Fee JPH (Ulster Hosp, Dundonald, Belfast, Northern Ireland; Queen's Univ of Belfast, Northern Ireland)
Br J Anaesth 87:415-420, 2001   11–12

Background.—Remifentanil is a selective mu opioid agonist with a rapid onset of peak effect (1.2-1.4 minutes), rapid clearance (40 mL/kg/min), and other characteristics that suggest it could be suitable for use in a patient-controlled analgesia system (PCA). This pilot study examined the efficacy and safety of remifentanil in a PCA device during labor.

Methods.—The subjects were 21 pregnant women (6 nulliparous, 15 multiparous; mean age, 29 years) expected to undergo normal labor. PCA was available at 3 "levels" with a lock-out time of 2 minutes between boluses. All patients received a remifentanil bolus of 0.25 or 0.5 µg/kg. At the second and third levels, bolus doses could be increased up to 1.0 µg/kg, and patients received a background infusion of 0.025 (level 2) or 0.05 (level 3) µg/kg/min. Patients rated their level of pain and adverse effects (nausea, anxiety, sedation) on a 10-cm visual analogue scale every 15 minutes. Safety parameters (arterial pressure, fetal heart rate, etc) were assessed every 5 minutes during labor.

Results.—Of the 21 patients, 13 (62%; 2 nulliparous and 11 multiparous) used remifentanil PCA up to and during delivery, and all had a normal delivery. Nineteen patients (90%) reported a significant reduction in pain score compared with baseline (median reduction, 3 cm). In 17 of these 19 responders, the level 1 dose (boluses up to 0.5 µg/kg) provided maximum pain relief, and thus a background infusion was not needed.

Anxiety scores were significantly lower, and sedation scores significantly higher at the level 1 dose compared with baseline. Ten patients (48%) experienced vomiting, 12 (57%) reported itch, and 9 (43%) reported dizziness during labor. Five patients (24%) had 1 or more episodes of significant oxygen desaturation during remifentanil PCA; all episodes occurred at remifentanil doses above the level 1 dose, and all episodes resolved rapidly after dose reduction. However, remifentanil did not significantly slow the fetal heart rate, and Apgar scores and cord blood gas levels remained normal.

Conclusion.—PCA with remifentanil at boluses of up to 0.5 µg/kg with a 2-minute lockout provided safe and effective analgesia during labor. Most patients did not require a background remifentanil infusion for pain control. Given that about one fourth of these patients experienced oxygen desaturation at higher doses, patients using remifentanil PCA should undergo pulse oximetry monitoring until further data are available.

▶ Additional studies are needed to assess the safety and efficacy of patient-controlled IV remifentanil analgesia in laboring women. Meanwhile, the authors have correctly recommended the use of pulse oximetry in laboring women receiving remifentanil PCA.

D. H. Chestnut, MD

Analgesia for Labor: Obstetric Outcome and Economic Issues

Intensity of Labor Pain and Cesarean Delivery

Alexander JM, Sharma SK, McIntire DD, et al (Univ of Texas, Dallas)
Anesth Analg 92:1524-1528, 2001   11–13

Background.—Labor pain intensity may be related to labor dystocia, which is characterized by abnormal progress. An analysis of previously published, randomized comparisons of the effects of epidural analgesia and of patient-controlled IV meperidine on cesarean delivery was presented.

Methods.—Data on 259 women receiving patient-controlled IV meperidine were analyzed. All were in spontaneous labor with singletons at term. Women needing 50 mg/h or more meperidine during labor were compared with women needing less than 50 mg/h. Pain scores, as measured on a visual analogue scale, were compared before and after analgesia.

Findings.—Women needing 50 mg/h meperidine or more had a significantly higher mean pain score than those requiring less meperidine (Table 2). The mean scores were 8.7 and 8.0, respectively. In addition, women requiring higher doses of meperidine tended to have longer labors, at 9 versus 5 hours. More cesarean deliveries were done for obstructed labor in the women needing higher meperidine doses. Fourteen percent of those requiring higher meperidine doses underwent cesearean delivery, compared with only 1.4% of those requiring lower doses. Neonatal outcomes in the 2 groups were comparable.

TABLE 2.—Method of Delivery Based on Hourly Meperidine Dosage Required for Pain Relief During Labor

| Method of Delivery | Hourly Meperidine Dose Required | | P Value |
	<50 mg/h ($n = 209$) (%)	≥50 mg/h ($n = 50$) (%)	
Spontaneous	197 (94)	39 (78)	0.001
Forceps	8 (4)	1 (2)	0.45
Cesarean delivery			
Total	4 (2)	10 (20)	0.001
Dystocia	3 (1.4)	7 (14)	0.001
Nonreassuring FHR tracing	1 (5)	2 (4)	0.04
Other	0	1	0.44

Abbreviation: FHR, Fetal heart rate.
(Courtesy of Alexander JM, Sharma SK, McIntire DD, et al: Intensity of labor pain and cesarean delivery. *Anesth Analg* 92:1524-1528, 2001.)

Conclusion.—Women who ultimately required cesarean delivery for difficult labor self-administered greater amounts of meperidine for labor pain relief. These women reported more intense pain before analgesia was offered.

▶ This study supports other studies that suggest that severe intrapartum pain predicts an increased risk of prolonged labor and cesarean section for dystocia.

D. H. Chestnut, MD

A Randomised Controlled Trial of Epidural Compared With Non-epidural Analgesia in Labour
Howell CJ, Kidd C, Roberts W, et al (North Staffordshire Hosp (NHS) Trust, Staffordshire, England; Keele Univ, Staffordshire, England)
Br J Obstet Gynaecol 108:27-33, 2001   11–14

Objective.—An epidural block may increase the risk of a chronic backache, a chronic headache, bladder problems, tingling and numbness, and sensory confusion. The short- and long-term side effects of epidural analgesia were compared with those of nonepidural analgesia in a randomized, controlled trial in laboring women.

Methods.—Between April 1992 and October 1996, primigravid laboring women were randomly allocated to epidural analgesia (n = 184) with 10 mL of 0.25% bupivacaine with top-ups as required or 50 to 100 mg intramuscular pethidine (n = 185). The outcome measures were backaches at 3 and 12 months, the incidence of instrument delivery, and pain relief.

Results.—In the epidural group, 33% did not receive epidural analgesia. In the nonepidural group, 28% required an epidural. There were no significant differences between groups with respect to low or middle backaches at 3 or 12 months (Fig 1). Although the route of administration of analgesia did not affect the first stage of labor, the second stage was

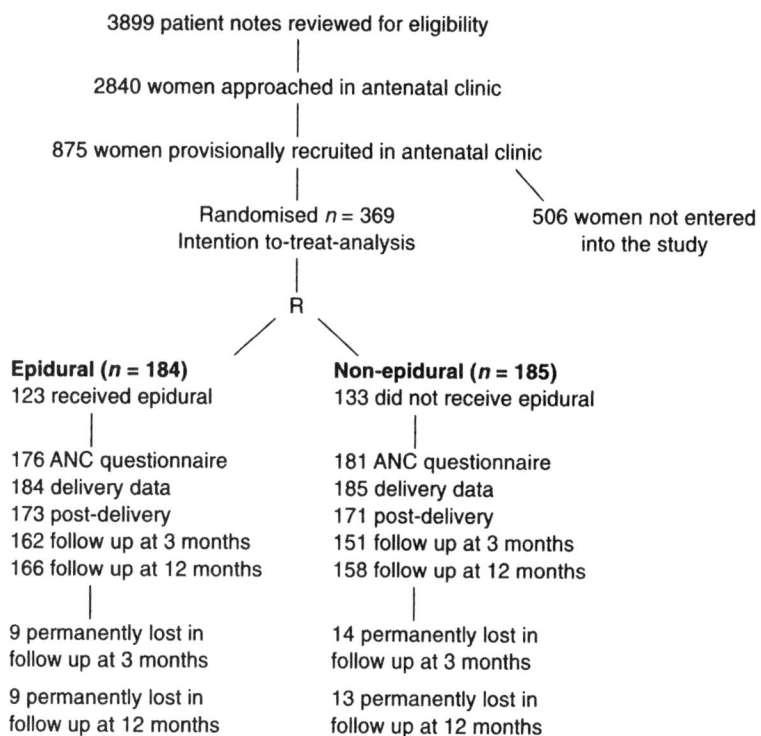

FIGURE 1.—Pain relief study entry flow chart. (Courtesy of Howell CJ, Kidd C, Roberts W, et al: A randomised controlled trial of epidural compared with non-epidural analgesia in labour. *Br J Obstet Gynaecol* 108:27-33, 2001. Published by Elsevier Science.)

significantly lengthened by an average of 19 minutes in the epidural group compared with the nonepidural group. The incidence of instrument deliveries was a significant 19% higher in the epidural group compared with the nonepidural group. The cesarean section rate was similar for the 2 groups. Satisfaction rates did not differ between the 2 groups.

Conclusion.—The use of epidural analgesia significantly increased the duration of the second stage of labor and significantly increased the rate of instrument delivery compared with nonepidural analgesia.

▶ This study provides further evidence that administration of epidural analgesia is *not* an independent risk factor for a long-term backache after delivery.

D. H. Chestnut, MD

Does Epidural Analgesia Prolong Labor and Increase Risk of Cesarean Delivery? A Natural Experiment

Zhang J, Yancey MK, Klebanoff MA, et al (Natl Inst of Child Health and Human Development, Bethesda, Md; Tripler Army Med Ctr, Honolulu, Hawaii)

Am J Obstet Gynecol 185:128-134, 2001   11–15

Objective.—More than 50% of pregnant women in the United States are using epidural analgesia for labor pain. However, whether epidural analgesia prolongs labor and increases the risk of cesarean delivery remains controversial.

Study Design.—We examined this question in a community-based, tertiary military medical center where the rate of continuous epidural analgesia in labor increased from 1% to 84% in a 1-year period while other conditions remained unchanged—a natural experiment. We systematically selected 507 and 581 singleton, nulliparous, term pregnancies with spontaneous onset of labor and vertex presentation from the respective times before and after the times that epidural analgesia was available on request during labor. We compared duration of labor, rate of cesarean delivery, instrumental delivery, and oxytocin use between these two groups.

Results.—Despite a rapid and dramatic increase in epidural analgesia during labor (from 1% to 84% in 1 year), rates of cesarean delivery overall and for dystocia remained the same (Fig 1) (for overall cesarean delivery:

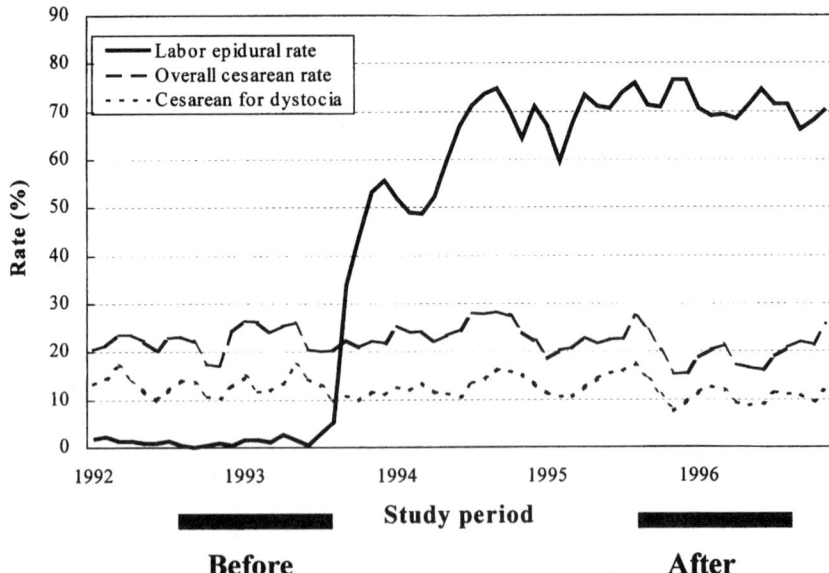

FIGURE 1.—Epidural analgesia use during labor and cesarean delivery rates both overall and for dystocia among nulliparous women, 1992-1996. (Courtesy of Zhang J, Yancey MK, Klebanoff MA, et al: Does epidural analgesia prolong labor and increase risk of cesarean delivery? A natural experiment. *Am J Obstet Gynecol* 185:128-134, 2001.)

adjusted relative risk, 0.8; 95% confidence interval, 0.6-1.2; for dystocia: adjusted relative risk, 1.0; 95% confidence interval, 0.7-1.6). Overall instrumental delivery did not increase (adjusted relative risk, 1.0; 95% confidence interval, 0.8-1.4), nor did the duration of the first stage and the active phase of labor (multivariate analysis; $P > .1$). However, the second stage of labor was significantly longer by about 25 minutes ($P < .001$).

Conclusion.—Epidural analgesia during labor does not increase the risk of cesarean delivery, nor does it necessarily increase oxytocin use or instrumental delivery caused by dystocia. The duration of the active phase of labor appears unchanged, but the second stage of labor is likely prolonged.

▶ Other studies have likewise demonstrated that the introduction of an epidural analgesia service has not resulted in an increase in the cesarean section rate in a given hospital. In contemporary obstetric practice, maternal-fetal factors and obstetric management—not epidural analgesia—are the most important determinants of the cesarean section rate.

D. H. Chestnut, MD

Effect of Low-Dose Mobile Versus Traditional Epidural Techniques on Mode of Delivery: A Randomised Controlled Trial
Shennan AH, for the Comparative Obstetric Mobile Epidural Trial (COMET) Study Group UK (Univ of Birmingham, England; et al)
Lancet 358:19-23, 2001   11–16

Background.—The most effective relief of labor pain is obtained from epidural analgesia, but it is associated with increased rates of instrumental vaginal delivery, prolonged labor, and oxytocin augmentation. However, the likelihood of cesarean section delivery does not appear to be affected by epidural analgesia. The effects may be related to the poor motor function that is associated with traditional epidural techniques. Newer forms of epidural analgesia have been developed by using combinations of opioid and less concentrated local anesthetic. This approach has been shown to preserve motor function and allow ambulation for the patient. However, these low-dose epidurals are not in wide use. A randomized trial

TABLE 3.—Mode of Delivery

Delivery	Traditional Epidural (n=353)	Combined Spinal Epidural (n=351)	Low-dose Infusion Epidural (n=350)
Normal vaginal	124 (35%)	150 (43%)	150 (43%)
Instrumental vaginal	131 (37%)	102 (29%)	98 (28%)
Caesarean section	98 (28%)	99 (28%)	102 (29%)

Note: P = .04, 1DF for normal versus other deliveries.
(Courtesy of Shennan AH, for the Comparative Obstructive Mobile Epidural Trial [COMET] Study Group UK: Effect of low-dose mobile versus traditional epidural techniques on mode of delivery: A randomised controlled trial. *Lancet* 358:19-23, 2001. Copyright, The Lancet Ltd., 2001.)

TABLE 4.—Neonatal Outcomes

	Traditional Epidural (n=353)	Combined Spinal Epidural (n=351)*	p	Low-Dose Infusion Epidural (n=350)	p
APGAR at 1 min					
≤7	38 (11%)	55 (16%)	0·07	64 (18%)	0·01
≥8+	315 (89%)	295 (84%)		286 (82%)	
APGAR at 5 min					
≤7	3 (1%)	7 (2%)	0·33	10 (3%)	0·09
≥8	350 (99%)	343 (98%)		340 (97%)	
Admission to neonatal unit	16 (5%)	10 (3%)	0·33	13 (4%)	0·72
Any resuscitation	88 (25%)	88 (25%)	0·98	98 (28%)	0·40
High-level resuscitation†	5 (1%)	5 (1%)	0·98	16 (5%)	0·02

Note: Values are numbers (percentages).
*One neonate delivered with known lethal congenital abnormality and missing APGAR scores.
†One or more of bag and mask, intubation, or naloxone.
(Courtesy of Shennan AH, for the Comparative Obstructive Mobile Epidural Trial [COMET] Study Group UK: Effect of low-dose mobile versus traditional epidural techniques on delivery: A randomised controlled trial. *Lancet* 358:19-23, 2001. Copyright, The Lancet Ltd., 2001.)

was conducted to compare the use of low-dose combined spinal epidural and low-dose infusion (mobile) techniques with traditional epidural technique.

Methods.—In a 14-month trial, 1054 nulliparous women requesting epidural pain relief were randomly assigned to traditional (353 patients), low-dose combined spinal epidural (351 patients), or low-dose infusion epidural (350 patients) analgesia. The primary outcome was mode of delivery, and the secondary outcomes were progress of labor, efficacy of the procedure, and the effect on neonates. Data were obtained during labor and women were interviewed postnatally.

Results.—In the traditional epidural group, the normal vaginal delivery rate was 35.1%, while the rate was 42.7% in the low-dose combined spinal group and 42.9% in the low-dose infusion group (Table 3). A reduction in instrumental vaginal delivery was responsible for these differences. Apgar scores of 7 or less at 5 minutes were more frequent with the low-dose technique. The low-dose infusion group had a higher rate of high-level resuscitation (Table 4).

Conclusion.—These findings indicate the benefits for delivery outcome with the use of low-dose epidural techniques for labor analgesia. The continued use of traditional epidurals may not be justified on the basis of these findings.

▶ I agree that epidural administration of dilute solutions of local anesthetic is preferable to administration of more concentrated solutions when providing epidural analgesia in laboring women. However, I question the author's conclusion that *this study* demonstrated "clear advantages in delivery outcome with low-dose techniques" when compared with "traditional" epidural techniques. The incidence of operative delivery—both cesarean section and instrumental vaginal delivery—was remarkably high in all 3 groups. The authors also observed an increased incidence of low 5-minute APGAR scores in the low-dose infusion group. Regrettably, the author did not determine umbilical cord blood gas and pH measurements in the 3 groups.

D. H. Chestnut, MD

Effect of Epidural Analgesia With Ambulation on Labor Duration
Vallejo MC, Firestone LL, Mandell GL, et al (Univ of Pittsburgh, Pa)
Anesthesiology 95:857-861, 2001   11–17

Introduction.—Ambulation during labor can be beneficial to both mother and infant. Using ambulatory epidural analgesia (AEA) for labor allows complete mobility and may promote a more natural progression of labor. A prospective, randomized study sought to determine whether ambulation with AEA shortens the duration of labor from the time of epidural insertion to complete cervical dilatation.

Methods.—The 160 women included in the study were nulliparous, at 36 to 42 weeks' gestation with a singleton pregnancy in the vertex position, and at 3- to 5-cm cervical dilatation at the time of epidural insertion. Randomization was to AEA with ambulation or AEA without ambulation. The AEA blocks were initiated with 15 to 20 mL ropivacaine (0.07%) plus 100 μg fentanyl, followed by a continuous infusion of 0.07% ropivacaine plus 2 μg/mL fentanyl at 15 to 20 mL/h. The 2 groups were compared for ambulation time, time to complete dilatation, stage II duration, pain scores, mode of delivery, and APGAR scores at birth.

Results.—Seventy-five patients in the ambulatory group and 76 in the nonambulatory group completed the study. The 2 groups were similar in demographic data. All patients in the ambulatory group met eligibility

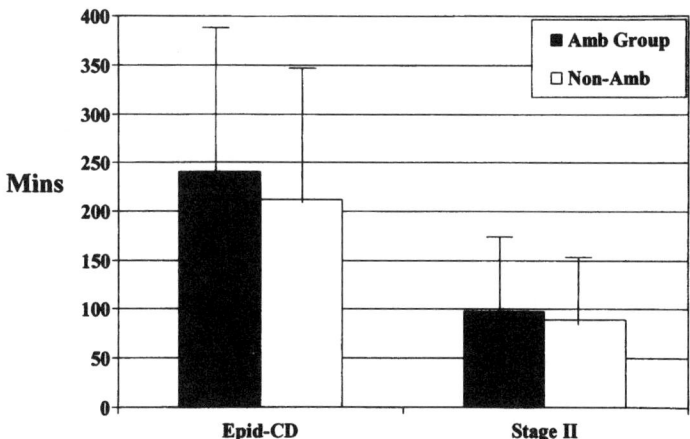

FIGURE 1.—Epidural insertion time to complete cervical dilatation (*Epid-CD*) and stage II labor duration. (Courtesy of Vallejo MC, Firestone LL, Mandell GL, et al: Effect of epidural analgesia with ambulation on labor duration. *Anesthesiology* 95:857-861, 2001. Copyright, American Society of Anesthesiologists, Inc. Used with permission of Lippincott-Raven Publishers.)

requirements for ambulation during labor. The time from epidural insertion to complete dilatation was 240.9 minutes in the ambulatory group versus 211.9 minutes in the nonambulatory group (Fig 1), not a significant difference. The 2 groups were also similar in stage II labor duration, mode of delivery, pain scores, and APGAR scores. The ambulatory group had a significantly higher total infusion volume of local anesthetic.

Conclusion.—Ambulatory epidural analgesia with walking or sitting in a chair did not shorten the duration of labor from the time of epidural insertion to complete cervical dilatation. Low-dose epidural analgesia, however, by allowing ambulation, may improve maternal comfort and satisfaction.

▶ A minority of parturients want to ambulate during active labor. However, the majority of parturients dislike the lower extremity paralysis that may occur with epidural analgesia. The authors correctly noted that "the ability to walk to the bathroom and change positions in bed are compelling enough as reasons in support of low-dose epidural analgesia." However, under the conditions of this study, ambulation did not shorten the duration of labor for women receiving epidural analgesia with low-dose ropivacaine and fentanyl.

D. H. Chestnut, MD

Epidural Analgesia and Fetal Head Malposition at Vaginal Delivery
Yancey MK, Zhang J, Schweitzer DL, et al (Tripler Army Med Ctr, Honolulu, Hawaii; Natl Inst of Child Health and Human Development, Bethesda, Md)
Obstet Gynecol 97:608-612, 2001   11–18

Objective.—Women who use epidural analgesia are reported to require more operative deliveries, possibly because of malpositioning of the fetal head. Whether the introduction of on-request labor epidural analgesia resulted in an increased frequency of malpositioning of the fetal vertex at vaginal delivery was investigated in a retrospective cohort study for nulliparous women.

Methods.—The frequency and consequences of epidural use were compared for 434 women who delivered between October 1992 and October 1993 (before epidural use on request) and 511 women who delivered between July 1995 and July 1996 (after epidural use on request). The outcome measure was the position of the fetal head.

Results.—Epidural use increased from 0.9% during the first period to 82.9% in the second period. Fetal head malpositioning occurred in 6.0% of births in the first period and in 5.7% of births during the second period.

Conclusion.—Although the use of epidural analgesia on request increased significantly from the first period to the second, there was no increased in fetal head malpositioning.

▶ Some obstetricians contend that epidural analgesia results in pelvic floor relaxation and thus predisposes to an increased incidence of fetal head malposition. In contrast, many anesthesiologists argue that patients with preexisting fetal head malposition are more likely to experience severe pain during labor, and thus are more likely to request epidural analgesia. Indeed, several studies have suggested that severe pain during early labor predicts an increased risk for prolonged labor and operative delivery.

Other studies have noted that the availability of on-demand epidural analgesia in a given hospital did not increase the incidence of cesarean section in that hospital. Using similar methodology, Yancey et al observed that the availability of on-demand epidural analgesia did not result in an increased incidence of fetal head malposition in nulliparous women who delivered vaginally at their hospital. The authors administered 0.0625% to 0.125% bupivacaine with fentanyl. Perhaps the epidural administration of such dilute solutions of local anesthetic is less likely to result in pelvic floor relaxation, and thus is less likely to predispose to fetal head malposition, than epidural administration of a more concentrated solution of local anesthetic.

D. H. Chestnut, MD

The Effect of Epidural Analgesia on Rates of Episiotomy Use and Episiotomy Extension in an Inner-City Hospital
Newman MG, Lindsay MK, Graves W (Emory Univ, Baton Rouge, La)
J Matern Fetal Med 10:97-101, 2001   11–19

Introduction.—Although there are well-defined obstetric indications for episiotomy, the education and bias of the individual practitioner and the patient's socioeconomic status are important nonmedical determinants of episiotomy usage. Trials addressing the relationship between epidural analgesia, episiotomy, and pelvic lacerations have conflicting results. Some trials have reported increased perineal traumas. The relationship between epidural analgesia and episiotomy was examined in an inner city population, as were the effects of epidural analgesia on the risk of episiotomy extension.

Methods.—A database of 20,888 women who underwent spontaneous vaginal delivery between 1990 and 1995 was assessed to identify patients receiving epidural analgesia. An epidural group was made up of women who underwent epidural catheter placement and had sufficient perineal anesthesia at delivery. All other patients comprised the control group. A comparison was made between demographic characteristics and obstetric outcomes. The association between epidural analgesia, rates of episiotomy, and episiotomy extension underwent univariate and multivariate analyses.

Results.—Of the 20,888 women who had spontaneous vaginal delivery, 6,785 (32.5%) had epidural analgesia. Women who received epidural analgesia were more likely than those who did not to be African American, nulliparous, and had infants with an occiput posterior presentation. Women who received epidural analgesia were also more likely to receive an episiotomy (27.8% vs 13.1%, odds ratio [OR], 2.56; 95% confidence interval [CI], 2.38-2.75) and were less likely to have a second-degree perineal laceration (11.6% vs 14.4%, OR, 0.75; 95% CI, 0.62-0.82) or a third- or fourth-degree extension (8.9% vs 12.4%, OR, 0.81; 95% CI, 0.68-0.97). After adjusting for nulliparity, posterior presentation, macrosomia, shoulder dystocia, and prolonged second stage, epidural analgesia remained independently correlated with episiotomy (OR, 1.97; 95% CI, 1.88-2.06) and decreased episiotomy extension (OR, 0.74; 95% CI, 0.54-0.94).

Conclusion.—The episiotomy rate is increased in women who undergo epidural analgesia, along with a reduced rate of episiotomy extension and independent of clinical factors related to episiotomy.

▶ Retrospective studies typically suffer from the potential for selection bias. Nonetheless, it seems intuitive that obstetricians might be more likely to perform an episiotomy in patients with excellent perineal anesthesia provided by epidural analgesia. Of interest, the authors also observed that women receiving epidural analgesia were less likely to experience a third- or fourth-degree episiotomy extension. The authors speculated that this may reflect a protective effect from perineal relaxation provided by epidural analgesia. Alternatively, this observation may reflect a decreased incidence of precipitous, traumatic delivery in patients with epidural analgesia. The authors acknowledged that their "findings of a protective effect of epidural analgesia on the occurrence of perineal trauma is in agreement with some studies but at variance with others."

D. H. Chestnut, MD

Fetal and Neonatal Considerations

Effect of Direct Fetal Opioid Analgesia on Fetal Hormonal and Hemodynamic Stress Response to Intrauterine Needling

Fisk NM, Gitau R, Teixeira JM, et al (Imperial College School of Medicine, London; Queen Mother's Hosp, Glasgow, Scotland)
Anesthesiology 95:828-835, 2001   11–20

Introduction.—Newborns are known to be capable of experiencing pain, but whether the fetus can experience pain remains controversial. There is evidence, however, that stress responses occur in the human fetus, and a number of studies advocate giving analgesia when diagnostic and therapeutic invasive procedures are performed. Fentanyl, widely used in neonatal anesthesia, was used to test the hypothesis that IV administration of the drug would reduce fetal hormonal and hemodynamic stress responses to intrahepatic vein needling.

Methods.—Women recruited for the study had singleton pregnancies and were undergoing clinically indicated serial intrauterine transfusions at between 20 and 35 weeks for alloimmune fetal anemia or thrombocytopenia. IV fentanyl (10 µg/kg estimated fetal weight × 1.25 placental correction) was given once at intrahepatic vein (IHV) transfusion in 16 fetuses. In 12 of these fetuses, a second IHV transfusion was performed without fentanyl. An additional 29 fetuses were transfused without fentanyl at either the placental cord insertion or the IHV. Fentanyl and control transfusions were compared for changes in β endorphin, cortisol, and middle cerebral artery pulsatility index.

Results.—In fetuses who had paired IHV transfusions with and without fentanyl, the administration of fentanyl reduced the β endorphin and middle cerebral artery pulsatility index response, but not the cortisol response. The magnitude of the β endorphin and cortisol response was halved with fentanyl. When compared with control fetuses transfused without analgesia, the β endorphin and cerebral Doppler response to IHV transfusion with fentanyl was close to that of nonstressful placental cord transfusions.

Conclusion.—Direct administration of 10 µg/kg fentanyl was found to blunt the fetal stress response to intrauterine needling. The analgesic dose used may have been too low to reduce the cortisol response.

▶ The clinical implications of this study are clear.

D. H. Chestnut, MD

Fetal Heart Rate Abnormalities After Regional Analgesia for Labor Pain: The Effect of Intrathecal Opioids

Van de Velde M, Vercauteren M, Vandermeersch E (Katholieke Univ Leuven, Belgium; Univ Hosp Antwerp, Edegem, Belgium)
Reg Anesth Pain Med 26:257-262, 2001   11–21

Objective.—A limited number of reports have described nonreassuring fetal heart rate (FHR) patterns immediately after spinal administration of opioids, possibly caused by uterine hyperactivity. A retrospective chart review of singleton, term, vertex-presenting women in labor who received neuraxial analgesia was performed to determine the occurrence of nonreassuring FHR tracings.

Methods.—Between May 1, 1997 and April 30, 1998, 1184 laboring women received conventional epidural analgesia with 10 mL of 0.125% bupivacaine and 0.75 µg/mL of sufentanil (EPI = 346); combined spinal and epidural analgesia (CSE_{suf} = 351) with 7.5 µg of intrathecal sufentanil; or CSE with 2.5 mg of bupivacaine and 1.5 µg of sufentanil (CSE_{LA} = 487). The incidence of nonreassuring FHR tracings and uterine hyperactivity, and neonatal and labor outcomes were compared between groups.

Results.—Labor characteristics and labor outcome were similar for the 3 groups. Although the CSE_{suf} group had significantly less hypotension and required significantly less ephedrine to relieve hypotension than the other 2 groups, significantly more fetuses had nonreassuring FHR tracings, and significantly more women required tocolysis for uterine hyperactivity. Neonatal outcome was similar in all 3 groups.

Conclusion.—CSE with 7.5 µg of intrathecal sufentanil induces significantly more nonreassuring FHR tracings and uterine hyperactivity in laboring women than do CSE_{LA} and EPI.

▶ Some studies have suggested that intrathecal opioid analgesia results in an increased risk of FHR abnormalities, including fetal bradycardia. The clinical significance of these FHR abnormalities remains unclear. Specifically, it is unclear whether the apparent increase in the occurrence of fetal bradycardia after administration of intrathecal opioid analgesia has an adverse effect on obstetric and neonatal outcome.

D. H. Chestnut, MD

Anesthesiologists' Interest in Neonatal Resuscitation Certification
Gaiser R, Lewin SB, Cheek TG, et al (Univ of Pennsylvania, Philadelphia)
J Clin Anesth 13:374-376, 2001   11–22

Introduction.—Published guidelines of both the American Society of Anesthesiologists and the American Society of Obstetricians and Gynecologists state that the responsibility of resuscitating a newborn belongs to someone other than the anesthesiologist, whose primary duty is the care of the mother. Anesthesiologists may occasionally become involved, however, in neonatal resuscitation. A survey was sent to anesthesiologists to assess their involvement and their interest in becoming certified in neonatal resuscitation.

Methods and Results.—The survey was mailed to graduates of the University of Pennsylvania Anesthesia Program between 1989 and 1999. Of the 212 individuals who completed the residency, 189 could be contacted and 156 responded. Among respondents with obstetric anesthesia responsibilities, 65% reported involvement in the resuscitation of the newborn. Only 16% of these anesthesiologists were certified in neonatal resuscitation, but 81% expressed interest in certification. Respondents whose practice was at hospitals with fewer than 1000 deliveries per year were more likely to be asked to resuscitate a newborn, compared with respondents at hospitals with more than 1000 deliveries per year. Most of the anesthesiologists with obstetric anesthesia responsibilities were in private practice.

Conclusion.—An individual with the skills required for neonatal resuscitation must be present at every delivery. Participation of the anesthesiologist should be a rare and unexpected event, but the findings of this survey indicate otherwise. Because of the interest expressed by anesthesiologists, the American Society of Anesthesiologists may need to establish programs in neonatal resuscitation.

▶ On occasion, it may be necessary for the anesthesiologist attending the mother to assist with resuscitation of the newborn infant. However, American Society of Anesthesiologists guidelines clearly state that this should not be routine practice.

D. H. Chestnut, MD

The Neurologic and Adaptive Capacity Score Is Not a Reliable Method of Newborn Evaluation
Halpern SH, Littleford JA, Brockhurst NJ, et al (Univ of Toronto)
Anesthesiology 9:958-962, 2001   11–23

Introduction.—The Neurologic and Adaptive Capacity Score (NACS) is a multi-item scale developed to identify central nervous system depression in term neonates exposed to intrapartum medications. This scoring system is used widely in obstetric anesthesia research, yet there are no published trials verifying its reliability. The NACS was examined for its reliability in measuring neurobehavior in the term neonate.

Methods.—Two teams of observers performed the NACS on 200 healthy, term neonates born in the vertex presentation. All neonates underwent 2 examinations within the first 2.5 hours of life. Simultaneous (or split-half) reliability was examined using the α coefficient. Test-retest reliability was evaluated using the intraclass correlation coefficient. The test was considered reliable if α was greater than 0.7 and the intraclass correlation coefficient was greater than 0.6.

Results.—Of 200 infants evaluated, 22 were excluded for various reasons. Local anesthetics as a group were the most commonly used drugs; fentanyl was the most commonly used opioid. One patient received a general anesthetic, 12 had unmedicated vaginal delivery, and 4 received only nitrous oxide. The α coefficient was 0.47 for total NACS, 0.42 for the adaptive component, and 0.48 for the neurologic component. The intraclass correlation coefficient was 0.38.

Conclusion.—The NACS demonstrated poor reliability on simultaneous testing and in the test-retest situation when used to assess term, healthy neonates. Other measures need to be created to ascertain the effect of intrapartum drug administration in the newborn. Health measurement scales need to undergo rigorous evaluation for reliability and validity before they may be used in clinical practice or for research purposes.

▶ The clinical relevance of tests that assess the subtle effects of intrapartum maternal drug administration on neonatal neurobehavior remains unclear.

D. H. Chestnut, MD

Anesthesia for Cesarean Section

Phenylephrine Added to Prophylactic Ephedrine Infusion During Spinal Anesthesia for Elective Cesarean Section

Mercier FJ, Riley ET, Frederickson WL, et al (Stanford Univ, Calif)
Anesthesiology 95:668-674, 2001   11–24

Objective.—Although prophylactic IV ephedrine (E) has been recommended to prevent hypotension after spinal anesthesia during cesarean section, clinical experience suggests that E may not always correct hypotension. Whether the addition of phenylephrine (P) can improve the efficacy of E was examined in a randomized, double-blind study comparing the effectiveness of infusions of E + P versus E alone.

Methods.—Women, with American Society of Anesthesiologists status I or II, scheduled for cesarean delivery of a singleton fetus under spinal anesthesia, received an infusion of E + P (n = 21) or E alone (n = 21) at a rate of 2 mg/min of 60 mg E ± 300 µg P. Blood pressure, umbilical cord blood pH values and Apgar scores were measured.

Results.—Two patients receiving P + E and 1 patient receiving E alone were excluded because of protocol violations. Severe and recurrent episodes of hypotension developed in 1 patient in the E group. Hemodynamic stability was restored after administration of 100 µg P. One patient in the E + P group experienced pronounced bradycardia that resolved in less than 1 minute. Compared with the E group, the E + P group had half the incidence of hypotension (75% vs 37%), although systolic blood pressure values were similar for both groups after initiation of spinal anesthesia (Fig 1). The maximum heart rate and the maternal heart rate were significantly

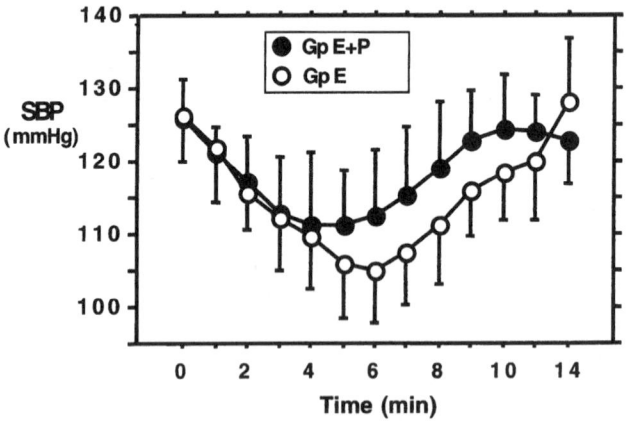

FIGURE 1.—Maternal systolic blood pressure (SBP) after onset of spinal anesthesia. Vasopressor infusions (ephedrine [E] ± phenylephrine [P]) were started at the end of spinal injection (time 0). Mean SBP values were not significantly different between the 2 groups (*P* = .3). Data are mean values with 95% CIs. (Courtesy of Mercier FJ, Riley ET, Frederickson WL, et al: Phenylephrine added to prophylactic ephedrine infusion during spinal anesthesia for elective cesarean section. *Anesthesiology* 95:668-674, 2001. Copyright American Society of Anesthesiologists, Inc. Used with permission of Lippincott-Raven Publishers.)

TABLE 3.—Neonatal Outcome

| | Group | | |
	Ephedrine + Phenylephrine	Ephedrine	P
Umbilical venous pH*	7.33 (7.18-7.46)	7.28† (7.11-7.38)	0.03
Umbilical arterial pH‡	7.24 (7.12-7.36)	7.19† (7.01-7.37)	0.05
Apgar score at 1 min	9 (7-10)	9 (8-10)	0.7
Apgar score at 5 min	10 (9-10)	10 (9-10)	0.7

Note: Values are median (range).
*One missing value for umbilical venous pH (in ephedrine group).
†Significantly different from ephedrine + phenylephrine group.
‡Four missing values for umbilical arterial pH (1 in ephedrine group and 3 in ephedrine + phenylephrine group).
(Courtesy of Mercier FJ, Riley ET, Frederickson WL, et al: Phenylephrine added to prophylactic ephedrine infusion during spinal anesthesia for elective cesarean section. *Anesthesiology* 95:668-674, 2001. Copyright American Society of Anesthesiologists, Inc. Used with permission of Lippincott-Raven Publisher.)

higher in the E group than in the E + P group. The E group required significantly more E and supplemental E and had a significantly higher incidence of nausea than did the E + P group (59% vs 30%). Umbilical pH values were significantly higher in the E + P group than in the E group, although Apgar scores were similar (Table 3).

Conclusion.—Addition of P significantly decreased the incidence of hypotension, reduced nausea and vomiting, and raised venous and arterial umbilical pH values for women undergoing cesarean delivery under spinal anesthesia.

▶ The authors have made an interesting observation, but their methods may be somewhat tedious for the solo anesthesiologist providing spinal anesthesia for cesarean section in clinical practice. I continue to favor the prophylactic administration of 5 or 10 mg of IV E immediately after administration of spinal bupivacaine, although I acknowledge that most published studies do not support the efficacy of this practice. If hypotension persists—despite the cumulative administration of 20 to 25 mg of prophylactic or therapeutic E—it seems reasonable to treat refractory hypotension with small bolus doses of P. Rarely, in cases of severe refractory hypotension, it may be necessary to administer epinephrine.

D. H. Chestnut, MD

Comparison of Two Oxytocin Regimens to Prevent Uterine Atony at Cesarean Delivery: A Randomized Controlled Trial

Munn MB, Owen J, Vincent R, et al (Univ of Alabama, Birmingham)
Obstet Gynecol 98:386-390, 2001   11–25

Objective.—Uterine atony can result in increased blood loss during cesarean delivery. Because oxytocin has been shown to reduce the risk of postpartum hemorrhaging after vaginal delivery, the effect of 2 high-dose oxytocin regimens on the incidence of clinically significant uterine atony was tested in a randomized, double-blind trial involving an at-risk population of women undergoing cesarean delivery.

Methods.—Between January 1997 and November 1999, 321 at-risk women in labor undergoing cesarean section were randomly allocated to receive a standard prophylactic (low-dose) oxytocin regimen (333 mU/min) (n = 163) or a high-dose oxytocin regimen (2667 mU/min) (n = 158) infused over a 30-minute period after delivery of their infants. The oxygen saturation level and blood pressure were monitored continuously, and clinically significant hypotension was recorded. Additional uterotonic agents were administered as needed.

Results.—No patient required a hysterectomy or a blood transfusion. Significantly more women in the low-dose group than in the high-dose group required an additional uterotonic agent (39% vs 19%; $P < .001$; relative risk [RR], 2.1; 95% CI, 1.4, 3.0). Significantly more women in the low-dose group than in the high-dose group required additional oxytocin (36% vs 19%; $P = .006$). Among women requiring additional oxytocin, 9% of the low-dose group and 2% of the high-dose group also required methylergonovine or 15-methyl prostaglandin $F_{2\alpha}$ for persistent atony ($P = .005$; RR, 4.8; 95% CI, 1.4, 16). One woman required treatment for hypotension. The mean blood loss and change in hematocrit level were similar for both groups. Women having labor arrest were significantly more likely to require additional uterotonic agents than were women with other indications (41% vs 22%; $P < .001$). Women with chorioamnionitis were also significantly more likely than women without chorioamnionitis to require additional uterotonic agents (50% vs 24%; $P < .001$). After these 2 diagnoses were controlled for, multiple logistic regression analysis showed that, compared with women in the low-dose group, fewer women in the high-dose group required additionally administered uterotonic agents (odds ratio, 0.38; 95% CI, 0.22, 0.64).

Conclusion.—Administration of high-dose oxytocin after cesarean delivery significantly reduces the incidence of uterine atony.

▶ Rapid IV administration of a bolus dose of oxytocin may result in maternal hypotension. In this study, patients in the high-dose group received 80 U of oxytocin over 30 minutes, via a continuous infusion pump. In my judgment, a smaller dose of oxytocin is effective in most patients undergoing cesarean delivery, provided that the oxytocin infusion is begun immediately after delivery of the infant. In fact, I prefer to begin the oxytocin infusion immediately after cesarean delivery of the fetal head.

Readers should note that this study (and my comments) applies to cesarean deliveries. In contrast, some controversy exists regarding the optimal timing of oxytocin administration after vaginal deliveries.

D. H. Chestnut, MD

Special Situations in Obstetric Anesthesia

The Effect of Intrathecal Analgesia on the Success of External Cephalic Version

Birnbach DJ, Matut J, Stein DJ, et al (Columbia Univ, New York)
Anesth Analg 93:410-413, 2001

11–26

Introduction.—Nearly 4% of term singleton pregnancies are in the breech position and require delivery by cesarean section. External cephalic version (ECV) may be done to convert the fetus from breech to vertex presentation to avoid an operative delivery. Success rates of ECV vary from 35% to 86% (average 58%). There is controversy regarding the potential benefits of epidural and spinal anesthesia for this procedure. Epidural anesthesia produced by sufentanil was evaluated to determine if it could safely improve the success of ECV at term.

Methods.—Twenty patients who received subarachnoid analgesia for ECV were compared with 15 patients who did not in terms of ECV success, level of pain during ECV, and satisfaction.

Results.—The ECV procedure was successful in 21 patients (60%). Success was observed more frequently in the spinal analgesia group vs the nonspinal analgesia group (80% vs 33%; $P = 0.005$). Patients who received spinal analgesia reported less pain and were more satisfied with the procedure. None of the women who received spinal analgesia developed a postdural puncture headache. The only occurrence of fetal bradycardia occurred in a patient who did not receive spinal analgesia.

Conclusion.—The success of ECV was higher after administration of spinal analgesia. The profound patient comfort afforded by spinal analgesia may have allowed greater manipulation of the abdomen during ECV, thus improving the success rates of ECV without increasing the risk.

▶ External cephalic version is often painful. Thus it is not surprising that effective analgesia would improve the rate of success. Some obstetricians have contended that the absence of anesthesia limits the force that the obstetrician can apply during external cephalic version. They have argued that the administration of anesthesia may allow the obstetrician to use excessive force, which might increase the risk of perinatal morbidity and mortality. However, in this study, the only case of fetal bradycardia occurred in a patient who did not receive spinal analgesia. Most obstetricians perform external cephalic version with real-time ultrasonographic guidance, which allows concurrent monitoring of the fetal heart rate.

D. H. Chestnut, MD

Oxytocics Reverse the Tocolytic Effect of Glyceryl Trinitrate on the Human Uterus

Lau LC, Adaikan PG, Arulkumaran S, et al (Natl Univ Hosp, Singapore; Univ of Nottingham, England)

Br J Obstet Gynaecol 108:164-168, 2001   11–27

Objective.—A growing body of evidence suggests that glyceryl trinitrate may be an effective inhibitor of preterm labor. It is unknown whether glyceryl trinitrate–induced uterine relaxation is reversible by currently used oxytocics. An in vitro study was performed to assess the effects of glyceryl trinitrate on isolated strips of pregnant human uterus and whether those effects could be reduced by common oxytocic drugs.

Methods.—The investigators obtained uterine myometrial strips from 18 women undergoing term cesarean section. In organs baths of Krebs-Henseleit solution aerated with oxygen in 5% carbon dioxide, the strips were preloaded at an initial tension of 1.5 g. Strips showing regular, spontaneous contractions under these conditions were used to study the effects of glyceryl trinitrate. Where uterine activity was inhibited by this treatment, the ability of oxytocin, ergometrine, and prostaglandin $F_{2\alpha}$ to re-induce contractions was assessed.

Findings.—The strips varied significantly in their sensitivity to glyceryl trinitrate. However, treatment did reduce contraction amplitude and frequency in concentration-dependent fashion. Complete inhibition of contractions was observed at glyceryl trinitrate concentrations of 44 to 705 µM. All 3 oxytocic drugs studied showed the ability to restore at least the initial level of contractility; they were oxytocin at a concentration of 20 mU/mL, ergometrine at 6.15 µM, and prostaglandin $F_{2\alpha}$ at 6.15 µM.

Conclusion.—These in vitro findings support the uterine-relaxing effects of glyceryl trinitrate. These effects appear to be reversible by commonly used oxytocic drugs. Glyceryl trinitrate is a promising agent for acute tocolysis in clinical obstetrics.

▶ The authors' observations support the rationale for IV or sublingual administration of nitroglycerin in obstetric emergencies (eg, fetal head entrapment, retained placenta, uterine inversion) when rapid-onset, transient uterine relaxation is needed. This report suggests that oxytocin effectively increases the tone of uterine smooth muscle that has been recently exposed to nitroglycerin. Thus, the anesthesiologist need not fear an increased risk of uterine atony in patients who have received small bolus doses of nitroglycerin.

D. H. Chestnut, MD

Platelet Count May Predict Abnormal Bleeding Time Among Pregnant Women With Hypertension and Preeclampsia

McDonagh RJ, Ray JG, Burrows RF, et al (McMaster Univ, Hamilton, Ont, Canada; Monash Univ, Clayton, Australia; Sunnybrook and Women's College Health Sciences Ctr, Toronto)
Can J Anesth 48:563-569, 2001   11–28

Background.—Laboratory data are often needed to estimate bleeding risk among hypertensive pregnant women before regional anesthesia is given. Many anesthesiologists rely on the bleeding time (BT) to make this determination. Whether the platelet count adequately predicts BT in a group of hypertensive parturients was investigated.

Methods.—Of 2051 hypertensive pregnant women, 87 underwent both a BT and platelet count before delivery. The association between platelet count and BT at 3 cut-off points was determined.

Findings.—Platelet count at delivery was significantly negatively correlated with BT. The sensitivity of all 3 platelet cut-off points was less than 66%. Negative predictive values were less than 75% for abnormal BT. A platelet count of $75 \times 10^9/L$ or greater had a 97.8% specificity for abnormal BT. The positive predictive value was 95.5%, and the positive likelihood ratio was 24.

Conclusion.—Platelet count appears to be very specific for predicting prolonged BT in hypertensive parturients. Thus, platelet count may be useful for determining the risk for bleeding from regional anesthesia.

▶ Epidural hematoma is a rare but catastrophic complication of spinal and epidural anesthesia. I acknowledge that published studies have not confirmed the predictive value of the platelet count in determining the risk of epidural hematoma. However, the preponderance of evidence and opinion suggests that the platelet count is the best single laboratory test for assessing the risk of abnormal bleeding during/after administration of spinal or epidural anesthesia in obstetric patients, especially in patients with pregnancy-induced hypertension.

D. H. Chestnut, MD

The Effect of Magnesium on Coagulation in Parturients With Preeclampsia

Harnett MJP, Datta S, Bhavani-Shankar K (Harvard Med School, Boston)
Anesth Analg 92:1257-1260, 2001   11–29

Objective.—Magnesium sulfate, used to prevent seizures in pregnant women with preeclampsia, also has anticoagulant and antiplatelet properties. The mechanism of magnesium sulfate's effect on coagulation has not been investigated. The effects of magnesium sulfate on several components of the coagulation system were studied in women with preeclampsia.

Methods.—Venous blood was collected before administration of a 6-g magnesium sulfate bolus and 30 and 120 minutes after bolus administration from 18 women (average age, 28.6 years) with preeclampsia. Samples were analyzed for time to first clot formation (*R* time), rate of clot strengthening (*K* time), rate of clot strengthening (α angle), maximum strength of clot (MA), and percent lysis at 30 minutes after MA is reached (LY30).

Results.—Although *R* time was significantly slower 30 minutes after bolus administration, the coagulation index did not change at either time point after bolus administration.

Conclusion.—Administration of magnesium sulfate to women with preeclampsia did not affect overall coagulation.

▶ For many years, obstetric anesthesiologists have safely administered epidural anesthesia to patients with preeclampsia, most of whom receive magnesium sulfate for seizure prophylaxis. Epidural hematoma is a rare but devastating complication of epidural anesthesia. Some physicians have expressed concern regarding the potential adverse effects of hypermagnesemia on coagulation and platelet function. This study demonstrated no effect of hypermagnesemia on overall coagulation and platelet function, as assessed by thromboelastography, and provides support for the common practice of administration of epidural anesthesia to preelamptic women who do not have thrombocytopenia or clinical evidence of abnormal bleeding.

D. H. Chestnut, MD

Combined Spinal and Epidural Anesthesia With Low Doses of Intrathecal Bupivacaine in Women With Severe Preeclampsia: A Preliminary Report

Ramanathan J, Vaddadi AK, Arheart KL (Univ of Tennessee, Memphis)
Reg Anesth Pain Med 26:46-51, 2001   11–30

Objective.—Although regional anesthesia may be risky in obstetric patients with severe preeclampsia, single-shot spinal and combined spinal and epidural (CSE) anesthesia can be used safely in these women. The quality of surgical anesthesia for cesarean delivery (CD), the quality of labor analgesia (LA), maternal hemodynamic changes, and neonatal effects were investigated after CSE with low intrathecal doses of bupivacaine and fentanyl in patients with severe preeclampsia.

Methods.—Women with severe preeclampsia were given an anesthetic for CD (n = 46) or for labor and delivery (LA, n = 39). Hemodynamic variables and the cephalad spread of sensory analgesia were recorded.

Results.—The CD group received intrathecal CSE (7.5 mg bupivacaine and 25 μg fentanyl) to obtain a T4 block. Four patients who did not sustain a T4 block also received 2% lidocaine. The LA group received 1.25 mg bupivacaine and 25 μg fentanyl intrathecally followed by a 12 to 15 mL/hour epidural infusion of 0.0625 to 0.125% bupivacaine and 2 to 4 μg

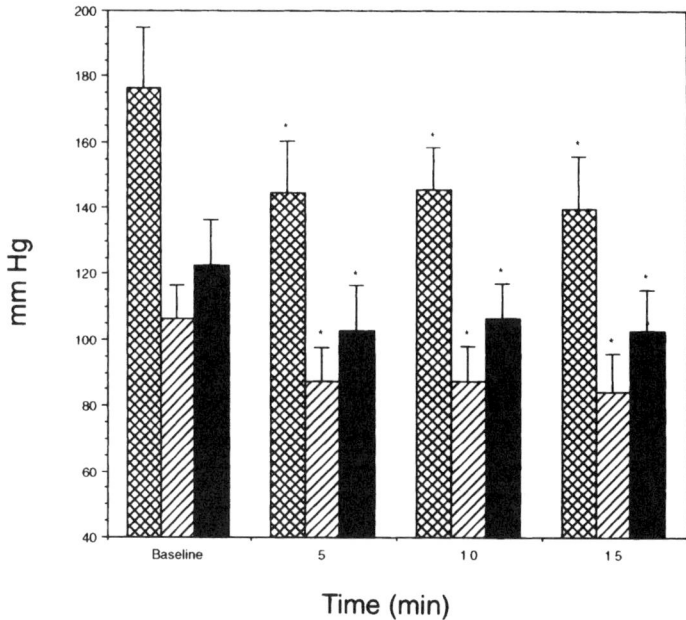

Time (min)

FIGURE 1.—The changes in maternal systolic blood pressure (*cross-hatched bar*), diastolic blood pressure (*hatched bar*), and mean arterial pressure (*black bar*) at 5, 10, 15 minutes compared with baseline in the CD group. *P<.05. (Courtesy of Ramanathan J, Vaddadi AK, Arheart KL: Combined spinal and epidural anesthesia with low doses of intrathecal bupivacaine in women with severe preeclampsia: A preliminary report. *Reg Anesth Pain Med* 26:46-51, 2001.)

fentanyl. After CSE, mean arterial pressure (MAP), decreased significantly in both groups within 5 minutes (Fig 1). Maximum MAP decreases, neonatal Apgar scores, and umbilical artery pH were similar in both groups. Umbilical artery pH was unrelated to lowest MAP or maximum percentage change in MAP before delivery in both groups.

Conclusion.—Patients with severe preeclampsia receive adequate surgical anesthesia for CD or LA when given CSE with low intrathecal doses of bupivacaine and fentanyl and show only modest hemodynamic changes.

▶ This observational study provides further support for the use of CSE anesthesia in women with severe preeclampsia. Among the 46 patients who received CSE anesthesia for cesarean delivery, 42 had a sensory level of at least T4 after the intrathecal administration of only 7.5 mg of hyperbaric bupivacaine with 25 µg of fentanyl. The anesthesiologist administered 2% lidocaine epidurally to extend the block in the remaining 4 patients. Others have suggested that the addition of an opioid to the solution of local anesthetic allows the anesthesiologist to administer a smaller-than-expected intrathecal dose of local anesthetic for cesarean section.

D. H. Chestnut, MD

Epidural Compared With General Anaesthesia for Caesarean Delivery in Conscious Women With Eclampsia

Moodley J, Jjuuko G, Rout C (Univ of Natal, South Africa)
Br J Obstet Gynaecol 108:378-382, 2001   11–31

Objective.—Whether epidural or general anesthesia is more appropriate for stable, conscious women with eclampsia undergoing cesarean section was retrospectively investigated.

Methods.—Records of all 533 women with eclampsia, who delivered between January 1995 and September 1999, were reviewed and 66 were defined as stable. Of these, 37 had epidural anesthesia, 27 had general anesthesia, and 2 had spinal anesthesia. The outcome after cesarean section was compared for women having epidural versus general anesthesia.

Results.—There were 2 stillbirths in the epidural group and 4 in the general anesthesia group. Significantly more newborns in the epidural group than in the general anesthesia group had 1-minute Apgar scores of more than 7. Four infants in the epidural group and 3 in the general anesthesia group required ventilatory support. One mother, who received epidural anesthesia, died from causes unrelated to anesthesia. One woman receiving epidural anesthesia had urinary retention, and 5 had hypotensive episodes that were treated successfully.

Conclusion.—The use of epidural anesthesia for stable women with eclampsia having a cesarean section did not increase the incidence of adverse events.

▶ Fortunately, few, if any, obstetric units in the United States will provide care for 533 women with eclampsia over a 5-year period. Readers should note that in this retrospective study, the authors reported outcome only for the 66 (12.4%) eclamptic women who were defined as "stable."

D. H. Chestnut, MD

Use of Inhaled Nitric Oxide for Emergency Cesarean Section in a Woman With Unexpected Primary Pulmonary Hypertension

Decoene C, Bourzoufi K, Moreau D, et al (Clinic of Anesthesiology and Reanimation in Cardiovascular Diseases, Lille, France)
Can J Anesth 48:584-587, 2001   11–32

Background.—Inhaled nitric oxide (iNO) may be useful in emergent primary pulmonary hypertension (PPH) in pregnant women during labor and delivery. It acts as a selective pulmonary bed vasodilator. Because of its ease of administration, systemic hemodynamic effects can be avoided. Pulmonary bed vasodilation directly improves right ventricular function and indirectly improves left ventricular function. A patient with unexpected PPH who required emergent cesarean delivery was reported.

Case Report.—Woman, 33, para 2, gravida 2, was brought to the hospital in active labor at 34 weeks' gestation. On admission, PPH was diagnosed. Because of fetal breech presentation, a cesarean section was necessary. Epidural anesthesia was induced. During labor and delivery and in the first 24 hours post partum, iNO was administered through a noninvasive ventilation device. The delivery was uneventful. At 12 hours after delivery, a severe pulmonary hypertensive crisis occurred, which resolved with an increase of iNO concentration and isoprenalin administration. The mother and infant were able to go home 10 days after admission.

Conclusion.—In this patient, iNO allowed optimal control of pulmonary arterial hypertension. There were no interactions with epidural anesthesia. The use of iNO may improve the management of emergent cesarean section in women with unexpected PPH.

▶ The good outcome observed in this case was unusual and gratifying.

D. H. Chestnut, MD

Hemodynamic Deterioration After Cardiopulmonary Bypass During Pregnancy: Resuscitation by Postoperative Emergency Cesarean Section

Baraka A, Kawkabani N, Haroun-Bizri S (American Univ of Beirut, Lebanon)
J Cardiothorac Vasc Anesth 14:314-315, 2000   11–33

Objective.—Cardiopulmonary bypass (CPB) surgery is necessary in 2% of pregnant women. A pregnant woman scheduled for a mitral valve replacement experienced severe hemodynamic deterioration after weaning from CPB. She improved dramatically after an emergency cesarean section.

Case Report.—Woman, 34, at 31 weeks' gestation, had progressive dyspnea and orthopnea. She had a history of closed mitral valve commissurotomy and was found to have severe mitral stenosis, mild tricuspid and aortic regurgitation, a moderately dilated right ventricle, and a 40% ejection fraction. Magnesium sulfate was used as a prophylactic tocolytic. The patient was anesthetized, her body temperature was lowered, and the mitral valve was replaced uneventfully. The aortic cross-clamping was released, and the patient was rewarmed. The fetal heart rate began to increase, and uterine contractions were recorded. The patient was stabilized, but 30 minutes later, the maternal blood pressure dropped to 70/30 mm Hg, the pulmonary artery pressure and pulmonary capillary wedge pressure increased to 90/50 mm Hg and 70 mm Hg, respectively, and cardiac output decreased to 2 L/min. Norepinephrine, epinephrine, and dobutamine infusions failed to improve hemodynamic variables. Transesophageal echocardiography revealed severe left ventricular dysfunction with an ejection fraction of less than 15%. Insertion of an intra-aortic balloon and counterpulsations failed to improve the hemodynamics. An emergency cesarean section was performed 12 hours postoperatively. The woman improved dramatically and was discharged on day 10. The baby had a ventricular hemorrhage at birth and died a week later.

Conclusion.—For pregnant women requiring CPB, it may be advisable to perform cesarean sections before CPB for fetuses with gestational ages older than 28 weeks.

▶ This is an interesting case that reminds me of other published cases of maternal cardiac arrest, in which perimortem performance of a cesarean section resulted in successful maternal resuscitation. Evacuation of the uterus significantly reduces aortocaval compression and results in improved venous return, which undoubtedly contributed to the successful outcome observed in these cases.

D. H. Chestnut, MD

Comparison of Cisatracurium-Induced Neuromuscular Blockade Between Immediate Postpartum and Nonpregnant Patients

Pan PH, Moore C (Virginia Commonwealth Univ, Richmond)
J Clin Anesth 13:112-117, 2001   11–34

Objective.—Pregnancy often changes the pharmacodynamics and pharmacokinetics of drugs, including muscle relaxants. Although cisatracurium is 4 times as potent as atracurium, it has minimal cardiovascular side effects, has an intermediate duration of action, undergoes Hofmann elimination, lacks a cumulative effect, and provides good to excellent intubating conditions in healthy nonpregnant adults. There have been no studies comparing the effects of cisatracurium between pregnant and nonpregnant patients. The cisatracurium-induced neuromuscular blockade and intubating conditions between nonpregnant (NP) patients and immediate postpartum (PP) patients were prospectively compared.

Methods.—Under general anesthesia with IV thiopental 5 mg/kg, fentanyl 2.0 to 3.0 µg/kg, midazolam 0.015 to 0.025 mg/kg, and cisatracurium 0.2 mg/kg, 22 immediate postpartum patients (group PP) underwent postpartum tubal ligation and 22 nonpregnant patients (group NP) underwent elective gynecologic surgery. Evoked electromyographic responses of the adductor pollicis muscle were obtained by stimulating the ulnar nerve with supramaximal, square wave impulses of 0.2 milliseconds in a train-of-four sequence of 2 Hz, repeated every 10 seconds with surface electrodes at the wrist on a Datex Relaxograph, interfaced serially to a computer. Airway conditions and responses were scored, and intubating conditions, time to successful intubation attempt, onset times to 50%,

TABLE 3.—Comparison of Onset Time and Recovery of Cisatracurium Between Group NO and Group PP

	Group NP (n = 21)	Group PP (n = 21)	p-Value
Time to 50% T_1 depression (seconds)	80 ± 17	68 ± 19	$p = 0.049$
Time to 90% T_1 depression (seconds)	131 ± 28	110 ± 26	$p = 0.019$
Time to maximal T_1	181 ± 44	147 ± 32	$p = 0.0073$
Time to 25% T_1 recovery (min)	69.1 ± 12.3	60.0 ± 6.3	$p = 0.0048$

Note: Data are expressed as mean ± SD for each group. $P < .05$ is considered significant.
Abbreviations: NP, Nonpregnant patients; PP, immediate postpartum patients.
(Courtesy of Pan PH, Moore C: Comparison of cisatracurium-induced neuromuscular blockade between immediate postpartum and nonpregnant patients. *J Clin Anesth* 13:112-117, 2001. Copyright 2001 by Elsevier Science Inc.)

90%, and maximal T1 depression, and time to 25% T1 recovery were recorded and compared for the 2 groups.

Results.—One patient in each group did not complete the study. Mean onset times and duration of action were significantly shorter in the PP group than in the NP group, even though there were no differences between groups for jaw relaxation, cord immobility, and overall intubating process (Table 3). More PP patients than NP patients had mild diaphragmatic movement after intubation.

Conclusion.—Cisatracurium had a significantly faster onset and shorter clinical duration in PP patients than in NP patients probably because of the combination of the physiologic changes of pregnancy and the unique organ-dependent Hofmann elimination of cisatracurium.

▶ Notwithstanding the results of the present study, I do not consider cisatracurium to be a first-line choice of muscle relaxants for patients undergoing postpartum tubal ligation.

D. H. Chestnut, MD

Complications in Obstetrics and Obstetrics Anesthesia

Informed Consent for Labour Epidurals: What Labouring Women Want to Know

Jackson A, Henry R, Avery N, et al (Queen's Univ, Kingston, Ont, Canada)
Can J Anesth 47:1068-1073, 2000   11–35

Objective.—Some anesthesiologists believe that obtaining informed consent for obstetric epidural analgesia is not possible during active labor. A real-time prospective survey, completed by actively laboring women, was used to determine what a woman in labor wants to hear about epidural analgesia before consenting and whether she feels able to understand the risks.

Methods.—Between May and October 1999, 60 women in labor who had requested epidural analgesia completed the survey. The average age of the women was 29 years. Each woman was interviewed immediately after the request. One-way analysis of variance was used to determine whether education or previous epidural analgesia and opioid premedication had an effect on comprehension.

Results.—Four women were unable to complete the survey because of labor pain or delivery. Four women did not understand the question about level of risk considered significant. Three women refused to disclose their level of education. Most (75%) had more than a high school education, 80% realized that epidural analgesia was not free of risk, and 75% knew about alternatives. At the time of the request for epidural analgesia, women had been in labor for an average of 12 hours and were experiencing a high degree of pain and anxiety. Women wanted all potential complications to be included in the consent form, but this knowledge did not dissuade them from consenting to epidural analgesia. The most important side effects were seizure, death, or paralysis or effects on the baby, but none of these changed the women's minds about consenting. The least important side effects were headache, confinement in bed, and prolonged labor. Although 21% of the women said that 1 in 10 was a significant risk, 52% said they did not want to be told the incidence of complications. The average ability to understand information was 4.9/10. Women wanted the risks of epidural analgesia explained to them (8/10). Women did not feel pressured to have epidural analgesia (0.2/10). Understanding was not correlated with any variable measured.

Conclusion.—Although women wanted all risks disclosed, they were not interested in the risk incidences. Women in labor appear to be able to give informed consent.

▶ The presence of labor does not preclude the requirement for the anesthesiologist to obtain informed consent for regional anesthesia. Others have concluded that women in labor are as able to give informed consent for anesthesia as are other patients who are not in labor. Further, the authors of this study observed that women in labor want to be informed about the potential complications of epidural anesthesia.

D. H. Chestnut, MD

Labor Epidural Analgesia and Intrapartum Maternal Hyperthermia
Yancey MK, Zhang J, Schwarz J, et al (Tripler Army Med Ctr, Honolulu, Hawaii; Natl Inst of Child Health and Human Development, Bethesda, Md)
Obstet Gynecol 98:763-770, 2001   11-36

Introduction.—Previous studies have found labor epidural analgesia to be associated with an increased incidence of maternal intrapartum fever, but patient crossover and self-selection bias may have affected outcomes. In a retrospective cohort analysis, women eligible for on-request labor

TABLE 5.—Neonatal Outcome by Study Period

Characteristics	Before On-Demand Epidural Analgesia (N = 498)	After On-Demand Epidural Analgesia (N = 572)	RR (95% CI)
Complete blood count*	67 (13.5%)	137 (24%)	1.52 (1.3, 1.8)
Chest radiograph	53 (10.6%)	59 (10.4%)	0.98 (0.8, 1.2)
Blood culture†	43 (8.6%)	86 (30.7%)	1.7 (1.2, 2.4)
Antibiotic therapy for presumed neonatal sepsis‡	23 (4.6%)	33 (5.8%)	1.15 (0.8, 1.6)
Median neonatal length of stay (days)*	2 (2, 4)	2 (2, 4)	
Mean	2.53	2.68	

Note: Data are presented as *n* (%), except length of stay, which is presented as median (10th, 90th percentile) and mean ± standard deviation. Analysis by Student *t*-test, χ^2 test, Fisher exact test, or Wilcoxon rank sum test, as appropriate.
*P < .01.
†P < .05.
‡P = .38.
Abbreviations: CI, Confidence interval; *RR,* relative risk.
(Courtesy of Yancey MK, Zhang J, Schwarz J, et al: Labor epidural analgesia and intrapartum maternal hyperthermia. *Obstet Gynecol* 98:763-770, 2001. Reprinted with permission from The American College of Obstetricians and Gynecologists.)

epidural analgesia were compared for intrapartum fever with women who did not have this option.

Methods.—Before October 1993, epidural analgesia in laboring women was available at the study institution only to those with a medical indication. After this date, round-the-clock on-demand labor epidural analgesia was provided. Women eligible for the study were nulliparous with term gestations and in spontaneous labor. During the year before the policy change, 498 eligible women delivered (Before group); 572 delivered in the first year of on-demand epidural analgesia (After group). The techniques and dosing used for labor epidural analgesia were similar in the 2 periods. Excluded from analysis were women admitted with a temperature of at least 99.5° F.

Results.—Labor epidural analgesia was used by 5 (1.0%) women in the Before group and by 475 (83.0%) in the After group. The mean maximal intrapartum temperature was higher in women who had labor epidural analgesia than in those who did not (99.1° F vs 98.4° F). A maximal temperature of at least 99.5° F was recorded in 30% of women with epidural analgesia, but in only 8.7% of those who did not receive epidural analgesia. In multivariable analysis, on-request labor epidural analgesia was significantly associated with an intrapartum temperature of at least 99.5° F and an intrapartum temperature of at least 100.4° F. In the After group there were statistically significant increases in the frequency of neonatal screening complete blood count and blood cultures (Table 5) and in median length of stay. No cases of culture-proven neonatal sepsis occurred, and the proportion of infants who received antibiotic therapy was similar in the Before (4.6%) and After (5.8%) groups.

Conclusion.—Labor epidural analgesia is associated with a clinically significant increase in the incidence of intrapartum fever. The precise etiology of this effect is unknown, but it may be related to alteration in maternal thermoregulatory physiology.

▶ It is unclear why women who receive epidural analgesia during labor are at increased risk for intrapartum fever. The authors noted that "there is currently no reliable means of accurately differentiating the woman with an infectious-mediated fever from the parturient with hyperthermia resulting from physiologic alterations induced by epidural analgesia." Nonetheless, in this hospital, there was no significant increase in the proportion of infants who received antibiotic therapy for presumed sepsis after the introduction of on-demand epidural analgesia for laboring women.

D. H. Chestnut, MD

Risk of Uterine Rupture During Labor Among Women With a Prior Cesarean Delivery

Lydon-Rochelle M, Holt VL, Easterling TR, et al (Univ of Washington, Seattle)
N Engl J Med 345:3-8, 2001   11–37

Introduction.—Every year in the United States, nearly 60% of women with a prior cesarean delivery who again become pregnant attempt labor. There are concerns that a trial of labor may increase the risk of uterine rupture. State-wide linked birth-certificate and hospital-discharge data were used to evaluate the risk of uterine rupture associated with spontaneous onset of labor, induction of labor not involving prostaglandins, induction of labor with prostaglandins, and repeated cesarean delivery without labor among women with 1 prior cesarean delivery.

Methods.—A population-based, retrospective analysis was performed using data from all primiparous women who gave birth to live singletons by cesarean section in civilian hospitals in Washington state between 1987 and 1996 and who delivered a second singleton child during the same period. A total of 20,095 women were assessed for the risk of uterine rupture in deliveries with spontaneous onset of labor, those with labor induced by prostaglandins, and those in which labor was induced by other means. These 3 groups of deliveries were compared in women who had repeated cesarean delivery without labor.

Results.—The rate of uterine rupture was 1.6/1000 among women with repeated cesarean delivery without labor (11 women), 5.2/1000 among women with spontaneous onset of labor (56 women), 7.7/1000 among women whose labor was induced without prostaglandins (15 women), and 24.5/1000 among women with prostaglandin-induced labor (9 women). Compared with the risk for women with repeated cesarean delivery without labor, uterine rupture was more likely among women with spontaneous onset of labor (relative risk, 3.3; 95% confidence interval, 2.4-9.7), and induction with prostaglandins (relative risk, 15.6; 95% confidence interval, 8.1-30.0).

Conclusion.—For women with 1 prior cesarean delivery, the risk of uterine rupture is higher among those whose delivery is induced versus those with repeated delivery without labor. The highest risk is among women whose labor is induced with prostaglandins.

▶ Recent studies have reevaluated the risk of a trial of labor and attempted vaginal birth after cesarean delivery (VBAC). These studies have suggested that earlier studies may have underestimated the risk of VBAC. The reason is unclear. Perhaps some hospitals have been unable to replicate the favorable results obtained in earlier, carefully controlled clinical trials. Perhaps the good outcomes obtained in earlier published studies reflect the natural bias toward publication of favorable results. Or perhaps familiarity with VBAC may breed complacency. Regardless, the American College of Obstetricians and Gynecologists (ACOG) has stated that institutions offering VBAC should have facilities and personnel *immediately* available to perform emergency cesarean delivery in cases of uterine rupture. To my knowledge, this represents the only circumstance in which the ACOG has established a standard that is more strict than the longstanding "30-minute rule" for cases of emergency cesarean delivery.

D. H. Chestnut, MD

Unexpected Hyperkalemia Following Succinylcholine Administration in Prolonged Immobilized Parturients Treated With Magnesium and Ritodrine

Sato K, Nishiwaki K, Kuno N, et al (Nagoya Univ, Japan)
Anesthesiology 93:1539-1541, 2000   11–38

Objective.—Magnesium prolongs the action of nondepolarizing neuromuscular blocking drugs. Cases of 3 obstetric patients, treated with continuous IV magnesium and ritodrine therapy, who experienced cardiac arrest or ECG abnormalities concomitant with hyperkalemia after induction of IV anesthesia are discussed.

Case 1.—Woman, 34, pregnant with triplets, had vaginal bleeding at 18 weeks' gestation. Chorioamnionitis was diagnosed, and she was treated with antibiotics. Treatment with continuous IV magnesium became necessary at 22 weeks' gestation. Delivery of 1 fetus with recerclage of the cervix became necessary at 25 weeks' gestation. Magnesium concentration was 9.0 mg/dL, plasma potassium level was 4.0 mm, and total calcium level was 5.9 mg/dL. The patient was given a general anesthetic and ritodrine and was intubated. She was given succinylcholine intravenously. After induction she became cyanotic and pulseless and went into ventricular fibrillation. She was successfully defibrillated and delivered 3 infants. She was stabilized and experienced no postoperative neurologic or ECG abnormalities.

Case 2.—Woman, 25, pregnant with twins, was hospitalized at 23 weeks' gestation because of preterm labor. She received a continuous IV administration of magnesium sulfate and ritodrine. She underwent a cesarean section at 26 weeks' gestation because of acute fetal distress. The magnesium concentration was 7.8 mg/dL. She was anesthesthetized and intubated. After succinylcholine administration, her ECG showed elevated T waves, and ECG abnormalities and ventricular tachycardia developed. She was injected with calcium chloride and recovered uneventfully.

Case 3.—Woman, 28, with bronchial asthma and pregnant with twins, was admitted at 25 weeks' gestation for preterm labor. She received IV ritodrine and magnesium sulfate. She was scheduled to undergo a cesarean section at 28 weeks' gestation because of twin-twin transfusion syndrome. The magnesium concentration was 5.3 mg/dL. She was anesthetized and intubated. After receiving succinylcholine, her plasma potassium level increased to 7.2 mm and an ECG showed widened QRS complexes and elevated T waves. Calcium chloride was injected, and the ECG became normal. The remainder of the procedure was uneventful.

Conclusion.—Succinylcholine should be used with caution in pregnant women who have been immobilized for a long time and have been given magnesium sulfate and ritodrine.

▶ The authors have made an observation of interest to anesthesiologists who provide care for pregnant women subjected to prolonged bed rest and tocolytic therapy for treatment of preterm labor. The authors offer speculation regarding the relative contributions of prolonged immobilization, hypermagnesemia, and β-adrenergic tocolytic therapy as predisposing factors to the occurrence of hyperkalemia and cardiac arrest after succinylcholine administration in these patients. It is difficult to determine the relative importance of these 3 factors as causes of the adverse events observed in these 3 patients.

D. H. Chestnut, MD

Rebound Perioperative Hyperkalemia in Six Patients After Cessation of Ritodrine for Premature Labor
Kotani N, Kushikata T, Hashimoto H, et al (Univ of Hirosaki, Japan)
Anesth Analg 93:709-711, 2001   11–39

Introduction.—Rebound hyperkalemia developed in 6 patients 60 to 150 minutes after cessation of IV ritodrine. A combined case report is presented.

Case Report.—All patients, aged 24 to 32 years, had normal plasma potassium levels before a continuous infusion of ritodrine. All patients underwent emergency cesarean deliveries under general anesthesia because their preterm labor could not be arrested. During postoperative recovery, patients' plasma potassium levels increased dramatically (>7.0 mmol/L) and concurrently with a peaked T wave on ECG. The PR interval was prolonged or the P wave was lost within 1 hour after emergence from anesthesia. Potassium levels of all patients gradually returned to normal after treatment with potassium-free fluid, furosemide, and calcium chloride.

Conclusion.—Rebound hyperkalemia can occur within 1 to 2 hours after cessation of ritodrine and may last as long as 8 hours.

▶ The authors have made an important observation. Fortunately, the use of continuous IV infusion of ritodrine for treatment of preterm labor has markedly declined in the United States.

D. H. Chestnut, MD

Maternal Anaphylactic Reaction to a General Anaesthetic at Emergency Caesarean Section for Fetal Bradycardia
Stannard L, Bellis A (Billinge Hosp, England)
Br J Obstet Gynaecol 108:539-540, 2001   11–40

Background.—Anaphylaxis to anesthetic agents, which has a variable incidence, is especially difficult to assess in obstetric populations. A case of maternal anaphylactic reaction to a general anesthetic at emergency cesarean delivery for fetal bradycardia was presented.

> *Case Report.*—Woman, 31, was a primigravida. Her pregnancy had been uneventful until 38 weeks' gestation, when spontaneous labor began. Her cervix was 4 cm dilated, and the fetal heart rate was 110 beats/min. Cardiotocography showed early decelerations. The membranes were ruptured artificially, and diamorphine was given for pain relief. Lack of change in cervical dilation at the next examination prompted an order for oxytocin infusion. The epidural catheter was inserted for analgesia without difficulty.
>
> After a test dose of 3 mL of 2% lignocaine, the patient's blood pressure was 166/74 mm Hg. Her pulse rate was 81 beats/min. During this time, the fetal heart rate declined to 70 beats/min, which persisted despite changing maternal position and oxygen administration. This prompted the decision to perform a cesarean section. Because there was insufficient time to establish adequate epidural anesthesia for the cesarean section, general anesthesia in the operating room was planned, and no further drugs were delivered through the epidural catheter.
>
> Thiopentone, 500 mg, and suxamethonium, 100 mg, were given IV. Endotracheal intubation was performed successfully. However, ventilation rapidly became progressively difficult. The patient's oxygen saturation dropped to 80% to 90%. Despite the delivery of 100% oxygen, her oxygen saturation declined to 60%. Auscultation of the chest revealed respiratory and expiratory rhonci. The diagnosis of anaphylaxis was considered. The patient's pulse became weak, her heart rate delined to less than 40 beats/min, and her blood pressure was unrecordable. Oxygen saturation was less than 50%, with end-tidal carbon dioxide of less than 10 mm Hg.

Adrenaline, 1 mg, was given IV, and cardiopulmonary resuscitation was begun.

Resuscitation was continued through the delivery. Adrenaline, 4 mg, was delivered through a central venous catheter, with hydrocortisone, 500 mg IV colloid, and infusion of aminophylline. IM chlorpheniramine, 20 mg, was also administered. The infant was delivered, with 1- and 5-minute Apgar scores of 3 and 9, respectively. Although cardiopulmonary resuscitation saved the mother's life, severe bronchospasm and hypertension persisted, and a supraventricular tachycardia developed.

The patient was transferred to the ICU, where pulmonary edema, adult respiratory distress syndrome requiring a tracheostomy, and acute renal failure developed. These complications were treated successfully, and the patient was able to go home at 4 weeks. Subsequent skin prick testing demonstrated a positive reaction to atracurium and suxamethonium and a negative reaction to rocuronium and latex.

Conclusion.—The survival of this patient relied on prompt resuscitation. Early delivery of the baby and early adrenaline administration probably played a significant role in her successful resuscitation.

▶ I recently encountered a case of severe anaphylactic shock during induction of general anesthesia in a young woman who was scheduled for renal transplantation. Subsequent skin testing suggested that cisatracurium was the triggering agent. Prompt administration of epinephrine is the mainstay of effective treatment of anaphylaxis.

D. H. Chestnut, MD

Cardiac Arrest and Myocardial Infarction Induced by Postpartum Intravenous Ergonovine Administration
Tsui BCH, Stewart B, Fitzmaurice A, et al (Univ of Alberta, Edmonton, Canada; Royal Alexandra Hosp, Edmonton, Alta, Canada; Caritas Health Group, Edmonton, Alta, Canada)
Anesthesiology 94:363-364, 2001   11–41

Introduction.—Ergonovine can induce coronary spasm, sometimes causing acute myocardial infarction. During cesarean delivery, ergot derivatives are sometimes given to promote uterine contractions. Few ischemic cardiac events related to ergonovine have been reported in this setting. A patient who went into cardiac arrest with myocardial infarction after ergonovine administration during cesarean delivery was reported.

Case Report.—Woman, 34, underwent cesarean delivery after premature rupture of the membranes and failed induction of labor. She had no history of cardiovascular disease and no cardiac risk factors. The uterus was atonic after delivery, even after oxytocin. Thus, a single IV injection of ergonovine, 0.25 mg, was given. The patient rapidly became unresponsive and severe bradycardia developed, followed by cardiac arrest with asystole. During resuscitation, she went into ventricular fibrillation.

The patient was resuscitated and transferred to a coronary care unit, where an ECG showed an acute anterior infarction with anterior ST depression. Urgent cardiac catheterization was performed. Coronary angiography showed diffuse spasm of the left anterior descending and circumflex coronary arteries, including subtotal occlusion of the left anterior descending artery. The left ventricular ejection fraction was estimated at 15%. The spasm responded to intracoronary injection of nitroglycerin, 200 µg; however, before IV nitroglycerin could be started, the patient had new ST changes consistent with inferoposterior injury. This resolved with IV nitroglycerin. The patient's peak creatinine phosphokinase level was 2,763 U/L. She was extubated after 2 days and taken off intra-aortic balloon pump support and inotropic agents at 3 days. By the fifth day, her ejection fraction had improved to 45%. She was discharged at 11 days with no neurologic deficits.

Discussion.—Coronary vasospasm is a rare complication of ergonovine administration after cesarean section. Early recognition and prompt treatment are essential to preserve myocardial function. The cardiac risks associated with ergot derivatives can be minimized through careful drug administration, timely evaluation, and nitroglycerin treatment.

▶ This case illustrates one of the hazards of IV administration of an ergot derivative for treatment of uterine atony. Methylergonovine is the semisynthetic ergot alkaloid available for parenteral treatment of uterine atony in the United States. The preferred route of administration is *intramuscular*. Methylergonovine should not be administered IV, except in cases of severe, life-threatening hemorrhage. Even in those circumstances, it seems wise to dilute 0.2 mg in 10 mL of saline and administer small incremental doses of 1 mL (ie, 0.02 mg), while carefully monitoring maternal blood pressure.

D. H. Chestnut, MD

Does Pregnancy Protect Against Intrathecal Lidocaine-Induced Transient Neurologic Symptoms?
Aouad MT, Siddik SS, Jalbout MI, et al (American Univ of Beirut, Lebanon)
Anesth Analg 92:401-404, 2001   11–42

Objective.—Intrathecal hyperbaric lidocaine can produce transient neurologic symptoms (TNS) in as many as 40% of patients. The incidence of TNS was investigated in parturients undergoing cesarean section under spinal anesthesia with hyperbaric lidocaine or hyperbaric bupivacaine.

Methods.—Women (n = 200) undergoing elective cesarean section were randomly allocated to receive spinal anesthesia with 75 mg of 5% hyperbaric lidocaine (n = 100) or 12 mg of 0.75% hyperbaric bupivacaine. On postoperative days 1 to 3 an anesthesiologist blinded to the anesthetic used interviewed patients regarding pain or strange sensations in locations other than the surgical site. The frequency of occurrences of symptoms was compared for the 2 groups.

Results.—Compared with the bupivacaine group, the lidocaine group had a significantly higher incidence of pain at the puncture site. Other symptoms were similar for both groups. The bupivacaine block lasted significantly longer than the lidocaine block.

Conclusion.—Neither group experienced any TNS after administration of intrathecal anesthesia.

Transient Neurologic Symptoms After Spinal Anesthesia With Lidocaine in Obstetric Patients
Philip J, Sharma SK, Gottumukkala VNR, et al (Univ of Texas, Dallas)
Anesth Analg 92:405-409, 2001   11–43

Objective.—Spinal anesthesia of nonobstetrical patients with lidocaine frequently results in transient neurologic symptoms (TNS). Because lidocaine is often used for obstetric patients, the occurrence of TNS with lidocaine versus bupivacaine was investigated in a select group of obstetric patients in a randomized, double-blind, controlled comparison study.

Methods.—Spinal anesthesia with either hyperbaric 5% lidocaine (n = 30) or 0.75% bupivacaine (n = 28) was administered to 58 ASA physical status I women undergoing postpartum tubal ligation. The sensory level of anesthesia and the degree of motor blockade were assessed. At 24 and 48 hours and 1, 2, and 3 weeks postoperatively, patients were interviewed about presence and severity of TNS, functional impairment, and pain at the injection site. Patients with severe symptoms were given a neurologic examination. Results were compared for the 2 groups.

Results.—One lidocaine patient was switched to general anesthesia because of inadequate block. Significantly more patients receiving lidocaine than those receiving bupivacaine achieved complete motor blockade (100% vs 82%). The incidences of TNS were 3% with lidocaine and 7% with bupivacaine. The 3 patients reporting TNS described a bilateral aching or burning pain in the buttocks or back of the thighs with no radiation within the first 24 hours. Pain severity was rated no higher than 3. One patient given lidocaine was treated for hypotension.

Conclusion.—The incidence of TNS with intrathecal lidocaine anesthesia in obstetric patients is small.

▶ These 2 articles (Abstracts 11–42 and 11–43) were accompanied by a thoughtful editorial.[1] Aouad et al have suggested that pregnancy might "protect against intrathecal lidocaine-induced transient neurologic symptoms." However, Schneider and Birnbach[1] concluded that "there is still insufficient safety evidence to suggest that spinal hyperbaric 5% lidocaine be routinely used in obstetrics."

D. H. Chestnut, MD

Reference

1. Schneider MC, Birnbach DJ: Lidocaine neurotoxicity in the obstetric patient: Is the water safe (editorial)? *Anesth Analg* 92:287-290, 2001.

Effectiveness of Epidural Blood Patch in the Management of Post-Dural Puncture Headache
Safa-Tisseront V, Thormann F, Malassiné P, et al (Université Pierre et Marie Curie, Paris)
Anesthesiology 95:334-339, 2001   11–44

Background.—To date, the only effective treatment for postdural puncture headache (PDPH) is lumbar epidural blood patch (EBP), and evidence regarding its effectiveness is mixed. The effectiveness of EBP for severe PDPH and the factors predictive of EBP failure were evaluated.

Methods.—The subjects were 504 patients (26% male) who underwent EBP for incapacitating PDPH at a single institution over a 12-year period. EBP was performed at the suggestion of the patient's attending physician, rather than per protocol. Results of EBP were classified as complete relief (resolution of all symptoms), incomplete relief (clinical improvement with resumption of normal daily activities), or failure (persistence of severe symptoms). Patients who experienced EBP failure were offered another attempt. Success rates were determined, and patient and procedural characteristics, the timing of EBP relative to puncture, and the volume of blood injected during EBP were examined to determine their ability to predict EBP failure.

Results.—Symptoms of CSF leak developed from 1 to 10 days (median, 1 day) after dural puncture, and EBP was performed 1 to 53 days (median, 4 days) after puncture. Mean blood volume during EBP was 23 mL. Of the 504 patients, 377 (75%) had complete relief after EBP, 93 (18%) had incomplete relief, and 34 (7%) had EBP failure (Fig 1). About half of the patients with a failed EBP underwent a second EBP, and about half of these patients experienced complete relief after the second attempt. Multivariate analysis identified 2 significant independent predictors of EBP failure: use of a needle < 20 gauge during dural puncture (odds ratio, 5.96) and a delay in EBP of <4 days (odds ratio, 2.63).

Conclusion.—EBP was effective in eliminating or relieving pain in most of these patients with incapacitating PDPH. The use of a large-bore needle during lumbar puncture dramatically increased the likelihood of EBP failure. Whether performing EBP early after puncture truly increases the risk of EBP failure remains controversial, as the relationship between early

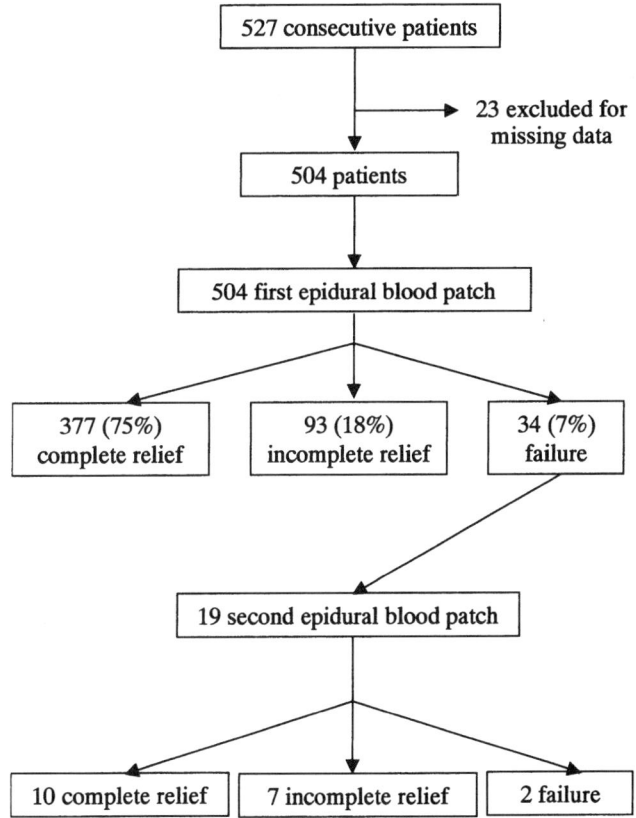

FIGURE 1.—Trial profile. (Courtesy of Safa-Tisseront V, Thormann F, Malassiné P, et al: Effectiveness of epidural blood patch in the management of post-dural puncture headache. *Anesthesiology* 95:334-339, 2001. Copyright, American Society of Anesthesiologists, Inc. Used with permission of Lippincott-Raven Publishers.)

EBP and failure may have been influenced by the fact that patients with more severe symptoms were treated earlier.

▶ In this prospective study, performance of early EBP (ie, within 3 days of dural puncture) was associated with an increased likelihood of failure. However, the authors correctly called attention to the potential for selection bias, and they noted that "it is likely that patients experiencing more pain were treated earlier, [and] . . . the diminished effectiveness of early EBP was more related to the size of the dural puncture and the severity of the CSF leak than with the fact of not delaying EBP." In my judgment, the evidence supporting a delay in performing EBP, until an arbitrary time interval after dural puncture, is tenuous.

D. H. Chestnut, MD

12 Pain Management

Acute Pain Management

Dextromethorphan Attenuation of Postoperative Pain and Primary and Secondary Thermal Hyperalgesia

Weinbroum AA, Gorodezky A, Niv D, et al (Tel Aviv Univ, Israel)

Can J Anesth 48:167-174, 2001   12–1

Background.—Dextromethorphan (DM) can function as an N-methyl-D-aspartate (NMDA) receptor antagonist that dose-dependently reduces slow temporal summation of electrically and thermally evoked secondary pain sensation. How the use of oral DM as a premedication affects patients' perception of pain, requirement for morphine, and subjective ratings of various parameters was evaluated.

Methods.—The 30 patients evaluated underwent either laparoscopic cholecystectomy or inguinal hernioplasty under general anesthesia. DM (90 mg) was given to 15 patients 90 minutes before anesthesia; the other 15 received placebo. Within the 6-hour period of observation, patient-controlled analgesia with morphine was available for 2 hours; doses of diclofenac (75 mg) were given later as needed for the first 24 hours. Visual analogue scales were used to assess pain. Among the other parameters measured were sedation level, morphine consumption, touch sensation, thermal thresholds for cold and hot sensation, and pain sensation, both at the site of the incision and distantly.

Results.—Patients who received DM had lower pain intensity and sedation levels and reported a greater sense of well-being. Only the DM patients had no primary or secondary hyperalgesia; similar pain sensation was produced by von Frey filaments in the 2 groups. None of the patients had adverse effects attributable to DM during the 24 hours immediately following surgery.

Conclusion.—DM effectively reduced pain intensity, reduced the amount of analgesic agents required postoperatively, and improved patients' sense of well-being over the results with placebo. In addition, the sedation rating was lower among those receiving DM than for the placebo group. Postoperative thermal-induced hyperalgesia and hyperpathia were eliminated. Thus, DM appears to be of value as a premedication.

▶ There are only a few clinically used compounds with demonstrated NMDA antagonist effects. These include ketamine, DM, and amantadine.

Preemptive administration of these compounds has had mixed success in reducing postoperative opioid requirements or pain levels. A number of other drugs have recently been shown to have some NMDA antagonist effects. These include methadone, propoxyphene, and amitriptyline.

S. E. Abram, MD

Large-Dose Oral Dextromethorphan As an Adjunct to Patient-Controlled Analgesia With Morphine After Knee Surgery
Wadhwa A, Clarke D, Goodchild CS, et al (Monash Univ, Clayton, Australia; Avenue Hosp, Melbourne, Australia)
Anesth Analg 92:448-454, 2001   12–2

Background.—Experimental evidence suggests that dextromethorphan, a weak antagonist of N-methyl-D-aspartate (NMDA) receptors, decreases spinal cord sensitization and inhibits the development of cutaneous secondary hyperalgesia after tissue trauma. Previous studies have shown that ketamine (another NMDA antagonist), when coadministered with an opioid, improves pain relief and reduces the dose of opioid needed for pain relief. However, previous studies in which dextromethorphan was coadministered with an opioid failed to show either improved pain control or opioid sparing. Whether the coadministration of a large oral dose of dextromethorphan (close to the maximum tolerated dose) would have a significant effect on postoperative pain or morphine requirement after knee surgery was tested.

Methods.—Two studies were performed. The first study involved 25 patients undergoing knee or hip surgery in whom the maximum tolerated dose of oral dextromethorphan was determined to be 750 mg. The second study involved 56 patients undergoing either knee reconstruction (29 patients; 22 men and 7 women, 18-41 years of age) or knee replacement (27 patients; 17 men and 10 women, 53-74 years of age). Patients were randomly assigned to receive 3 doses of either placebo (34 patients) or 200 mg of oral dextromethorphan (22 patients). Postoperatively, a continuous passive movement machine was used to move the operated knee through an angle of flexion of 50° 1 to 5 times per minute for 24 hours after the first placebo or dextromethorphan dose. Additionally, patients were given a patient-controlled analgesia device for morphine self-medication. Postoperative morphine requirements, pain with movement, and side effects were compared between the 2 groups.

Results.—Patients in the dextromethorphan group required significantly less morphine than patients taking placebo (37.2 vs 52.6 mg per patient at 24 hours; a 29.3% difference). Patients taking dextromethorphan also experienced significantly more episodes of mild-to-moderate nausea (there were no episodes of severe nausea). The severity of postoperative pain with movement did not differ significantly between the 2 groups up to 24 hours after placebo or dextromethorphan administration.

Conclusion.—Dextromethorphan has a morphine-sparing effect compared with placebo. However, the extent of the morphine-sparing effect with this 600-mg dose was not significantly different from that reported in other trials in which 20 to 40 mg of dextromethorphan was administered every 6 to 8 hours. Additionally, the modest morphine-sparing effect with the large dose came at the cost of increased nausea. Dextromethorphan did not significantly improve pain with movement. Therefore, even when administered near the maximally tolerated dosage, oral dextromethorphan is not clinically useful in managing pain after knee surgery.

▶ This study utilized the maximum dextromethorphan dose that failed to produce substantial side effects. While it did produce some sparing of opioid use, it did not significantly improve analgesia. The morphine-sparing effect was associated with a slight reduction in the incidence of nausea, but there was no decreased incidence of other side effects.

S. E. Abram, MD

Intrathecal Bupivacaine With Morphine or Neostigmine for Postoperative Analgesia After Total Knee Replacement Surgery

Tan P-H, Chia Y-Y, Lo Y, et al (Chang-Gung Mem Hosp, Kaohsiung, China; Natl Yang-Ming Univ, Taiwan, Republic of China)
Can J Anesth 48:551-556, 2001   12–3

Introduction.—Few comparative data are available demonstrating how postoperative analgesic effects differ between neostigmine and conventional intrathecal (IT) opioid agents. The analgesic effects of IT neostigmine and IT morphine, measured by analgesic demand and visual analog scale (VAS) pain scores, were compared in 60 patients scheduled for elective total knee replacement under spinal anesthesia. Patients were randomized to 1 of 3 equal groups receiving IT 0.5% hyperbaric bupiv-

TABLE 2.—Spinal Anesthesia Characteristics and Postoperative Data

Group	Saline	Morphine	Neostigmine	
Number of patients	20	20	20	
Maximal level of sensory block	T 3.5 ± 0.3	T 3.8 ± 0.2	T 3.6 ± 0.3	NS
Duration of absolute analgesia (min)	320.7 ± 24.6	615.3 ± 64.7†	443.2 ± 35.4‡	
First diclofenac (hr)	6.1 ± 1.2	12.5 ± 2.6†	9.3 ± 2.2‡	
Number of *im* 75 mg diclofenac injections	2 (1-2)	2 (0-2)	2 (1-2)	NS
24-hr VAS assessment	3.6 ± 0.9	1.6 ± 0.5*	2.2 ± 0.7‡	
Duration of motor block (hr)	4.7 ± 0.3	4.5 ± 0.2	5.7 ± 0.4‡	

Number of 75 mg diclofenac IM injections is expressed as mean (25% to 75%). Other data are expressed as mean ± SEM.
*Absolute analgesia, time of neostigmine administration to the time when the VAS pain score became greater than zero.
†P < .05 compared with the other 2 groups.
‡P < .05 compared with saline solution group.
Abbreviations: VAS, Visual analog scale; *NS,* not significant.
(Courtesy of Tan P-H, Chia Y-Y, Lo Y, et al: Intrathecal bupivacaine with morphine or neostigmine for postoperative analgesia after total knee replacement surgery. *Can J Anesth* 48:551-556, 2001.)

TABLE 3.—Incidence of Side Effects and Satisfaction Rate

	Saline	Morphine	Neostigmine	
Nausea/vomiting	1/20	5/20	7/20*	
Pruritus	0/20	14/20†	0/20	
Dizziness	0/20	5/20	4/20	NS
Anxiety	0/20	0/20	3/20	NS
Respiratory depression	0/20	0/20	0/20	NS
Satisfaction	1/20	4/20	11/20†	

*$P < .05$ compared with saline solution group.
†$P < .05$ compared with the other 2 groups.
Abbreviation: NS, Not significant.
(Courtesy of Tan P-H, Chia Y-Y, Lo Y, et al: Intrathecal bupivacaine with morphine or neostigmine for postoperative analgesia after total knee replacement surgery. *Can J Anesth* 48:551-556, 2001.)

---

acaine 15 mg with either normal saline solution, 0.5 mL, neostigmine 50 µg, or morphine 300 µg. Five measures were recorded for 24 hours after drug administration: maximal level of sensory block, duration of analgesia, time to use of rescue analgesic, overall 24-hour and 4-hour-interval VAS pain score, and incidence of adverse effects.

Results.—All groups were similar in maximal level of sensory block. The morphine group had later onset of postoperative pain and longer time to first rescue analgesic compared with the neostigmine group ($P < .05$). Overall 24 VAS pain scores were significantly higher in the saline solution group than the morphine and neostigmine groups ($P < .05$). Motor block lasted significantly longer in the neostigmine group compared with the morphine and saline solution groups ($P < .05$) (Table 2). The incidence of adverse effects was similar in the neostigmine and morphine groups, with the exception of pruritis (70%), which was more common in the morphine group than in the neostigmine and saline solution groups (0%; $P < .05$). Patients in the neostigmine group had higher rates of satisfaction than did those in the morphine and saline solution groups ($P < .05$) (Table 3).

Conclusion.—Administration of IT neostigmine 50 µg provides postoperative analgesia that lasts about 7 hours, with fewer side effects and better satisfaction ratings than IT morphine 300 µg and placebo in patients with total knee replacement surgery.

▶ Nausea and vomiting have limited the utility of IT neostigimine in most studies that have assessed its perioperative effects. IT neostigmine may be a reasonable alternative to spinal morphine in patients at high risk for respiratory depression or in those with known intolerance to opioids. It may also have additive or synergistic analgesic effects when combined with other spinal analgesics. It would be helpful to have a variety of drugs for neuraxial intraoperative and postoperative use that affect different receptors, particularly for patients who have become tolerant to opioids.

S. E. Abram, MD

PCA Ketamine and Morphine After Abdominal Hysterectomy

Burstal R, Danjoux G, Hayes C, et al (John Hunter Hosp, Newcastle, New South Wales)
Anaesth Intensive Care 29:246-251, 2001   12–4

Introduction.—Postoperative analgesia with opioid agents is a significant factor in postoperative nausea and vomiting in patients who have undergone gynecologic surgery. The addition of ketamine to morphine patient-controlled analgesia (PCA) may be beneficial because of significantly decreased opioid usage and opioid-related side effects. The effect of combined morphine-ketamine PCA for postoperative analgesia after abdominal total hysterectomy was examined in 70 women.

Methods.—Patients were randomized in double-blind fashion to a PCA group with either morphine 1 mg/mL (group M, n = 33) or morphine 1 mg/mL plus ketamine 2 mg/mL (group K; n = 37) for 48-hours. In the first 43 women, the area of allodynia around the incision was measured on day 2.

Results.—A significant reduction in the area of allodynia was observed in group K (42 cm^2; interquartile range [IQR], 57) compared with group M (57 cm^2; IQR, 82; $z = -2.0$; $P = .04$). Both groups were similar in age and weight, as were subgroups in which the area of allodynia was measured with respect to length of incision. Thirty women used PCA for the entire 48 hours (group K, n = 10; group M, n = 19); 29 stopped PCA before 48 hours (group K, n = 16; group M, n = 13). Eleven patients withdrew because of side effects (group K, n = 10; group M, n = 1; $P = .006$; Table 2). Significant differences were observed in the duration each group used PCA ($P = .003$). The total dose of PCA was similar. The median IQR area of allodynia in group M and group K was 57 cm^2 and 42 cm^2 ($P = .04$), respectively.

TABLE 2.—Patients Withdrawn From Study Because of Side Effects

Recruitment Number	Group	Total PCA Dose (ml)	Time (h) at Withdrawal	Reason for Withdrawal
5	K	78	20	Pruritus
17	K	25	22	Dysphoria
18	K	40	22	Nausea
19	K	38	22	Pruritus
24	K	30	10	Dysphoria
36	K	80	40	Dysphoria
50	M	8	15	Nausea
54	K	36	22	Dysphoria
60	K	44	22	Nausea
61	K	10	20	Pruritus
69	K	93	43	Pruritus

Median (interquartile range) dose (ketamine 2 mg/mL) for patients in group K 39 (48) mL.
Median (interquartile range) time for patients in group K 22 (48) hours.
(Courtesy of Burstal R, Danjoux G, Hayes C, et al: PCA ketamine and morphine after abdominal hysterectomy. *Anesth Intensive Care* 29:246-251, 2001.)

Conclusion.—The potential usefulness of ketamine after hysterectomy was offset by a high rate of adverse effects and lack of opioid-sparing effects, to the extent that combined IV ketamine and morphine PCA in the doses used in this trial cannot be recommended for routine use.

▶ While ketamine does not appear to be useful for routine management of postoperative pain, it can be helpful in postoperative patients who have been given opioids chronically and are opioid tolerant or in patients with coexisting neuropathic pain. The psychotomimetic effects of ketamine may preclude the use of dosages that are adequate to effectively block *N*-methyl-D-aspartate receptors.

S. E. Abram, MD

Adding Ketamine to Morphine for Patient-Controlled Analgesia After Major Abdominal Surgery: A Double-Blinded, Randomized Controlled Trial
Reeves M, Lindholm DE, Myles PS, et al (Alfred Hosp, Prahran, Victoria, Australia; Monash Univ, Australia)
Anesth Analg 93:116-120, 2001   12–5

Introduction.—A drug that could improve pain scores and decrease the adverse effects related to large doses of opioids would have great clinical usefulness. Ketamine decreases pain after laparotomy. The addition of ketamine to morphine for patient-controlled analgesia (PCA) was examined in a double-blind controlled trial of 76 patients who underwent major abdominal surgery.

Methods.—Patients were randomized to receive PCA consisting of either morphine 1 mg/mL (group M) or morphine with ketamine 1 mg/mL (group MK). Patients were stratified according to whether they had upper or lower abdominal surgery. Preoperative and 48-hour postoperative quality of recovery scores and trail-making tests (cognitive tests of attention and perception) were performed. Patients were evaluated at regular intervals postoperatively for pain scores at rest and during movement, PCA use, sedation scores, heart rate, blood pressure, and respiratory rate. Patients were asked to rate pain using a 5-point verbal rating score. Side effects were recorded. No other analgesics and no regional blocks were administered during the 48-hour evaluation.

Results.—Groups were similar postoperatively in subjective evaluations of analgesic efficacy, pain scores at rest and during movement (Fig 1), opioid use, and adverse effects. Patients in group MK had worse cognitive testing scores ($P = .037$), and were at increased risk for vivid dreaming (relative risk, 1.8; 95% confidence interval, 0.78-4.2).

Conclusion.—Small-dose ketamine combined with PCA morphine offers no benefit to patients undergoing major abdominal surgery.

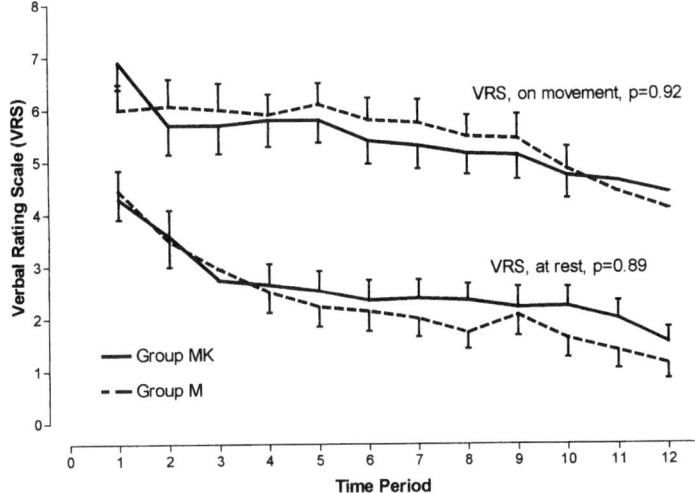

FIGURE 1.—Pain verbal rating scale (VRS) (0 = no pain, 10 = worst pain imaginable) in patients receiving patient-controlled analgesia after major abdominal surgery. Postoperative time periods: 1 = 4 h, 2 = 8 h, 3 = 12 h, 4 = 16 h, 5 = 20 h, 6 = 24 h, 7 = 28 h, 8 = 32 h, 9 = 36 h, 10 = 40 h, 11 = 44 h, 12 = 48 h. (Courtesy of Reeves M, Lindholm DE, Myles PS, et al: Adding ketamine to morphine for patient-controlled analgesia after major abdominal surgery: A double-blinded, randomized controlled trial. *Anesth Analg* 93:116-120, 2001.)

▶ While the rationale for adding an N-methyl-D-aspartate antagonist to morphine for postoperative pain relief is compelling, the addition of ketamine at doses that do not produce significantly increased psychotomimetic effects does not provide significant benefit. While the routine use of ketamine may not be indicated, the drug may be useful in certain clinical situations. I have found intermittent low doses helpful in patients with chronic nonmalignant or cancer pain that is difficult to control with opioid therapy alone. Regional anesthetic techniques are ideal for such patients, but when they are inappropriate or contraindicated, ketamine can be extremely helpful. A bolus dose of 20 to 40 mg every 2 to 3 hours often provides significant relief with minimal side effects.

S. E. Abram, MD

The Injectable Cyclooxygenase-2-Specific Inhibitor Parecoxib Sodium Has Analgesic Efficacy When Administered Preoperatively
Desjardins PJ, Grossman EH, Kuss ME, et al (Scirex Corp, Austin, Tex; GD Searle, Skokie, Ill)
Anesth Analg 93:721-727, 2001   12–6

Background.—Preventing or ameliorating pain after surgery, inhibiting inflammation, and reducing hyperalgesia are reasons for administering analgesics preoperatively. The conventional nonsteroidal anti-inflammatory drugs (NSAIDs) inhibit cyclo-oxygenase (COX)-1 and COX-2 non-

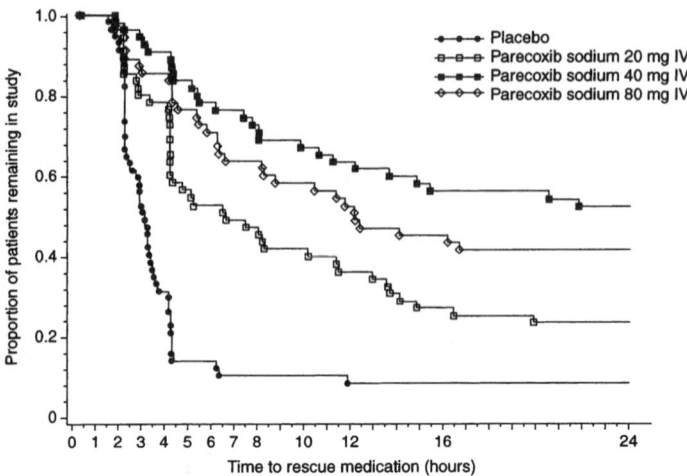

FIGURE 1.—Survival plot of time to rescue medication. *P* < .05 by log-rank test for each dose of parecoxib sodium versus placebo. (Courtesy of Desjardins PJ, Grossman EH, Kuss ME, et al: The injectable cyclooxygenase-2-specific inhibitor parecoxib sodium has analgesic efficacy when administered preoperatively. *Anesth Analg* 93:721-727, 2001.)

specifically, which then inhibits prostaglandin production. These agents have clinically important adverse side effects, however. Newer, specific COX-2 inhibitors such as parecoxib sodium seem to have fewer of these side effects and are well tolerated when used to manage moderate to severe pain. Preoperative parecoxib sodium was studied for its analgesic efficacy and safety when used for oral surgery pain.

Methods.—This placebo-controlled trial used single intravenous doses of parecoxib sodium (20, 40, and 80 mg) or placebo given randomly before oral surgery in 214 patients ages 18 to 45. Efficacy was assessed during the 24 hours after surgery. Patients completed visual analogue scale evaluations of pain at 2-hour intervals beginning 30 minutes after surgery. Rescue medication was given when the patient requested it; pain evaluations were not obtained after rescue medication had been administered. Efficacy of analgesia was evaluated based on median time to rescue medication, proportion of patients requiring such agents, intensity of pain, and patient's assessment of the efficacy of parecoxib sodium or placebo.

Results.—The effects of placebo were consistently inferior to those of parecoxib sodium, regardless of dose. Placebo patients' median time to rescue medication was 2 hours, 15 minutes, and 93% of these patients requested it. Patients in the parecoxib 20-mg group requested rescue medication after a median of 6 hours, 17 minutes. Comparable times were more than 24 hours after surgery in the 40- and 80-mg groups, and only 48% of these patients requested it. At all doses, the median time difference to rescue medication between placebo and parecoxib sodium was statistically significant (Fig 1). In addition, the proportion of patients taking parecoxib sodium who requested rescue medication, regardless of dose, was significantly smaller than the proportion of patients taking placebo

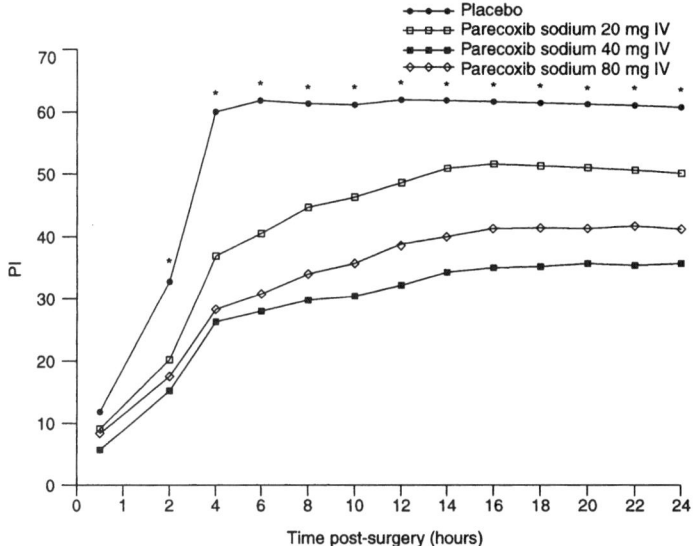

FIGURE 3.—Mean pain intensity scores (visual analogue scale) over time. *Abbreviation: PI*, pain intensity. (Courtesy of Desjardins PJ, Grossman EH, Kuss ME, et al: The injectable cyclooxygenase-2-specific inhibitor parecoxib sodium has analgesic efficacy when administered preoperatively. *Anesth Analg* 93:721-727, 2001.)

who made such requests. The mean pain intensity scores increased for all groups in the first 4 hours after surgery, but 2 hours after surgery, those receiving parecoxib sodium had statistically significant lower mean time-specific pain intensity scores than those receiving placebo. Significant differences occurred between those receiving 40 mg and those receiving 20 mg; the 40- and 80-mg groups were similar (Fig 3). Thirty-nine percent of the placebo group had adverse effects (generally mild to moderate) during the first 3 days after surgery; 30% of those taking 20 mg, 34% of those taking 40 mg, and 25% of those taking 80 mg of parecoxib sodium had such effects.

Conclusions.—The preoperative administration of parecoxib sodium was able to effectively manage postoperative pain and was both safe and well tolerated in these patients undergoing oral surgery.

▶ This study indicates, as have several previous studies, that preoperative administration of COX-2 inhibitors has analgesic and opiate-sparing effects. The major advantage of these drugs over conventional NSAIDs is the reduced effect on platelet function and lower incidence of gastrointestinal side effects. While the authors state that COX-2 inhibitors are less likely to produce renal dysfunction, I believe that this remains to be seen. The other unanswered questions are whether the COX-2 inhibitors are as effective as ketorolac, and whether they are more effective when given preoperatively than postoperatively.

S. E. Abram, MD

Acute Pain Induces Insulin Resistance in Humans

Greisen J, Juhl CB, Grøfte T, et al (Aarhus Univ, Denmark)
Anesthesiology 95:578-584, 2001   12–7

Background.—Trauma that produces pain may disturb metabolic function. Specifically, impaired insulin sensitivity relative to the magnitude of the trauma can result. Insulin resistance is preventable in part by the use of epidural anesthesia, which indicates a role for neural input. Ten healthy men volunteered to test whether pain itself is sufficient to induce insulin resistance, undergoing 2 randomly sequenced hyperinsulinemic-euglycemic clamp studies.

Methods.—Nontraumatic painful transcutaneous electrical stimulation was used in vivo on the men, who ranged in age from 20 to 36 (mean, 27). Each man participated in a pain experiment using self-controlled electrical stimulation and a control experiment using the same procedures without painful electrical stimulation. Four weeks separated the studies. The maximum pain intensity was 8 on a visual analogue scale of 0 to 10.

Results.—The whole-body insulin-stimulated glucose uptake fell from 6.37 mg/kg/min during the control study to 4.97 mg/kg/min in the pain study. Indirect calorimetry showed a decline in nonoxidative glucose disposal from 3.41 to 2.47 mg/kg/min between the 2 studies. Isotopically determined endogenous glucose output during hyperinsulinemia was suppressed less after the pain experience, falling from 2.04 to 1.67 mg/kg/min. Serum cortisol levels, free fatty acids, and plasma epinephrine increased twofold to threefold in response to the pain (Fig 4), and circulating concentrations of glucagon and growth hormone also increased.

Conclusions.—Insulin sensitivity declined with the experience of acute, severe, nontraumatic pain, leading to the conclusion that pain is a sufficient stimulus for this alteration. Rates of nonoxidative glucose disposal declined an average of 28%, with no effect on glucose oxidation rates. Insulin's ability to suppress endogenous glucose output decreased with pain, and the circulating concentrations of epinephrine, cortisol, growth hormone, and free fatty acids all rose, indicating that these substances may play a role in the glucose homeostatic alterations that occur with pain. Thus, controlling pain for patients who undergo trauma and stress may improve glucose metabolism.

▶ This study indicates that pain per se can induce the hormonal changes associated with tissue injury. Previous studies have indicated that analgesic interventions carried out in the perioperative period can reduce such changes. This study goes a step further, showing that pain induced by a stimulus that does not cause tissue injury can produce insulin resistance and increase levels of cortisol, catecholamines, glucagons, growth hormone, and free fatty acids. The researchers showed in a separate study that local anesthetic infiltration abolished these responses, indicating that it was the

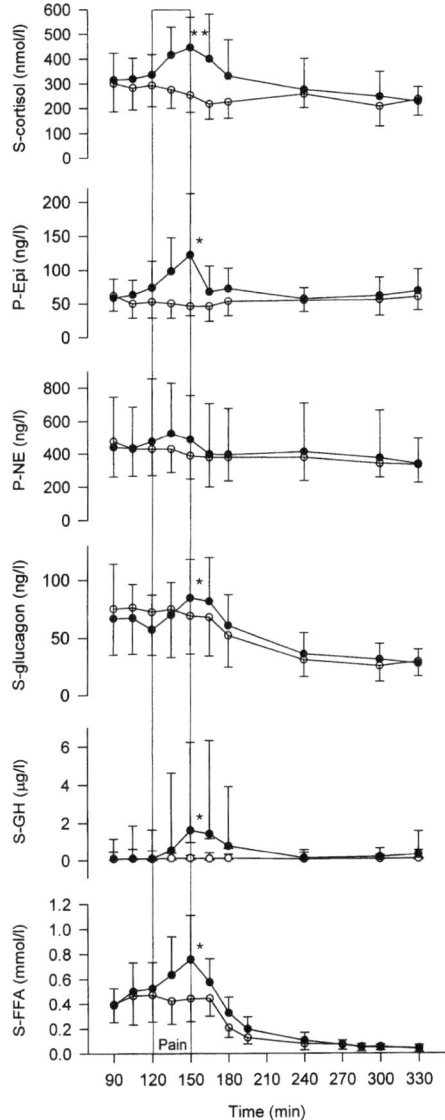

FIGURE 4.—Mean concentrations of serum cortisol, plasma epinephrine, plasma norepinephrine, serum glucagon, and serum free fatty acids (± SD) during the control study (*open circles*) and after painful electric stimulation of the abdominal skin for 30 minutes (*filled circles*). Serum growth hormone data are medians (25th, 75th percentiles). The pain was stimulated at 120-150 minutes. *P < .05, †P < .01 between the 2 studies. *Abbreviations: S-cortisol*, serum cortisol; *P-Epi*, plasma epinephrine; *P-NE*, plasma norepinephrine; *S-glucagon*, serum glucagon; *S-FFA*, serum free fatty acids; *S-GH*, serum growth hormone. (Courtesy of Greisen J, Juhl CB, Grøfte T, et al: Acute pain induces insulin resistance in humans. *Anesthesiology* 95:578-584, 2001. Copyright American Society of Anesthesiologists, Inc. Used with permission of Lippincott-Raven Publishers.)

pain, not other possible effects of electrical stimulation, that produced these hormonal changes.

S. E. Abram, MD

Magnesium Sulfate Does Not Reduce Postoperative Analgesic Requirements

Ko S-H, Lim H-R, Kim D-C, et al (Chonbuk Natl Univ, Chonju, South Korea)

Anesthesiology 95:640-646, 2001   12–8

Background.—The activation of N-methyl-D-aspartate (NMDA) receptors begins a process that leads to calcium's entering the cell and central sensitization, which is manifested as lowered pain threshold after injury and increased sensitivity of the withdrawal reflex. Magnesium blocks this response, possibly preventing central sensitization. Normal humans are limited in their ability to transport magnesium from blood to CSF via the blood-brain barrier. Whether perioperative intravenous magnesium sulfate infusion can influence postoperative pain was studied in a randomized, double-blind, placebo-controlled assessment.

Methods.—An intravenous bolus dose of 50 mg/kg of magnesium sulfate was administered to 60 women having an abdominal hysterectomy, followed by either a continuous infusion of 15 mg/kg/h over a period of 6 hours or an equal amount of isotonic saline solution over the same period. Serum and CSF magnesium concentrations were measured after surgery. To assess the effect on pain, a patient-controlled epidural analgesia device measured the cumulative postoperative analgesic consumption. Six, 24, 48, and 72 hours after surgery, pain intensity was determined at rest and during forced expiration.

Results.—Results were analyzed for 58 women, all of whom completed the 72-hour follow-up period with adequate relief of pain. Patients who received magnesium sulfate consumed significantly lower doses of vecuronium than the control group. The mean dosage of magnesium given to women in the magnesium group was 8038 mg. Serum magnesium concentrations were similar preoperatively, but those in the control group were significantly less than those of the magnesium group when surgery was completed. The magnesium levels of the magnesium group were significantly higher than those of the control group or the preoperative measurements. However, CSF magnesium concentrations did not differ significantly at the end of surgery between the 2 groups. The cumulative postoperative analgesic doses were comparable. Both groups had an inverse relationship between cumulative postoperative analgesic consumption and CSF magnesium concentration. The pain scores of the 2 groups (taken both at rest and during forced expiration) were both less than 4 and similar.

Conclusions.—CSF magnesium concentrations did not increase when perioperative intravenous magnesium sulfate was given, and no effect on postoperative pain resulted. An inverse relationship existed between CSF magnesium concentration and cumulative postoperative analgesic consumption, suggesting that CSF magnesium levels modulate pain postoperatively, but they do not respond to the administration of magnesium sulfate.

▶ Animal studies have shown that NMDA antagonists can block spinal sensitization induced by noxious stimulation. However, the ability of preemptive administration of NMDA antagonists to reduce postoperative analgesic requirements or to reduce postoperative pain has been disappointing. As the authors point out, it is spinal concentrations of magnesium that are important in producing an antihyperalgesic effect, and the CSF magnesium concentrations were essentially the same in both groups. They also point out that higher CSF Mg++ concentrations were associated with reduced analgesic requirements, suggesting that there may well be a beneficial effect if increased spinal cord concentrations can be achieved.

S. E. Abram, MD

A Systematic Review of the Peripheral Analgesic Effects of Intraarticular Morphine
Gupta A, Bodin L, Holmstrøm B, et al (Örebro Univ, Sweden)
Anesth Analg 93:761-770, 2001   12–9

Background.—Morphine's effects on peripheral receptors remain elusive. Morphine's analgesic effect was compared with that of placebo in a systematic review to see if the effect is dose dependent, and to determine whether it is systemic or dependent on peripheral receptors.

Methods.—The literature was systemically surveyed and data gleaned from the Cochrane Foundation database and EMBASE, seeking studies evaluating the peripheral analgesic effects of morphine in patients undergoing arthroscopic knee procedures under local, regional, or general anesthesia. The visual analogue scale (VAS) score at 3 postoperative time periods (early, intermediate, and late phases) and the amount of analgesic consumed were identified. Meta-analysis used a weighted-analysis technique. The χ^2 test evaluated the essential homogeneity assumption.

Results.—Nineteen studies were suitable for meta-analysis, culled from 45 prospective randomized studies of the effects of morphine that were reduced to 32 using a placebo control. Analgesia was improved over placebo by 12 to 17 mm on the VAS. This held for all 3 postoperative phases. Smaller improvements occurred in studies that had high quality scores. Statistical analysis of total analgesic consumption was not possible. Six studies showed that analgesic consumption decreased, and 6 showed no difference between groups. When the area under the curve was used to indicate pain, a dose-response effect was clear. This was not true when VAS was used. Because the data were extremely limited, no systemic effect of peripherally administered morphine could be excluded.

Conclusions.—At all the postoperative phases, morphine reduced the intensity of pain postoperatively when compared with placebo. The mean reduction in pain intensity was 12 to 17 mm on the VAS. Dose dependency was incalculable, and systemic effects could not be ruled out.

▶ While the available data indicate that there is probably a peripheral opiate effect, the response is clearly not very robust. One potential problem with the model of intra-articular opioid application is that pain from extra-articular sources would not be affected. On the basis of these and other studies, the development of opioids that work only peripherally seems reasonable.

S. E. Abram, MD

Regional Block and Mexiletine: The Effect on Pain After Cancer Breast Surgery
Fassoulaki A, Sarantopoulos C, Melemeni A, et al (St Savas Hosp, Athens, Greece; Med College of Wisconsin, Milwaukee)
Reg Anesth Pain Med 26:223-228, 2001   12–10

Background and Objectives.—Breast surgery for cancer is associated with chronic pain and sensory abnormalities. The present study investigates the effect of regional block, oral mexiletine, and the combination of both, on acute and chronic pain associated with cancer breast surgery.

Methods.—One hundred patients scheduled for cancer breast surgery received either regional block with 18 mL of 1% ropivacaine intraoperatively and oral mexiletine for the first 6 postoperative days (R + M group), or regional block and placebo (R + PL), or normal saline instead of ropivacaine and mexiletine (PL + M), or normal saline and placebo (PL + PL). Postoperative analgesic requirements were recorded daily. Pain was assessed 0, 3, 6, 9, and 24 hours in the postanesthesia care unit (PACU) and on the second to sixth day postoperatively, at rest, and after movement using the visual analog scale (VAS). Three months after surgery, patients were interviewed for the presence and intensity of pain, abnormal sensations, and analgesic requirements.

Results.—Regional block reduced the number of intramuscular (IM) injections required the first 24 hours (*P* = .05), the R + PL group requiring less injections versus the PL + M group (*P* = .037). Lonarid tablet (paracetamol and codeine) consumption from the second to the fifth postoperative day differed among the 4 groups (*P* = .0304), the R + M group requiring fewer tablets than the PL + PL group (*P* = .009). Three hours postoperatively, the R + PL group had less pain at rest when compared with all other groups (*P* < .05 for all comparisons). On the second postoperative day, VAS at rest and after movement was less in the R + M versus the R + PL group (*P* < .01 and *P* < .05, respectively). Three months after surgery, the 4 groups were similar with regard to incidence or intensity of pain or analgesic requirements. The R + PL group had a lower incidence (77%) of reduced or absent sensation (*P* = .016).

Conclusions.—Regional block reduced the analgesic requirements in the early postoperative period, while mexiletine combined with regional block reduced the total analgesic requirements during the next 5 postoperative days. Although chronic pain was not affected by these treatments late-abnormal sensation may be diminished by combination of these treatments.

▶ The issue of prevention of chronic postoperative pain has been largely ignored by the research community. Mastectomy, thoracotomy, and limb amputation are associated with high rates of chronic pain, mainly neuropathic in nature. The role of intraoperative and postoperative noxious stimulation in the development of acute pain has been studied fairly extensively, but the issue of its role in chronic pain development has not been studied very much. Bach et al[1] demonstrated a substantial decrease in the incidence of phantom limb pain among patients with chronic preoperative limb pain when epidural anesthesia was initiated 3 days preoperatively. The incidence of phantom limb pain after 6 months was 0/10 among patients who had the 3-day preoperative infusions versus 5/13 for patients who had epidural anesthesia initiated on the day of surgery. Fassoulaki et al have asked the questions regarding the effect of perioperative interventions on the development of chronic pain in an effective manner. Much more research of this type is needed.

S. E. Abram, MD

Reference

1. Bach S, Noreng MF, Tjellden NU: Phantom limb pain in amputees during the first 12 months following limb amputation, after preoperative epidural blockade. *Pain* 33:297-301, 1988.

More Epidural Than Intravenous Sufentanil is Required to Provide Comparable Postoperative Pain Relief
Menigaux C, Guignard B, Fletcher D, et al (Hôpital Ambroise Paré, Boulogne-Billancourt, France; Univ of Louisville, Ky; Univ of Vienna; et al)
Anesth Analg 93:472-476, 2001   12–11

Background.—Sufentanil, a lipophilic opioid, is often used in postoperative epidural analgesia, on the theory that it acts on opioid receptors in the dorsal horn of the spinal cord to provide analgesia in the affected dermatomes with fewer supraspinal side effects. However, there is controversy as to the extent of sufentanil's direct action on spinal opioid receptors when administered epidurally. One critical factor would appear to be the size of the dose. Sufentanil has a preferential spinal effect when administered in boluses exceeding 10 μg, whereas analgesia with continuous infusions of small-dose sufentanil is primarily mediated by systemic absorption of the drug and subsequent recirculation to supraspinal centers. Epidural patient-controlled analgesia (PCA) enables patients to titrate small doses of analgesia to meet their specific needs. However, because the doses of sufentanil given with PCA are usually less than 5 µg, epidural PCA administration of sufentanil may not have any advantage over IV administration. The following 2 hypotheses were tested: (1) at similar analgesic levels, plasma sufentanil concentrations are similar with epidural and IV administration; and (2) more epidural than IV sufentanil is needed for comparable analgesia because the lipophilicity of sufentanil makes it likely to be absorbed into the fat surrounding the epidural space.

Methods.—Twenty postoperative patients were randomly assigned to either PCA epidural or IV sufentanil, and analgesia and plasma sufentanil concentrations were evaluated.

Results.—Epidural and IV sufentanil administration produced similar levels of analgesia, and plasma sufentanil concentrations in the 2 groups were virtually identical. However, epidural administration required significantly larger doses of sufentanil (238 ± 50 µg vs 160 ± 32 µg). Systemic absorption of sufentanil with subsequent recirculation to the supraspinal receptors appeared to be the primary mechanism by which small-dose boluses of sufentanil administered epidurally produce analgesia.

Conclusions.—An approximately 50% greater cumulative dose of sufentanil is needed when administered as a small epidural bolus to achieve analgesia comparable with that obtained through IV administration. It would appear that a large proportion of the drug may be absorbed by the epidural fat.

▶ There is overwhelming evidence that infusions of epidural fentanyl or sufentanil are no more effective than IV infusions. This study shows that a small epidural bolus of sufentanil is actually less effective than a comparable IV dose. Although epidural infusions of local anesthetic plus fentanyl or sufentanil are more effective than local anesthetic alone, the opioid effect appears to be entirely systemic.

S. E. Abram, MD

Buprenorphine Added to the Local Anesthetic for Brachial Plexus Block to Provide Postoperative Analgesia in Outpatients
Candido KD, Franco CD, Khan MA, et al (Cook County Hosp, Chicago)
Reg Anesth Pain Med 26:352-356, 2001   12–12

Background and Objectives.—Over the past 10 years, several studies have suggested that the addition of certain opiates to the local anesthetic used for brachial block may provide effective, long-lasting postoperative analgesia. One of these studies indicated that the agonist-antagonist, buprenorphine, added to bupivacaine provided a longer period of postoperative analgesia than the traditional opiates, but in this study, it is impossible to determine the relative contributions of the local anesthetic and the opiate to the postoperative analgesia because of the extremely long duration of the anesthesia provided by the local anesthetic, bupivacaine.

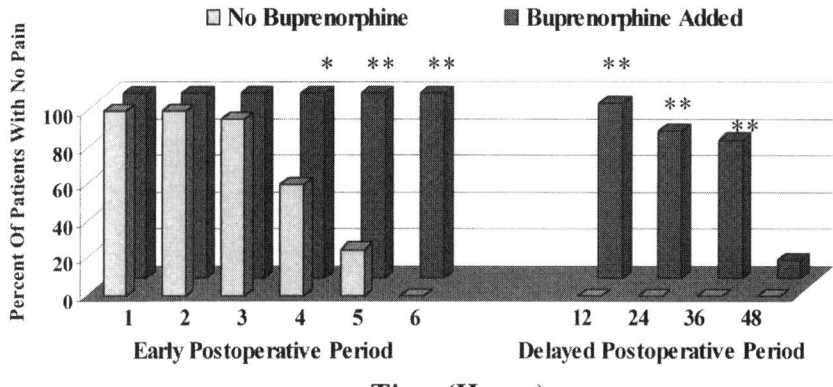

FIGURE 1.—Graphic representation of the data comparing the differences in the duration of complete analgesia provided by local anesthetic mixture alone (group I) and local anesthetic mixture with buprenorphine (group II). *Asterisk*, $P < .01$; *double asterisk*, $P < .0001$. (Courtesy of Candido KD, Franco CD, Khan MA, et al: Buprenorphine added to the local anesthetic for brachial plexus block to provide postoperative analgesia in outpatients. *Reg Anesth Pain Med* 26:352-356, 2001.)

By repeating the study using a local anesthetic of a shorter duration, the present study delineates more clearly the contribution of the buprenorphine to postoperative analgesia when added to a shorter-acting local anesthetic.

Methods.—Forty, healthy, consenting adult patients scheduled for upper extremity surgery were enrolled in the study. Premedication was provided by intravenous midazolam 2 mg/70 kg and anesthesia by a subclavian perivascular brachial plexus block. The patients were assigned randomly to 1 of 2 equal groups based on the agents used for the blocks. The patients in group I received 40 mL of a local anesthetic alone, while those in group II received the same local anesthetic plus buprenorphine 0.3 mg (Fig 1). The study was kept double-blind by having 1 anesthesiologist prepare the solutions, a second anesthesiologist perform the blocks, and a third anesthesiologist monitor the anesthesia and analgesia thereafter, up to and including the time of the first request for an analgesic medication. The data were reported as means ($\pm$ SEM), and differences between groups were determined using repeated measures of analysis of variance (ANOVA) and χ^2, followed by the Fisher exact test for post hoc comparison. A P value of less than .05 was considered to be statistically significant.

Results.—The mean duration of postoperative pain relief following the injection of the local anesthetic alone was 5.3 ($\pm$ 0.15) hours as compared with 17.4 ($\pm$ 1.26) hours when buprenorphine was added, a difference that was statistically (and clinically) significant ($P < .0001$).

Conclusions.—The addition of buprenorphine to the local anesthetic used for brachial plexus block in the present study provided a 3-fold increase in the duration of postoperative analgesia, with complete analgesia persisting 30 hours beyond the duration provided by the local anesthetic alone in 75% of the patients. This practice can be of particular benefit to patients undergoing ambulatory upper extremity surgery by providing prolonged analgesia after discharge from the hospital.

▶ There is growing interest in the peripheral effects of opioids. Peripheral opioid receptors are activated by opioid peptides released from leukocytes during inflammation.[1] A number of strategies have been devised to activate the peripheral opioid receptors that participate in this natural response, including perineural and intra-articular injection and the development of opioids that do not cross the blood-brain barrier. The long duration of buprenorphine is a major advantage, and the technique described here provides prolonged analgesia without motor or sensory block. One might envision the development of very long-acting drugs with high receptor affinity that do not cross into the CNS. Such drugs might be useful for both perineural injection and systemic administration.

S. E. Abram, MD

Reference

1. Rittner HL, Brack A, Machelska H, et al: Opioid peptide–expressing leukocytes: Identification, recruitment, and simultaneously increasing inhibition of inflammatory pain. *Anesthesiology* 95:500-508, 2001.

Amantadine, a *N*-Methyl-D-Aspartate Receptor Antagonist, Does Not Enhance Postoperative Analgesia in Women Undergoing Abdominal Hysterectomy

Gottschalk A, Schroeder F, Ufer M, et al (Univ Hosp Hamburg-Eppendorf, Germany; Westfälische Wilhelms-Universität, Münster, Germany)
Anesth Analg 93:192-196, 2001
12–13

Background.—It is known that N-methyl-D-aspartate (NMDA) antagonists will improve postoperative pain when administered before surgery. However, the clinical formulations of NMDA antagonists will only allow an oral delivery or are associated with psychotropic side effects. Amantadine, a noncompetitive NMDA antagonist, has been used in the treatment of patients with Parkinson disease, dementia, and spasticity. Amantadine can be delivered either orally or IV, and the side effects, when the drug is administered in appropriate dosages, appear to be nonharmful. In 2 previous clinical reports, the IV administration of amantadine to patients with cancer resulted in decreased neuropathic pain and less chronic pain up to 5 months after administration in comparison with the control group. Whether amantadine could improve postoperative analgesia when administered before surgically induced trauma, specifically in women undergoing elective abdominal hysterectomy, was determined.

Methods.—Thirty women undergoing elective abdominal hysterectomy were randomly assigned to receive either 500 mL of saline IV or 200 mg of amantadine IV in 500 mL of saline before the induction of standardized general anesthesia. Intravenous patient-controlled analgesia with piritramide was provided for postoperative pain control. Pain perception in the first 48 hours after tracheal extubation was assessed by visual analogue scales. All analgesic requirements were documented.

Results.—The 2 groups did not differ significantly in pain scores, postoperative requirements for analgesia, and the incidence of side effects.

Conclusions.—There were no differences in postoperative pain or opioid consumption between patients who received amantadine preoperatively and those who received placebo. Postoperative analgesia is not enhanced by 200 mg of amantadine IV administered preoperatively to patients undergoing elective abdominal hysterectomy.

▶ Although NMDA antagonists are nearly uniformly capable of producing preemptive analgesic effects in experimental animal models such as the formalin test, results with this class of drugs in human perioperative studies are disappointing. Ketamine and dextromethorphan, and now amantadine, appear to provide minimal benefit in terms of reduction of postoperative pain or reduction in analgesic requirement.

S. E. Abram, MD

Comparison of Patient-Controlled Epidural Analgesia With and Without Night-Time Infusion Following Gastrectomy

Komatsu H, Matsumoto S, Mitsuhata H (Akita Univ, Hiraka Gen Hosp, Juntendo Univ, Akita City, Japan)
Br J Anaesth 87:633-635, 2001   12–14

Objective.—Pain is the most common cause of sleep disturbance, and analgesia is the most effective way of treating sleep problems. Whether patient-controlled epidural analgesia (PCEA) alone or PCEA with a supplemental nighttime infusion is more effective at controlling postgastrectomy pain was investigated in a prospective, randomized, double-blind study.

Methods.—An epidural catheter was inserted through the T9 to T10 interspinous space into the epidural space in 40 patients who had distal or total gastrectomy. The patient-controlled analgesia (PCA) pump contained 5 g/mL fentanyl and 0.1% bupivacaine. The PCEA group received a 5-mL bolus on demand with a 15-minute lockout period. The PCEA + infusion group received 2 mL/hr of the bupivacaine/fentanyl mixture at night on the day of surgery and the day after. Three to 5 mL of 1% mepivacaine was available as rescue medication.

Results.—Patients receiving the infusion had fewer pain episodes, less sleep disturbance, and less pain on coughing than patients who received PCEA alone. The incidence of pruritus was similar in both groups. No excessive sedation or respiratory distress was observed.

Conclusion.—Nighttime infusion with PCEA after gastrectomy provided better pain relief, improved sleep, and less pain on coughing than PCEA alone.

▶ It would seem logical that PCEA with a continuous infusion would be more efficacious than PCEA without infusion. However, one might say the same for IV PCA opioids. Most data suggest that with IV PCA, a background infusion does not improve sleep or analgesia, and is associated with higher drug use and more side effects.

S. E. Abram, MD

The Effect of Preoperative Epidural Morphine on Postoperative Analgesia in Children

Kiffer F, Joly A, Wodey E, et al (Université Rennes 1, France)
Anesth Analg 93:598-600, 2001   12–15

Background.—When epidural morphine is given to adults before surgery, they experience better analgesia postoperatively with less morphine than when patient-controlled analgesia (PCA) with intravenous morphine is used. Whether this holds true for children undergoing major abdominal and orthopedic surgery was examined in a randomized, double-blind study.

Methods.—Twenty-one ASA I children over age 6 years were given 0.3 mg/kg of midazolam rectally 60 minutes before undergoing elective major

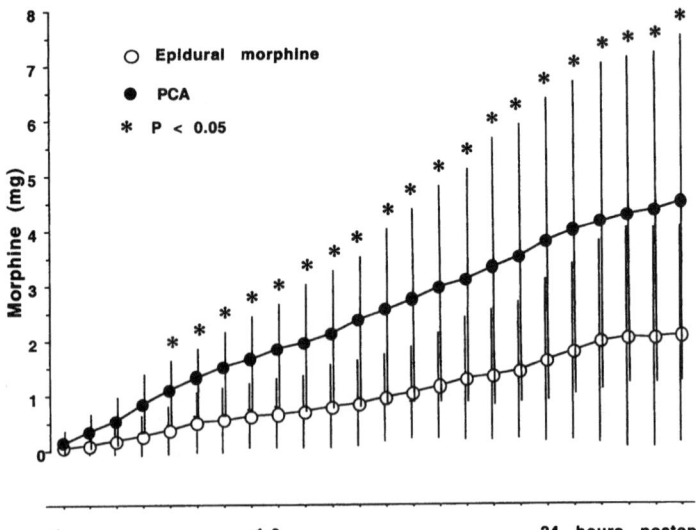

FIGURE 1.—Evolution of VAS pain scores in both groups (mean ± SD). *Abbreviation:* PCA, patient-controlled analgesia. (Courtesy of Kiffer F, Joly A, Wodey E, et al: The effect of preoperative epidural morphine on postoperative analgesia in children. *Anesth Analg* 93:598-600, 2001.)

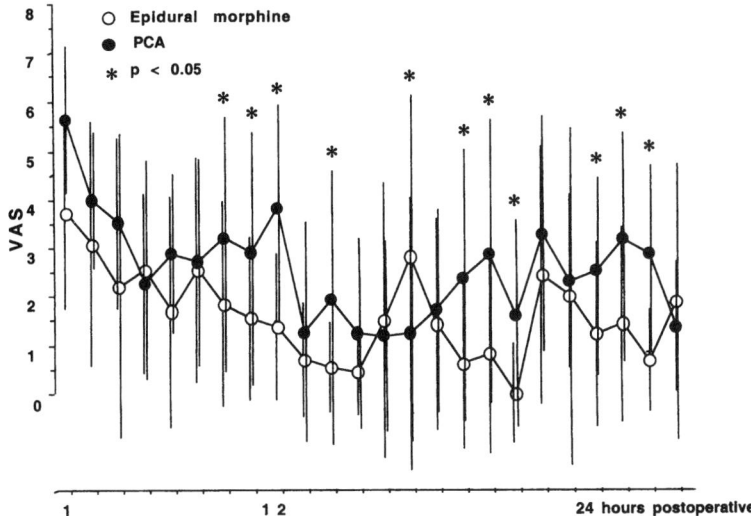

FIGURE 2.—Evolution of morphine requirements in both groups (mean ± SD). *Abbreviation: PCA*, patient-controlled analgesia. (Courtesy of Kiffer F, Joly A, Wodey E, et al: The effect of preoperative epidural morphine on postoperative analgesia in children. *Anesth Analg* 93:598-600, 2001.)

abdominal operations or orthopedic surgery of the lower limbs. After general anesthesia induction, 11 received 30 μg/kg of morphine epidurally (epidural group), and 10 had no puncture but had a dressing applied similar to that of the epidural group (control group). Children received instruction regarding use of the PCA device and were encouraged to use it to maintain pain relief. In addition, they were told how to indicate pain on a visual analogue scale (VAS). VAS pain scores, morphine consumption, and incidence of opioid side effects were assessed hourly for 24 hours postoperatively.

Results.—Patient factors were essentially equal between the 2 groups, as were type and duration of surgery, the total dose of sufentanil given intraoperatively, and the incidence of opioid side effects. The epidural group's time between end of anesthesia and use of the PCA device was 5.4 ± 7.2 hours; the control group's time was 3.4 ± 5.6 hours. The epidural group required significantly less morphine and had significantly lower VAS pain scores than the control group (Fig 1 and Fig 2).

Conclusions.—Better postoperative analgesia resulted from use of a preoperative epidural bolus of morphine along with PCA than was produced with PCA alone in these children undergoing major abdominal or orthopedic surgery. VAS scores were significantly better in the epidural group and remained so for 24 hours; these children also required less morphine than members of the control group. Time to the first postoperative intravenous morphine did not differ significantly between the 2 groups.

▶ The fact that the analgesic effect of epidural morphine lasted beyond 24 hours suggests that preoperative epidural morphine may have a preemptive effect in this population. It would have been interesting to follow these patients for longer periods.

S. E. Abram, MD

The Dose-Response Relationship for Clonidine Added to a Postoperative Continuous Epidural Infusion of Ropivacaine in Children

De Negri P, Ivani G, Visconti C, et al (IRCCS H "Casa Sollievo della Sofferenza" S Giovanni Rotondo [FG], Italy; Regina Margherita Children's Hosp, Turin, Italy; Karolinska Hosp, Stockholm)
Anesth Analg 93:71-76, 2001   12–16

Introduction.—Several clinical trials have reported the successful use of ropivacaine, a new local anesthetic correlated with decreased risk for systemic toxicity, for epidural or caudal blockade in children. Adjuncts to local anesthetics, including opioids, clonidine, and ketamine, have been used to further enhance the quality of epidural analgesia. The optimal adjunct dose of clonidine for continuous epidural administration in children has not been determined. The dose-response relationship and possible side effects of clonidine when added to postoperative continuous epidural ropivacaine were examined in 55 boys in a randomized, blinded investigation.

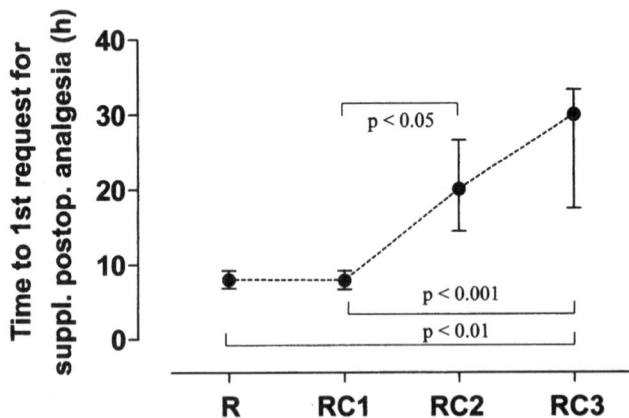

FIGURE 1.—Time to first request for supplemental postoperative analgesia, displayed as median and 95% confidence interval. Group R versus Group RC3, P < .01; Group RC1 versus Group RC2, P < .05; and Group RC1 versus Group RC3, P < .001. (Courtesy of De Negri P, Ivani G, Visconti C, et al: The dose-response relationship for clonidine added to a postoperative continuous epidural infusion of ropivacaine in children. *Anesth Anal* 93:71-76, 2001.)

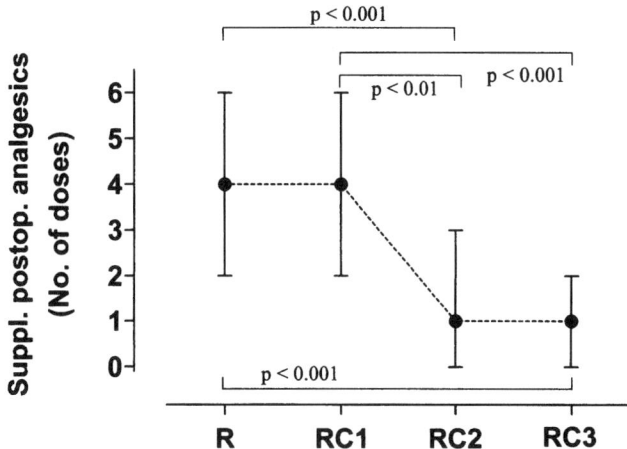

FIGURE 2.—Total number of doses of supplemental postoperative analgesics, displayed as median and 95% confidence interval. Group R versus Group RC2, P < .001; Group R versus Group RC3, P < .001; Group RC1 versus Group RC2, P < .01; and Group RC1 versus Group RC3, P < .001. (Courtesy of De Negri P, Ivani G, Visconti C, et al: The dose-response relationship for clonidine added to a postoperative continuous epidural infusion of ropivacaine in children. *Anesth Anal* 93:71-76, 2001.)

Methods.—Patient age range was 1 to 4 years. All patients had ASA physical status I, and underwent hypospadias repair. Patients were randomized to receive postoperative epidural infusion of either plain ropivacaine 0.1%, 0.2 mg/kg/h (group R); ropivacaine 0.08%, 0.16 mg/kg/h, plus clonidine, 0.04 µg/kg/h (group RC1); ropivacaine 0.08%, 0.16 mg/kg/h, plus clonidine, 0.08 µg/kg/h (group RC2); or ropivacaine 0.08%, 0.16 mg/kg/h, plus clonidine, 0.12 µg/kg/h (group RC3).

Results.—A clear dose-response relationship was observed for continuous infusion of epidural clonidine. Doses of 0.08 to 0.12 µ/kg/h provided improved postoperative analgesia (decreased Children's Hospital of Eastern Ontario pain score, increased time to first supplemental analgesic demand (Fig 1), and decreased number of total doses of supplemental analgesic (Fig 2) during the first 48 hours after surgery), with no signs of increased sedation, motor block, or other side effects.

Conclusion.—Adjunctive epidural clonidine in the dose range of 0.08 to 0.12 µg/kg/h added to a postoperative continuous epidural infusion of ropivacaine is effective and safe in children.

▶ These data should be helpful for programs initiating protocols for postoperative analgesia with combinations of local anesthetics and clonidine. Fear of respiratory depression has confined the use of combined epidural opioids and local anesthetics to ICUs in some institutions. This technique should help pediatric acute pain services to promote the use of epidural analgesia for patients at those centers.

S. E. Abram, MD

Pharmacokinetics of Bupivacaine After Continuous Epidural Infusion in Infants With and Without Biliary Atresia

Meunier J-F, Goujard E, Dubousset A-M, et al (Université Paris-Sud, France)
Anesthesiology 95:87-95, 2001   12–17

Objective.—Long-acting local anesthetics, such as bupivacaine, can cause adverse reactions in pediatric patients primarily because of a lower clearance and a lower serum protein binding in infants compared with children and adults. Although studies have examined the pharmacokinetics of bupivacaine in infants after a single injection, the complex reactions between age, α-1 acid glycoprotein (AAG), and human serum albumin (HSA) have not been fully investigated, particularly in patients with biliary atresia. Whether the association of cholestasis and mild hepatic dysfunc-

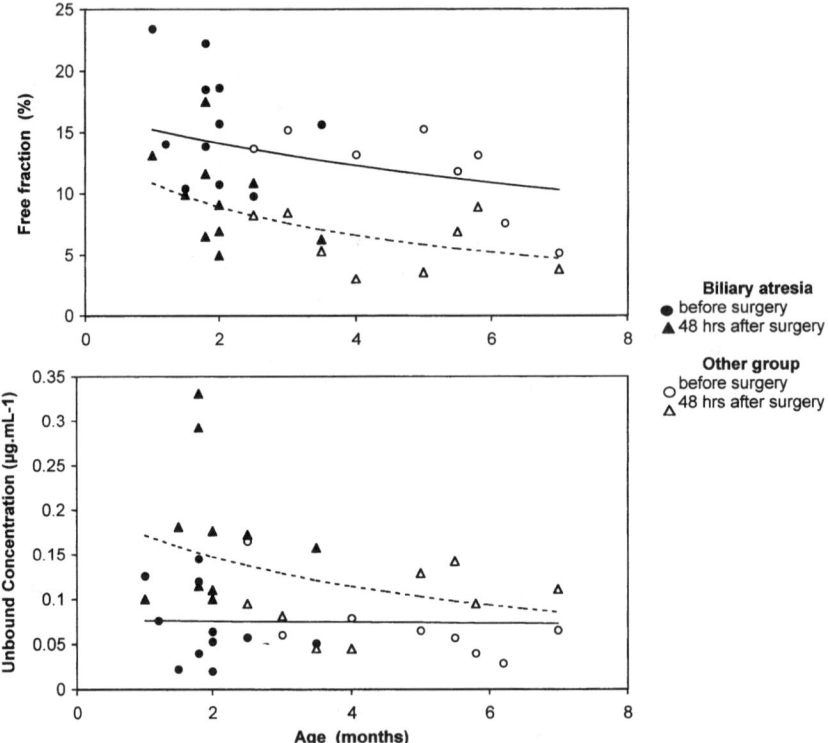

FIGURE 3.—Free fraction (*top*) and unbound concentration (*bottom*) versus age in the biliary atresia group (*closed symbols*) and the other group (*open symbols*) before surgery (*circles*) and 48 hours after the operation (*triangles*). The solid lines are the fitted free fraction (unbound concentration) 30 minutes after the beginning of infusion and the dashed lines are the fitted free fraction (unbound concentration) 48 hours after infusion initiation. The free fraction decreases with time because of the increase in α-1 acid glycoprotein concentration, but the unbound concentration (which is considered as the toxic moiety) increases. Note that 2 infants had unbound concentrations higher than 0.2 μg/mL. (Courtesy of Meunier J-F, Goujard E, Dubousset A-M, et al: Pharmacokinetics of bupivacaine after continuous epidural infusion in infants with and without biliary atresia. *Anesthesiology* 95:87-95, 2001. Copyright, American Society of Anesthesiologists, Inc. Used with permission of Lippincott-Raven Publishers.)

tion might modify the kinetics of bupivacaine was examined in infants with biliary atresia receiving bupivacaine epidurally for 2 days.

Methods.—Bupivacaine (0.375 mg/kg/hr) was administered to 12 infants, aged 1 to 3.5 months, with biliary atresia and to 10 infants, aged 2.5 to 7 months, without cholestasis, undergoing a urology procedure, by continuous epidural infusion for 2 days during and after surgery. Serum AAG and HSA were measured at 0.5, 4, 24, and 48 hours after bupivacaine administration. In vitro erythrocyte binding was determined in 8 additional infants, aged 0.6 to 7 months. Preoperative and postoperative hemoglobin concentrations in blood, and preoperative AAG and HSA serum content were compared for the 2 groups. Pharmacokinetic analyses were performed using a 4-point sampling design, and data were fitted using a 1-compartment model of unbound concentration. Effects of covariates were investigated using regression analysis.

Results.—Bupivacaine provided good postoperative analgesia. The significant increase in postsurgical AAG concentration in both groups was correlated only with age and preoperative AAG level. HSA levels were similar before and after surgery, and preoperative levels were significantly correlated with age. Free bupivacaine concentration increased with AAG concentration and with age (Fig 3). In vitro addition of bupivacaine has little effect on the proportion of molecules trapped by erythrocytes.

Conclusion.—Bupivacaine showed first-order absorption with a linear relationship between bound and unbound bupivacaine concentrations. Unbound bupivacaine, which increased to more than 0.2 μg/mL in 2 infants younger than 2 months, was associated with low levels of AAG. Neither the postsurgical increase in AAG nor erythrocyte binding was able to compensate for this increase in unbound bupivacaine. Bupivacaine dosages in infants younger than 4 months should be limited to 0.25 mg/kg/hr and to 0.3 mg/kg/hr in infants older than 4 months.

▶ This study provides some practical guidelines for postoperative epidural infusions based on very good science. It provides an excellent discussion of the role of metabolism of bupivacaine by the cytochrome P450 isoform CYP3A4 and the role of binding of bupivacaine to α-1 acid glycoprotein, albumin, and erythrocytes in infants. It also demonstrates the role of certain disease states in altering the clearance of the drug.

S. E. Abram, MD

Gender and the Placebo Analgesic Effect in Acute Pain
Averbuch M, Katzper M (Food and Drug Administration, Rockville, Md)
Clin Pharmacol Ther 70:287-291, 2001   12–18

Objective.—Our objective was to examine the placebo arms from a series of clinical trials in which the post-third molar extraction dental pain model was used to elucidate the time course of the placebo effect and the proportion of the population that are responders, as well as to evaluate

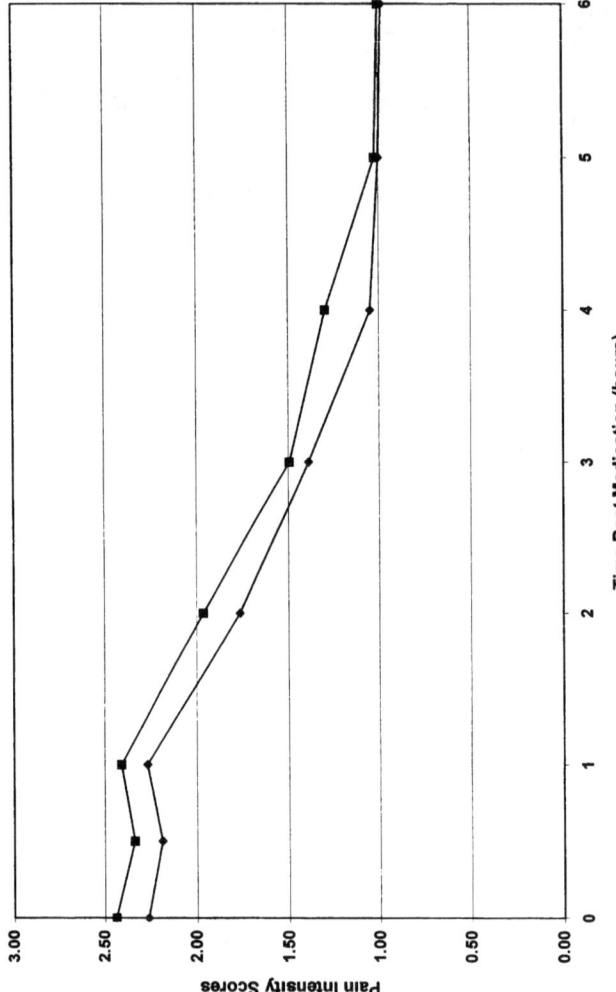

FIGURE 2.—Average pain intensity of unremedicated patients by sex. *Diamonds,* Average for male subjects; *squares,* average for female subjects. (Courtesy of Averbuch M, Katzper M: Gender and the placebo analgesic effect in acute pain. *Clin Pharmacol Ther* 70:287-291, 2001.)

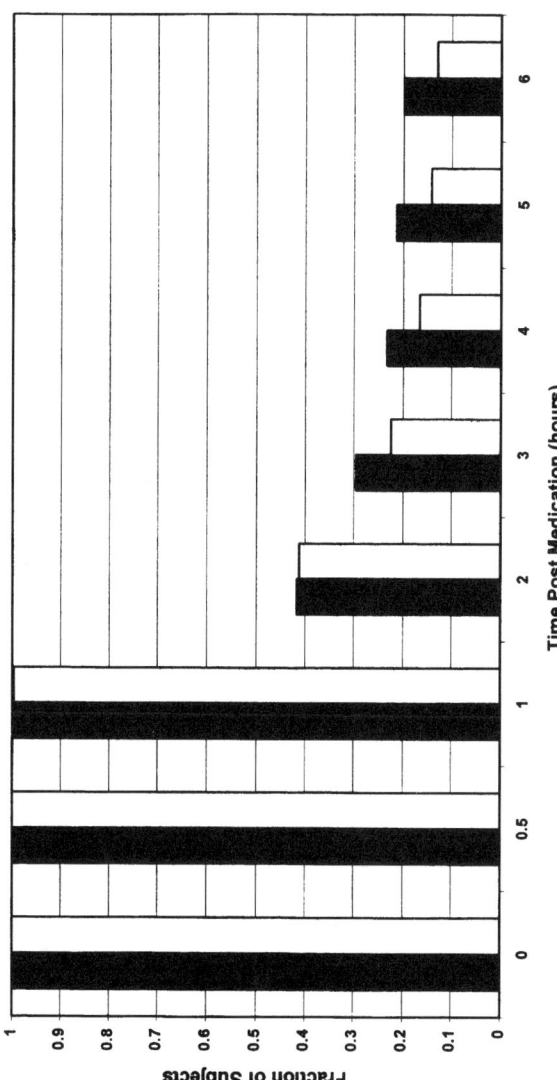

FIGURE 3.—Fraction of unremedicated subjects *vs* postmedication time by sex. *Solid bars,* Male subjects; *open bars,* female subjects. (Courtesy of Averbuch M, Katzper M: Gender and the placebo analgesic effect in acute pain. *Clin Pharmacol Ther* 70:287-291, 2001.)

whether the placebo analgesic response of female subjects may differ from that of male subjects.

Methods.—We performed a meta-analysis of 596 subjects included in the placebo treatment arm of 16 double-blind, post-third molar extraction dental pain (moderate to severe) studies submitted to the Food and Drug Administration electronically. The inclusion and exclusion criteria were practically identical in all studies. Pain relief and pain intensity measurements used the same metrics in all studies. The measurements were recorded just before drug administration and at least at postdose hours 0.5, 1, 1.5, 2, 3, 4, 5, and 6.

Results.—There were 325 female subjects and 271 male subjects. They were all otherwise healthy, with a mean age of 21.6 years for female subjects and 22.3 years for male subjects. The postoperative baseline pain was greater in female subjects than in male subjects, and this difference was statistically significant. Both pain intensity and pain relief scores demonstrate the well-established placebo effect in 10% of the pooled subjects, as well as in all the individual studies. Over time, however, the mean pain intensity and pain relief scores for the female and male treatment groups were not noticeably different at any time point after medication (Fig 2). Further analysis of the data showed no gender difference in duration of action of the placebo (Fig 3).

Conclusions.—The results demonstrated no gender difference in response to placebo. These results were obtained from the post-third molar extraction situation, in which the least possible confounding factors were present. To fully establish the generality of this phenomenon, studies should be carried out in other pain models.

▶ There has been much discussion as to whether gender affects pain response over the last 5 years. This study shows importantly that there are no gender differences in response to placebo. This could be key for the interpretation of clinical trials seeking to show a gender difference in pain response.

M. Wood, MD, FRCA

Chronic Pain Management

Gray Ramus Communicans Nerve Block: Novel Treatment Approach for Painful Osteoporotic Vertebral Compression Fracture
Chandler G, Dalley G, Hemmer J Jr, et al (Specialty Clinics of Georgia Research Ctr, Gainesville; Northeast Georgia Diagnostic Clinic, Gainesville; Gainesville Orthopaedic Associates, Ga)
South Med J 94:387-396, 2001   12–19

Background.—Osteoporotic vertebral compression fractures (OVCF) can occur in either men or women and may be associated with chronic or acute pain. Treatment generally involves analgesia and bed rest, although prolonged immobilization can introduce additional risks. The use of gray ramus communicans nerve block (GRCNB) to achieve pain relief was assessed.

Methods.—Fifty-two cases of OVCF treated with GRCNB were retrospectively evaluated. A 2% lidocaine and 2% sterile triamcinolone diacetate injection was given into the gray ramus tract of the somatic nerve root, which corresponded radiographically to the OVCF. Pain scores (patient- and physician-reported), use of analgesic medication, and overall patient satisfaction were noted. The follow-up was 9 months.

Results.—Dramatic improvements in pain scores were achieved, with 92% of patients and 88% of physicians reporting a 1-point improvement. Sixty-three percent of patients had a 4-point improvement, and 58% of physicians reported this degree of relief. While physicians believed that pain increased in 2 cases, none of the patients felt this way. There was no correspondingly dramatic reduction in the use of pain medication, with only 42% reporting a decline in analgesic requirement. Fifty percent of patients believed that their level of satisfaction was high and 25% rated it as medium. No complications were noted.

Conclusion.—The use of GRCNB was safe, effective, and cost effective in a large number of patients, with the improvements both prompt and sustained.

▶ Vertebroplasty is being used with increasing frequency to control the pain associated with vertebral compression fracture. It is effective in some patients with vertebral metastases as well as in some with OVCFs. The technique described in this study is less invasive, less expensive, and less risky. It seems reasonable to use the GRCNB as the primary treatment and to reserve neurolytic ramus communicans block or vertebroplasty for patients who have a temporary response to the local anesthetic block.

S. E. Abram, MD

Endoscopic Ultrasound-Guided Celiac Plexus Block for Managing Abdominal Pain Associated With Chronic Pancreatitis: A Prospective Single Center Experience
Gress F, Schmitt C, Sherman S, et al (Indiana Univ, Indianapolis; Univ of Tennessee, Chattanooga)
Am J Gastroenterol 96:409-416, 2001   12–20

Background.—Celiac plexus block has successfully treated pain in some patients with chronic pancreatitis. Until recently, CT has supplied the guidance for placement of the block, but the development of endoscopic US (EUS) for this purpose carries few risks and can be performed in a short time. The efficacy of EUS-guided and CT-guided celiac plexus block for controlling the abdominal pain occurring in chronic pancreatitis were compared.

Methods.—Ninety individuals underwent EUS-guided celiac plexus block. All had chronic abdominal pain that had not responded to various treatment options. A visual analogue scale was used to rate pain before the block and 2, 7, and 14 days after its placement, continuing monthly thereafter. Overall comfort level during the EUS procedure was also rated.

Results.—Fifty-five percent of patients reported a significant improvement in pain, with the mean pain score falling from 8 to 2 by 4 to 8 weeks following EUS celiac block. The benefit persisted longer than 12 weeks for 26%, longer than 24 weeks for 10%, and for 35 and 48 weeks for 3 patients. Age under 45 years and a history of previous pancreatic surgery were factors associated with a lessened likelihood of response to the EUS procedure. The EUS celiac block appeared to cost less and perhaps was more cost efficient in some patients. CT and EUS were performed in 12 patients, with 67% preferring the EUS technique and 33% the CT technique.

Conclusion.—The EUS-guided celiac block was found to be safe and easy to use. Few side effects were noted, and the majority of patients preferred it to CT celiac block. Some patients who do not respond to various therapies for abdominal pain caused by chronic pancreatitis may benefit from this technique.

▶ Obviously, celiac plexus block produces a temporary beneficial effect in patients with chronic pancreatitis. Unanswered questions about the technique include the following: Do repeated blocks produce the same benefits? What is the risk of repeated steroid blocks? Is a neurolytic block indicated for patients who experience temporary relief?

In my own experience, this procedure is not without risk. I am aware of 2 cases of retroperitoneal abscess occurring after celiac plexus block with steroids. Again, in my experience, neurolytic blocks are rarely successful in chronic pancreatitis. The only patients I have treated who experienced prolonged benefit did not have associated alcohol abuse problems.

S. E. Abram, MD

Twelve Month Follow-Up of a Controlled Trial of Intradiscal Thermal Anuloplasty for Back Pain Due to Internal Disc Disruption
Karasek M, Bogduk N (Northwest Spine Group, Eugene, Ore; Univ of Newcastle, Australia)
Spine 25:2601-2607, 2000   12–21

Background.—Internal disk disruption (IDD) is a condition in which the anulus fibrosus is intact but the nucleus pulposus has degraded, with radial fissures extending into the peripheral anulus that cause pain when the disk is stressed. A new approach to treating IDD is intradiskal electrothermal anuloplasty (IDTA), in which a flexible electrode is introduced into the nucleus and threaded circumferentially through the anulus at the region of the fissure. The electrode delivers heat to the anulus to coagulate the collagen and any nociceptive nerve fibers therein. Although IDTA is gain-ing in popularity, there have been no controlled trials of its efficacy. This is the first controlled trial to examine the efficacy of IDTA for IDD.

Methods.—The subjects were 53 patients, 31 to 50 years of age, with back pain caused by IDD at 1 or 2 levels, as confirmed by diskography and CT. Insurance carrier approval for IDTA was obtained for 36 patients (11 men and 20 women; mean age, 39 years) who became the test group. The remaining 17 patients (6 men and 11 women; mean age, 45 years) were included as controls and attended a rehabilitation program that included physical therapy, strengthening and conditioning exercises, education, and counseling. Before and at 3, 6, and 12 months after treatment, all subjects rated their level of pain on a 10-point visual analogue scale and indicated whether they had returned to work or used any opioids for pain relief.

Results.—At 3 months after treatment, 1 patient in the control group had dramatic pain relief, 3 had modest improvement, 4 had no improvement, and 9 had deterioration. Only 1 of the 5 patients who had not been working before treatment returned to work, and 3 patients who had been working before treatment were no longer working at 3 months. Five patients stopped using opioids, 4 began using opioids, and 7 continued using opioids. In contrast, at 3 months after treatment, 23 patients in the IDTA group achieved a significant degree of pain relief, and the median pain score on the visual analogue scale was significantly improved. Furthermore, this response was maintained at 6 and 12 months after treatment.

At 6 months, all 18 of the patients in the IDTA group who had been working before treatment continued to work, and 8 of the 15 patients (53%) who had not been working before treatment had returned to work. (Three patients were homemakers and did not seek outside employment.) All patients who did not achieve complete pain relief continued to use opioids. However, of the 19 patients who achieved 50% pain relief or greater, at 12 months, 11 had discontinued opioids, 5 had reduced their opioid dosage, and 3 were still using opioids for other conditions. Depending on the stringency of criteria used to define success, the IDTA success rate ranged from 23% (complete relief) to 60% (more than 50% reduction of pain to a level of 4 or 3).

Conclusion.—IDTA was significantly superior to physical rehabilitation in reducing and even eliminating back pain caused by IDD. The achievement of pain relief via IDTA was associated with an improvement in disability, a 53% return-to-work rate, and a reduced use of opioids. Furthermore, the effects were long lasting. Thus, the results of this first controlled trial of IDTA for IDD are encouraging.

▶ A number of new technologies for back pain have come into widespread use. It is surprising and distressing that these procedures have been introduced with minimal outcome studies. While this study is suggestive of a beneficial effect, it is not vigorously controlled, and the outcome measures are quite soft.

S. E. Abram, MD

Evaluation of Glucosamine Sulfate Compared to Ibuprofen for the Treatment of Temporomandibular Joint Osteoarthritis: A Randomized Double Blind Controlled 3 Month Clinical Trial

Thie NMR, Prasad NG, Major PW (Univ of Alberta, Edmonton, Canada)
J Rheumatol 28:1347-1355, 2001   12–22

Introduction.—Glucosamine is a naturally occurring aminosaccharide in the human body that is biosynthesized from glucose and used to produce glycosaminoglycan, a constituent of proteoglycans, which is an important component of the extracellular matrix of articular cartilage. Several trials have reported on maintenance of the therapeutic effects of glucosamine sulfate (GS) for treatment of osteoarthritis for weeks after discontinuation of therapy. The treatment potential of GS and ibuprofen were compared in patients with temporomandibular joint (TMJ) osteoarthritis (OA).

Methods.—Forty women and 5 men received either GS (500 mg tid) or ibuprofen (400 mg tid) for 90 days in a randomized, double-blind trial. Patients were evaluated for TMJ pain with function, pain-free, and voluntary maximum mouth opening. After a 1-week washout period and on day 90, the Brief Pain Inventory (BPI) questionnaire was administered and masticatory muscle tenderness was assessed. Acetaminophen tablets (500 mg), dispensed for breakthrough pain, were counted every 30 days to day 120.

Results.—Of 176 adults interviewed, 45 (26%) qualified for inclusion in the study, and 39 completed the trial (21 GS, 18 ibuprofen). Four patients dropped out because of stomach upset (3 ibuprofen, 1 GS), 1 because of dizziness (GS), and 1 because of inadequate pain control (ibuprofen). Within-group analysis showed significant improvement, compared with baseline of all variables in both treatment groups. Groups were similar in use of acetaminophen. Using a 20% reduction in primary outcome (TMJ pain with function), 15 and 11 patients, respectively, in the GS and ibuprofen groups had positive clinical response ($P = .73$). Between-group comparisons showed that patients in the GS group had a significantly greater reduction in TMJ pain with function, effect of pain, and acetaminophen used between days 90 and 120, compared with those in the ibuprofen group.

Conclusion.—Both GS and ibuprofen diminish pain in patients with TMJ degenerative joint disease. In the subgroup of patients who met the initial efficacy criteria, GS had a significantly greater effect in decreasing pain produced during function and effect of pain with daily activities. A carryover effect was seen with GS.

▶ It is encouraging to see outcomes studies that compare efficacy of dietary supplements with that of accepted medical therapies. If such substances are effective, we should be using them appropriately. If they are not, we should be advocating their abandonment, because their cost to the public is substantial. This study suggests that GS compares favorably with ibuprofen, both in terms of efficacy and side effects. The study would have been more useful if a placebo arm had been added, inasmuch as the response rate with both treatments is similar to that seen with placebo in many studies.

S. E. Abram, MD

Opioids and the Treatment of Chronic Pain in a Primary Care Sample

Adams NJ, Plane MB, Fleming MF, et al (Univ of Wisconsin, Madison)
J Pain Symptom Manage 22:791-796, 2001   12–23

Background.—Health care professionals are challenged by caring for patients with chronic pain. This widespread problem can have a myriad of causes, and numerous strategies are used in its management. How chronic pain is managed medically was studied in 12 primary care practices, with data gathered on the characteristics of the patients receiving opioids, the primary pain diagnoses, any comorbid mental health disorders, the types and dosages of opioids used, and whether opioid contracts, pain scales, and urine toxicology screens were used.

Methods.—Data were obtained on 209 adults (76% women; average age, 53) by using medical record audits covering the previous 12 months. Diagnostic codes identified patients with various chronic pain syndromes, and their billing records were reviewed. Physicians, physician assistants, and nurses identified patients receiving opioids for their pain.

Results.—Diagnoses differed by sex and age. Men over age 60 most frequently had diagnoses of lumbar/lower back pain and arthritis/joint pain. Men from age 22 to 39 had headaches/migraines more often than either men 40 to 60 or those over 60. A generally equal distribution across age groups was found for neck/upper back pain, which affected 16% of men. Women reported lumbar/low back pain most often (42%), and women over age 60 had this problem more often than men did. Arthritis/joint disease was reported in 35% of women, generally those over age 60. Thirty-four percent of women under 60 reported headache/migraine pain, 16% reported fibromyalgia, and 19% had neck/upper back pain. An equal distribution across age groups occurred for neuropathic/diabetic pain (3%). The most common diagnoses overall were lumbar/low back pain (44%), joint disease/arthritis (33%), and headache/migraine (28%). Oxycodone/acetaminophen was used in 31% of cases, morphine ERT in 19%, Tylenol #3 in 15%, and hydrocodone/acetaminophen in 14%. Forty-seven percent of the patient charts listed a comorbid mental health concern, with those under age 40 most likely to be so affected. Among these concerns were depression/affective disorders (seen in 36% of patient charts), anxiety/panic disorders (15%), drug abuse (6%), and alcohol abuse (3%). Women were more likely to have anxiety/panic disorders than men (21% vs 9%). Depression affected 32% of men and 41% of women. Thirty-one practitioners (42%) used written drug contracts, 29 (25%) used pain scales, and six (8%) used urine toxicology screens.

Conclusions.—While research has found that some patients with chronic pain benefit from opioid treatment, the practices outlined show that this is an underused tool in the armamentarium of primary care practitioners. A moderate number of individuals had comorbid mental health disorders that were being treated in the primary care setting.

▶ A common problem among pain clinic physicians is the need to provide long-term management of large numbers of patients who are stable on oral medications, thus limiting the physicians' ability to see new patients or manage more-difficulty problems. It is often difficult to convince primary care physicians that they can care for such patients successfully. Fear of regulatory scrutiny is 1 barrier, as identified in this study. Another problem is that primary care physicians are unwilling to schedule these patients often enough to adequately monitor their progress. A major advantage to primary care physicians' managing chronic pain patients is that they are often very skillful at managing these patients' comorbidities. Many primary care physicians bemoan the fact that they serve mainly a triage function. Here is an opportunity for them to serve as physicians.

S. E. Abram, MD

The Sequelae of Reflex Sympathetic Dystrophy
Zyluk A (Pomeranian Med Univ, Szczecin, Poland)
J Hand Surg [Br] 26B:151-154, 2001   12–24

Background.—Early treatment of reflex sympathetic dystrophy (RSD) can yield satisfactory results, even if normal function is not restored. Impaired hand function and discomfort can persist. Late sequelae may affect dexterity and hand function as well as quality of life. Functional and quality of life issues were assessed in a retrospective study 11 months after treatment for RSD.

Methods.—Ninety-six women and 48 men ranging in age from 29 to 78 (mean, 60) were diagnosed with RSD after upper limb trauma, with symptoms including diffuse pain, swelling, hand discoloration, abnormal skin temperature relative to the opposite limb, and limited range of motion. Various treatments were used, and 94 patients reported a good outcome at follow-up 11 months later. The results in these 94 patients provided the study data.

Results.—Twenty-seven patients had complete freedom from pain, 50 had pain related to weather conditions, and 32 had slight pain on use. Both use-related and weather-related pain afflicted 15 patients, and occasional analgesics eased the pain for 56 patients. Among the other effects were nail and hair growth changes (affecting 34% of patients), sensory alterations (34%), morning finger stiffness (28%), reduced ability to extend the finger, pain and loss of shoulder joint movement, and swelling of the hand after use. Reduced grip strength occurred in 78% of patients.

Conclusions.—Despite apparently good results from treatment, a significant number of patients experienced long-term adverse effects of RSD. These effects hindered hand function and reduced quality of life for many patients.

▶ While some treatments used by the authors are not mainstream, at least in the United States, the message of this study is that many patients who respond favorably to early intervention treatment fail to achieve long-term resolution of their symptoms. It is likely that patients with more chronic complex regional pain syndrome will have still worse outcomes.

S. E. Abram, MD

The Use of a Computer-Based Decision Support System Facilitates Primary Care Physicians' Management of Chronic Pain
Knab JH, Wallace MS, Wagner RL, et al (Anesthesia Services Med Group, San Diego, Calif; Univ of California, San Diego; VA San Diego Healthcare System)
Anesth Analg 93:712-720, 2001 12–25

Background.—Chronic pain patients consume significantly more resources than other patients in the managed care setting. When care for the pain fails, added costs can be incurred for drug side effects, adverse reactions to treatment, waste of health care resources, and the patients' lost faith in the health care system. Primary care physicians (PCPs) may undertreat pain because they lack clinical knowledge about diagnosing and caring for chronic pain. Frequent visits to the physician, re-evaluations, and adjustments to medications are often required, since chronic pain is rarely cured but rather daily function is enhanced and quality of life improved despite the presence of pain. The hypothesis that use of computer-based decision support (CBDS) could help the PCP manage chronic pain more effectively was tested.

Methods.—The participants had already "failed" primary care management and been referred to a pain clinic. Charts for 50 patients were carefully reviewed and data relevant to pain abstracted. A decision support system supplied data to a pain specialist for use in choosing appropriate therapy for the patients' pain, which the pain specialist recommended to referring physicians. "Treatment" of the 50 cases based on a CBDS system was carried out by 5 board-certified PCPs. A successful outcome was defined as use of a new or adjusted therapy that the software had recommended (meaning that the PCP would have prescribed it to an actual patient). Medical appropriateness scores ranged from 0 (totally inappropriate) to 10 (totally appropriate); these scores were determined by 2 pain specialists who reviewed the PCPs' outcomes. Actual outcomes were recorded in the hospital database and reviewed after a year, with focus on actual pain management used and the number of patients referred to the pain clinic again by their PCP.

Results.—In over half the cases, the PCPs all chose the same algorithm used by the pain specialist; at least 4 of the 5 chose the same algorithm in 72% of cases. Usually, the algorithm chosen differed when there was diffuse pain, multiple pain sites, or a contributing disease present. Neither the success rate nor the appropriateness of therapy was affected by choice of a different algorithm. A total of 793 new or altered therapies were prescribed by the PCPs, with nonpharmacologic therapies used much more often than pharmacologic ones. The CBDS system did not directly recommend 39 of the prescribed therapies, although all were found among the software's algorithms. Eighty-five percent of cases had successful outcomes. Overall, 77.6% and 57.5% of the PCPs' outcomes were rated by the 2 pain specialists as more appropriate than nonappropriate.

Conclusions.—Use of the CBDS system may augment PCPs' ability to successfully manage patients with chronic pain. The treatment recommendations generated were acceptable in 85% of cases. In addition, staff members of the pain clinic may be able to use the software to prescreen pain consults and suggest standard management algorithms for use by the PCP so that specialist referral is not needed.

▶ This study indicates that the use of a CBDS system lets PCPs successfully manage the large majority of referred chronic pain patients. The system encourages PCPs to provide care for chronic pain patients and provides them with algorithms and suggestions for ongoing management. This is a far better system than simply "dumping" patients back on the primary physician.

S. E. Abram, MD

Lumbar Sympathetic Block for Pain Relief in Two Patients With Interstitial Cystitis

Doi K, Saito Y, Nikai T, et al (Shimane Med Univ, Izumo, Japan)
Reg Anesth Pain Med 26:271-273, 2001   12–26

Background and Objectives.—Interstitial cystitis (IC) is characterized clinically by lower abdominal pain, pain during urination, and increased frequency of urination. Treatment of the symptoms in IC remains challenging. We report effective treatment using lumbar sympathetic block for 2 patients with IC.

> *Case Report.*—A 63-year-old and 78-year-old woman were diagnosed with IC. Medical therapy with nonsteroidal anti-inflammatory drugs (NSAID), anticholinergics, and hydrodistention of the bladder failed to improve their symptoms. Subsequently, a continuous lumbar epidural block using 1% mepivacaine was used in these patients. A transient reduction of the symptoms in both patients was achieved. A lumbar sympathetic block with a neuro-

lytic agent produced almost complete, and long-lasting relief of their symptoms.

Conclusion.—Lumbar sympathetic block using a neurolytic agent produced long-lasting pain relief in 2 patients with IC.

▶ These case reports remind us that much of the visceral afferent traffic from the pelvis travels cephalad in the sympathetic chain, returning via the white rami communicantes to the dorsal horn between T10 and L2. Alternative neurolytic procedures include superior hypogastric plexus block and selective sacral root blocks. Sacral root blocks would denervate visceral afferents that enter the spinal cord with the S2, S3, and S4 nerve roots, whereas the superior hypogastric plexus block would denervate the sacral visceral afferents as well as those that travel in the sympathetic chain.

S. E. Abram, MD

The Morbidity, Time Course and Predictive Factors for Persistent Post-thoracotomy Pain
Gotoda Y, Kambara N, Sakai T, et al (Osaka Med Ctr of Cancer and Cardiovascular Disease, Japan; Hannan Central Hosp, Osaka, Japan)
Eur J Pain 5:89-96, 2001   12–27

After thoracotomy, patients often suffer from a persistent pain syndrome called post-thoracotomy pain. To elucidate morbidity, time course, and predictive factors for this syndrome, we analyzed follow-up data for 85 post-thoracotomy patients (Table 2). We used a 4-point scale to assess pain: none, slight, moderate and severe. Of 85 patients, 50 reported pain (39 slight, 11 moderate) one day after surgery. A year after surgery, the patients were polled using a simple questionnaire received by the mail. Sixty patients reported persistent pain (34 slight, 14 moderate, 12 severe) a month after surgery, and 35 patients reported persistent pain (33 slight, 2 moderate) around the time of the poll (1 year after surgery). Although pain deterioration was observed in 40% (34/85) of patients during month 1 after surgery, pain alleviation was seen in 48% (41/85) of patients during

---

TABLE 2.—Demographic Characteristics and Pain Rating at Post-thoracotomy Day 1 (*PTD1*), Post-thoracotomy Month 1 (*PTM1*), and Post-thoracotomy Year 1 (*PTY1*)

Pain Rating	PTD1	PTM1	PTY1
(0) Pain free	35 (41%)	25 (29%)	50 (59%)
(1) Slight pain	39 (46%)	34 (40%)	33 (39%)
(2) Moderate pain	11 (13%)	14 (17%)	2 (2%)
(3) Severe pain	0 (0%)	12 (14%)	0 (0%)
Total	85 (100%)	85 (100%)	85 (100%)

(Courtesy of Gotoda Y, Kambara N, Sakai T, et al: The morbidity, time course and predictive factors for persistent post-thoracotomy pain. *Eur J Pain* 5:89-96, 2001. Reprinted with permission from the Society of Thoracic Surgeons.)

months 2 to 12. Stepwise regression analysis revealed that female gender and pain at postoperative day 1 were predictive for persistent pain both 1 month and 1 year after thoracotomy. Among 35 patients with persistent pain 1 year after surgery, 24 cases reported paresthesia-dysesthesia, and 14 cases reported hypoesthesia. The present data thus suggests that persistent pain is common and often severe 1 month after surgery but is alleviated after 1 year. Clinical time course and symptoms indicate that nerve impairment rather than simple nociceptive impact may be involved in this syndrome.

▶ Postamputation and postthoracotomy pain are serious clinical problems that can persist for months or years. Their incidence is probably greatly underestimated. A few studies of postamputation pain suggest that patients with preoperative pain are more likely to have persistent postoperative pain. There is some evidence that presurgical control of that pain may reduce the incidence of persistent postoperative pain. In this study, severe early postoperative pain was predictive of persistent pain. It remains to be determined whether aggressive control of pain in the early postoperative period will prevent long-term pain.

S. E. Abram, MD

Using Gabapentin to Treat Failed Back Surgery Syndrome Caused By Epidural Fibrosis: A Report of 2 Cases

Braverman DL, Slipman CW, Lenrow DA (Univ of Pennsylvania, Philadelphia)
Arch Phys Med Rehabil 82:691-693, 2001   12–28

Failed back surgery syndrome (FBSS) is a long-lasting, often disabling, and relatively frequent (5%-10%) complication of lumbosacral spine surgery. Epidural fibrosis is among the most common causes of FBSS, and it is often recalcitrant to treatment. Repeated surgery for fibrosis has only a 30% to 35% success rate, whereas 15% to 20% of patients report worsening of their symptoms. Long-term outcome studies focusing on pharmacologic management of chronic back pain secondary to epidural fibrosis are lacking in the literature. This report presents 2 cases of severe epidural fibrosis managed successfully with gabapentin monotherapy. In both cases, functional status improved markedly and pain was significantly diminished. Gabapentin has an established, favorable safety profile and has been shown to be effective in various animal models and human studies of chronic neuropathic pain. Clinicians should consider gabapentin as a pharmacologic treatment alternative in the management of FBSS caused by epidural fibrosis.

▶ Gabapentin produces effective analgesia in patients with a variety of neuropathic conditions. It is not surprising that it produced pain relief in patients with chronic radiculopathy. There is considerable variability in dose requirements, and some patients may require 3600 to 4800 mg/d to achieve optimal benefit. At higher doses, it is beneficial to administer the drug in at least 4 divided doses.

S. E. Abram, MD

Methadone Maintenance Patients Are Cross-Tolerant to the Antinociceptive Effects of Morphine
Doverty M, Somogyi AA, White JM, et al (Adelaide Univ, Australia; Drug and Alcohol Services Council of South Australia, Parkside; Royal Adelaide Hosp, Australia; et al)
Pain 93:155-163, 2001   12–29

Background.—The use of opioids such as methadone in substitution treatment for dependence is increasing. Patients receiving methadone maintenance are likely to experience acute and chronic pain to the same degree and with the same frequency as occurs in the general population. However, studies have suggested that heroin addicts have a disproportionately higher rate of traumatic injuries and medical disorders compared with the general population. Information concerning the antinociceptive effects of additional opioids in these patients is conflicting and sparse. Patients receiving methadone maintenance have been shown to be hyperalgesic to pain induced by a cold pressor (CP) test, a finding that could have clinical implications for pain management in this population. The antinociceptive effects of additional opioids in patients receiving methadone maintenance were examined.

Methods.—Four patients receiving stable, once-daily doses of methadone and 4 matched control subjects were studied. The intensity and duration of antinociceptive responses at 2 pseudo-steady-state plasma morphine concentrations (C_{SS1} and C_{SS2}) were measured in both methadone patients and controls. In methadone patients, the possibility that the antinociceptive effects of morphine are affected by changes in plasma $R(-)$-methadone concentration at the 2 extremes of methadone concentration, the peak (2 hours after the dose) and trough (23.5 hours after the dose), was investigated. The nociceptive stimuli used included a CP test and electrical stimulation (ES). Morphine was administered intravenously to achieve the consecutive plasma concentrations, and blood samples were collected, concurrently with nociceptive responses, to determine plasma morphine concentrations.

Results.—Methadone patients reached a mean C_{SS1} of 16 ng/mL and a mean C_{SS2} of 55 ng/mL, compared with 11 ng/mL and 33 ng/mL, respectively, for controls. The methadone patients were hyperalgesic to pain from CP but not ES. Methadone patients experienced minimal antinociception in comparison with controls, despite significantly greater plasma morphine concentrations. In these patients, the antinociceptive effects ended when the infusion ended; in the controls, however, antinociception lasted for 3 hours. The patients' responses to morphine were not significantly affected by the fluctuations that occurred in plasma R(−)-metha-done concentration.

Conclusions.—These findings suggest cross-tolerance in methadone pa-tients to the antinociceptive effects of morphine; conventional doses of morphine are not likely to be effective in managing acute pain in these patients. Additional research is necessary to determine whether other drugs are more effective than morphine in the management of acute pain among patients receiving methadone maintenance.

▶ This study provides documentation in human beings of a phenomenon that is well recognized in experimental animals: that chronic opioid admin-istration leads to hyperalgesia and cross-tolerance to the analgesic effect of other opioids. This study confirms the effect among patients without under-lying pain who have a history of opioid abuse.

The implications of these results are obvious. Patients receiving chronic opioid therapy for any reason require substantially higher opioid doses to control acute pain associated with surgery or trauma. Nonopioid regional analgesic techniques and nonopioid analgesics are extremely helpful for such patients.

The implications of these findings for chronic pain management are not as obvious. Large numbers of patients with chronic pain receive substantial doses of opioids and continue to report poor pain control, but are unwilling to reduce or discontinue their medication. Some of these patients experi-ence improvement in pain after discontinuation of their opioids. Others report worsening of pain. It is unclear how much time is required to reverse the hyperalgesic effect of chronic opioid administration when medication is stopped, so we don't know how long a drug holiday should be continued in such patients. This is a question that requires serious investigation.

There is currently a popular movement to liberalize the use of opioids for chronic pain management. Although certain patients benefit greatly from opioids, others are made worse, and we must be willing to discontinue opioids when they are clearly detrimental. The concept that all patients will obtain relief from opioids if we simply give a high enough dose is a danger-ous one.

S. E. Abram, MD

Abuse of Combinations of Carisoprodol and Tramadol
Reeves RR, Liberto V (Univ of Mississippi, Jackson)
South Med J 94:512-514, 2001   12–30

Background.—Carisoprodol (Soma) is a commonly prescribed skeletal muscle relaxant. Tramadol (Ultram) is a nonopioid, nonsteroidal agent commonly prescribed for pain control. Neither carisoprodol nor tramadol is considered a controlled substance by the federal government. However, several reports have indicated that there may be a potential for abuse of carisoprodol, most likely because one of its active metabolites, meprobamate, has abuse potential and has been designated a controlled substance. Data for the first 3 years of tramadol use indicate that a low rate of abuse has been reported; however, there have been cases of abuse and dependence reported in the literature. Tramadol should not be used by opioid-dependent patients. Three cases of abuse of a combination of carisoprodol and tramadol by patients seeking psychotropic effects were reported.

> *Case Reports.*—Woman, 28, being treated in a mental health clinic for anxiety had not responded to medication. She had a history of anxiety beginning in her early 20s, with related symptoms of irritability, muscle tension, and insomnia. She had also abused alcohol beginning in her late teens and later abused diazepam. She had a poor response to several antianxiety medications and was taking buspirone, 20 mg 3 times per day. Her medical history was not significant except for tension headaches and neck and back pain. Treatment with carisoprodol was initiated and improved the headache symptoms. The patient asked for extra carisoprodol prescriptions on 2 occasions, saying that she had lost either her prescription or her medication. She also requested tramadol for headaches. It was later discovered that she was refilling the carisoprodol prescriptions about 10 days after receiving a month's supply of the medication. When confronted about her misuse of the medication, the patient indicated that she had been obtaining carisoprodol and tramadol from a number of different physicians and taking the combination for about a year to produce a profoundly relaxing, euphoric effect. She had been introduced to the combined use of these drugs by 2 friends, a 32-year-old man and a 31-year-old woman. The man reported use for about 2 years, taking as many as 12 carisoprodol and 8 tramadol tablets per day. The woman had been using the combined drugs for 18 months, taking 2 carisoprodol tablets and 1 tramadol tablet 4 times daily. Both the man and the woman related feelings of euphoria and sedation and indicated that they used this combination because these drugs were easier to obtain than controlled substances. The first patient agreed to enter treatment for substance abuse, but the 2 friends refused. With abrupt withdrawal of carisoprodol and tramadol, the patient complained of extreme nervousness, irritability, insomnia, paravertebral muscular pain, headache, and craving for the medications, so a tapered withdrawal was begun and was well tolerated. The patient has been lost to follow-up.

Conclusions.—Three cases were presented involving the illicit use of a combination of carisoprodol and tramadol to obtain psychotropic effects. These medications should be prescribed with caution in patients who are at risk for substance abuse, and extreme caution is warranted in the prescription of both drugs simultaneously in any patient.

▶ That carisoprodol is one of the abused drugs in this report is not surprising. Patients with chronic pain who take this drug rarely state that it helps relieve their pain, but they often indicate that it "helps me relax." I have been unimpressed with the analgesic effects of either of these drugs among patients with chronic pain.

S. E. Abram, MD

Impact of Spinal Cord Stimulation on Sensory Characteristics in Complex Regional Pain Syndrome Type I: A Randomized Trial
Kemler MA, Reulen JPH, Barendse GAM, et al (Maastricht Univ, The Netherlands)
Anesthesiology 95:75-80, 2001   12–31

Objective.—The effects of spinal cord stimulation (SCS) on sensory symptoms were investigated in patients with chronic complex regional pain syndrome type I (CRPS I) in a randomized controlled trial.

Methods.—Seventy patients, aged 18 to 65 years, with CRPS I for at least 6 months, restricted to 1 extremity, and unresponsive to standard therapy, were randomly assigned to receive standardized physical therapy (PT) ($n = 18$) or PT + SCS ($n = 36$). PT + SCS patients underwent 1 week of test stimulation, and 24 patients who responded successfully underwent SCS implantation. Patients were assessed 6 times during the 12-month trial for pressure sensibility, warmth and cold sensibility, and mechanical hyperanalgesia. One patient in the PT only group did not complete the study.

Results.—Four PT patients and 1 SCS+PT patient were lost to follow-up after the 6-month assessment. Although SCS did not change warmth and cold detection thresholds, SCS patients experienced significant hypoesthesia at 1 and 3 months. Pressure thresholds returned to normal levels thereafter. SCS had no effect on pain thresholds for any sensation at the 12-month follow-up. Mechanical hyperanalgesia was not reduced significantly in the SCS group compared with the control group, although both patients and controls experienced a significant reduction of both dynamic and static hyperanalgesia.

Conclusion.—SCS has no effect on pain thresholds and does not appear to decrease sensitivity in either affected or contralateral limbs.

▶ Early studies of the mechanism of action of SCS indicated that analgesia was probably the result of a combination of activation of large afferent fibers with resultant central modulating effects plus blockade of spinal cord afferent pathways. Evoked potential studies indicated that there was some reduction in transmission of afferent traffic in the spinal cord. This study indicates that there is probably little effect of this modality on spinal cord transmission of afferent impulses responsible for pain perception. One difference between these and earlier findings is the fact that, in earlier studies,[1] electrode placement was different (anterior and posterior) and much larger electrodes were used. At any rate, using current equipment and technology, it appears that the majority of analgesic effects of spinal cord stimulation are mediated central to the site of electrode placement. A practical piece of information is the absence of effect on allodynia, which is important in informing patients of the potential benefits of the therapy.

S. E. Abram, MD

Reference

1. Larson SJ, Sances A, Riegel DH, et al: Neurophysiological effects of dorsal column stimulation in man and monkey. *J Neurosurg* 41:217-223, 1974.

Retrospective Review of Eighteen Patients Who Underwent Transtibial Amputation for Intractable Pain
Honkamp N, Amendola A, Hurwitz S, et al (Univ of Iowa, Iowa City; Univ of Virginia, Charlottesville)
J Bone Joint Surg Am 83-A:1479-1493, 2001   12–32

Objective.—Whether patients with intractable foot and ankle pain experienced relief and an increase in functional capability after transtibial amputation was investigated.

Methods.—A questionnaire was sent to 18 patients (4 women, 14 men), aged 26 to 61, who had below-the-knee amputation for intractable foot or ankle pain unrelated to diabetes mellitus, peripheral vascular occlusive disease, or peripheral neuropathy. The questionnaire assessed level of pain, need for analgesia, days missed from work, recreational status, satisfaction, and willingness to have the procedure again under similar circumstances.

Results.—Patients were assessed at an average of 41 months after amputation. Sixteen patients would have the procedure again under similar circumstances, 1 was unsure, and 1 would not undergo amputation again. Disability decreased from 8.4 to 3.7. Three of 13 patients who worked before the procedure were able to return to work. The remaining 10 did not return to work because of unrelated health problems (5 patients), increased and continuous pain and disability related to the amputated limb (2 patients), prosthetic complications (2 patients), and inability to walk long distances (1 patient). Five patients previously unable to work before amputation were able to find full employment after surgery. Two patients required additional treatment after surgery. The most difficult problem encountered by postamputation patients was maintaining an adequately fitted prosthesis. Degree of pain improved significantly from 8.8 to 1.3, pain frequency from 9.8 to 1.7, and pain intensity from 8.4 to 2.6. Office visits in the 6 months before and after amputation improved from an average of 6.6 to 1.9. Narcotic and other analgesic use declined or ceased after amputation in all patients. Fifteen patients experienced phantom limb sensations at an average of 3.1 on a 10-cm visual analog scale. The ability to walk and function improved significantly after amputation from a score of 6.4 to 2.0. Three patients participated in sports before amputation, and 9 did so after amputation. Distance walked increased from 0.3 mile before surgery to 0.8 mile after surgery. Seventeen patients were able to drive before amputation, and 18 were able to drive after amputation.

Conclusion.—These patients experienced less pain, took less medication, and had improved function after transtibial amputation for intractable ankle or foot pain.

▶ We have become sensitized to the possibility that amputation can worsen existing chronic pain in an extremity, or can lead to new, sometimes more distressing pain, such as phantom limb pain. Part of this sensitization is likely due to the fact that those of us working in pain clinics see only the postoperative failures—those with persistent postamputation pain. This study demonstrates that amputation may be a viable alternative for certain patients, particularly those whose limb is nonfunctional because of deformity or injury as well as pain.

It would be interesting to know how many of these patients had regional anesthetics versus general anesthesia, as there is the perception that perioperative regional anesthesia, particularly if begun some time before surgery and continued into the postoperative period, may reduce the incidence and duration of phantom limb pain.

S. E. Abram, MD

Are Cannabinoids an Effective and Safe Treatment Option in the Management of Pain? A Qualitative Systematic Review
Campbell FA, Tramèr MR, Carroll D, et al (Queen's Med Centre, Nottingham, England; Höpitaux Universitaires, Genève, Switzerland; Oxford Radcliffe Hosp, England)
BMJ 323:13-16, 2001   12–33

Background.—The central and peripheral nervous system in human beings are equipped with cannabinoid receptors, but the functions of these receptors and the endogenous ligands may be unclear. In animal models, cannabinoids have been shown to reduce the hyperalgesia and allodynia associated with formalin, capsaicin, carrageenan, nerve injury, and persistent visceral pain. It is hoped that exogenous cannabis or cannabinoid may function as analgesics in pain syndromes that are poorly managed, such as the spasms of multiple sclerosis and resistant neuropathic pain. Whether cannabis is an effective and safe treatment option for pain management was evaluated by reviewing the literature.

Methods.—The Medline, Embase, Oxford Pain database, and Cochrane Library electronic databases, references from identified papers, and hand searches were used in a systematic review of randomized controlled trials of cannabis administered by any route with any analgesic or placebo in patients with acute, chronic nonmalignant, or cancer pain. The main outcomes were pain intensity and pain relief scores and adverse effects. The validity of the trials was independently assessed with the Oxford score.

Results.—From 20 randomized controlled trials, 9 were included in the final analysis. A total of 222 patients were included. Five trials involved cancer pain whereas 2 trials each concerned chronic nonmalignant pain and acute postoperative pain, respectively. All the trials tested cannabinoids but not cannabis. Oral delta-9-tetrahydrocannabinol, 5 to 20 mg, and intramuscular levonantradol, 1.5 to 3 mg, were found to be about as effective as codeine, 50 to 120 mg. Oral benzopyranoperidine, 2 to 4 mg, was found to be no better than placebo and less effective than codeine, 60 to 120 mg. Adverse effects were common and usually involved psychotropic effects.

Conclusions.—Cannabinoids were found to be no more effective than codeine in controlling pain. In addition, cannabinoids exert depressant effects on the CNS, limiting their use. Further valid randomized controlled trials are needed before cannabinoids can be considered for use in the treatment of spasticity and neuropathic pain. They should not be used to treat acute postoperative pain.

▶ There is considerable political pressure to make marijuana and cannabinoids available for medical use. Although there may be other therapeutic uses for these substances, their analgesic effects are not impressive. However, as Campbell et al point out, there may be more reasonable applications in conditions for which opioids are relatively ineffective, such as opioid tolerance and neuropathic pain.

S. E. Abram, MD

Experimental Pain Management

Antinociceptive Properties of Neurosteroids IV: Pilot Study Demonstrating the Analgesic Effects of Alphadolone Administered Orally to Humans

Goodchild CS, Robinson A, Nadeson R (Monash Univ, Clayton, Australia)
Br J Anaesth 86:528-534, 2001   12–34

Background.—Gamma aminobutyric acid (GABA) receptors fall into 2 categories: $GABA_A$ and $GABA_B$. $GABA_A$ receptors are found in the dorsal horn of the spinal cord and may be the target of inhalational general anesthetics. Neuroactive steroids have been used on the spinal cord to produce antinociception in animals. Among these agents are alphaxalone and alphadolone. The efficacy, tolerability, and safety of alphadolone in humans were evaluated in a pilot study.

Methods.—This prospective, randomized, double-blind study evaluated 14 patients scheduled for orthopedic knee reconstruction surgery. All received oral doses of either alphadolone (9 patients; dose, 25 to 500 mg) or placebo (5 patients; lactose) 1 hour after operation. Each had a standardized general anesthetic and the same type of surgery. Then physiotherapy was undertaken with the use of a continuous passive movement machine. Patient-controlled analgesia was used to administer morphine IV after surgery. Over a period of 6 hours, verbal rating and visual analogue scales were used to evaluate the patients' pain experience.

Results.—The morphine dosages received in the operating room, recovery ward, and ward before capsules were administered did not differ significantly between the placebo and the alphadolone groups. As alphadolone dose increased from 25 to 100 mg, morphine dose decreased. One hundred milligram doses or more of alphadolone were associated with patient-controlled morphine administration lower than the lowest level used by patients receiving placebo. Alphadolone doses of up to 500 mg produced no increased sedation, respiratory depression, nausea, or vomiting. Alphadolone-treated patients had significantly lower pain scores on both the verbal and the visual analogue scales.

Conclusion.—Oral alphadolone may be a useful analgesic for humans. This study revealed a significant reduction in pain, no major side effects, and lessened need for morphine.

▶ IV neurosteroids have been used as IV anesthetics but have been largely abandoned because of poor water solubility and problems with their vehicle. The fact that these drugs have antinociceptive activity as well as low toxicity makes them interesting candidates for perioperative sedative/analgesic agents. Further exploration of their spinal analgesic properties, which are related to GABA receptor agonist effects, may be warranted as well.

S. E. Abram, MD

μ-Opioid Receptor Desensitization by β-Arrestin-2 Determines Morphine Tolerance but Not Dependence
Bohn LM, Gainetdinov RR, Lin F-T, et al (Duke Univ, Durham, NC)
Nature 408:720-723, 2000   12–35

Background.—While morphine produces impressive pain relief, it also induces tolerance and dependency, the former developing as the drug is continued, so that greater and greater amounts are needed to achieve pain relief. The decreased responsiveness may include desensitization of G-protein–coupled receptors through phosphorylation and subsequent binding of regulatory proteins (β-arrestins). This study in mice evaluated the contribution of desensitization of the μ-opioid receptor to morphine antinociceptive tolerance and eventual physical dependency.

Methods.—A group of wild-type mice and another of β-arrestin 2 (βarr2$^{-/-}$) mice were given a moderate dose of morphine or placebo, then assessed for nociceptive response latencies 24 hours later. Next, the mice were given daily doses of morphine and the paw-withdrawal latencies were noted. Finally, morphine pellets were implanted subcutaneously in the mice to simulate chronic administration.

Results.—The βarr2$^{-/-}$ mice maintained their responsiveness to morphine in the first part of the study. With chronic exposure, significantly reduced responsiveness to morphine developed in the wild-type mice after 5 days, but the βarr2$^{-/-}$ mice experienced no desensitization of the μ-opioid receptor with chronic morphine treatment. Thus, antinociceptive tolerance did not develop. It was noted that the βarr2$^{-/-}$ mice maintained the chronic morphine-induced upregulation of adenylyl cyclase activity and still became physically dependent on morphine.

Conclusion.—The antinociceptive response was maintained in these βarr2$^{-/-}$ mice, whether the exposure to morphine was acute or chronic. It was also shown that the mechanisms that produce tolerance differ from those that produce physical dependency.

▶ Prolonged exposure of opioid receptors on postsynaptic neurons leads to loss of responsiveness (tolerance) to the antinociceptive effects of the drug as well as to a hyperalgesic state. Both the tolerance and the hyperalgesia appear to be mediated by protein kinase C. β-arrestin 2, a regulatory protein, is involved in the development of tolerance but not in the development of physical dependence. It would be interesting to know whether in βarr2$^{-/-}$ mice, opioid mediated sensitization of postsynaptic dorsal horn neurons develops as well.

S. E. Abram, MD

Analgesic Effect of Bisphosphonates in Mice
Bonabello A, Galmozzi MR, Bruzzese T, et al (SPA - Societa' Prodotti Antibiotici SpA, Milan, Italy; Univ of Turin, Italy)
Pain 91:269-275, 2001   12–36

Background.—Bisphosphonates are an important therapeutic tool in various diseases, such as tumor-induced hypercalcemia, Paget's disease, and metastatic bone disease. They are able to control calcium phosphate formation and dissolution as well as mineralization and bone resorption. They help to reduce skeletal complications, relieve pain, and improve patients' quality of life. Using mice, this study evaluated the analgesic effect of 4 bisphosphonates (clodronate, alendronate, pamidronate, and etidronate) with respect to those of morphine and acetylsalicylic acid. In addition, these bisphosphonates' effect on gastrointestinal transit time was also noted.

Methods.—The 2 tests used (the tail-flick and abdominal constriction [writhing] tests) determined the nociceptive properties of the bisphosphonates. First, the predose tail response latency was noted. Then a dose was administered and the tail response latency at 30 minutes was measured, with a final calculation of the difference between postdose and predose latency times. Gastrointestinal transit time was determined as the distance traveled by a test meal as a percentage of the total length of the animal's small intestine.

Results.—In the tail-flick test, the antinociceptive effect of IV acetylsalicylic acid was dose-dependent and statistically significant for all 3 of the doses used. Clodronate given IV had a statistically significant effect at all 4 doses used, and pamidronate had a significant dose-dependent increase in tail-flick latency in all but the lowest dose. Alendronate and etidronate produced only a modest effect with IV doses of 30 mg/kg, a pronounced and statistically significant effect at 60 mg/kg, and serious toxicity at 80 mg/kg. After an intracerebroventricular injection, morphine's effect was dose dependent, and clodronate and pamidronate had significant, potent dose-dependent effects on tail-flick latency values for all of the doses used except the lowest dose of clodronate. No statistically significant effect occurred with the use of etidronate (Fig 2).

In testing abdominal constriction, a statistically significant dose-dependent effect was produced by acetylsalicylic acid when 30 and 60 mg/kg doses were used. All 3 doses of morphine produced a potent, dose-dependent effect. For all doses, IV clodronate and pamidronate significantly reduced the number of abdominal contractions. With intramuscular injections, clodronate significantly reduced contractions at doses of 2.5 and 5 mg/kg, but pamidronate's nociception was limited to the 5-mg/kg dose. No effect on gastrointestinal transit time was noted for doses of clodronate and pamidronate up to 5 mg/kg, but a statistically notable effect was produced by morphine at a dose of 1.25 mg/kg.

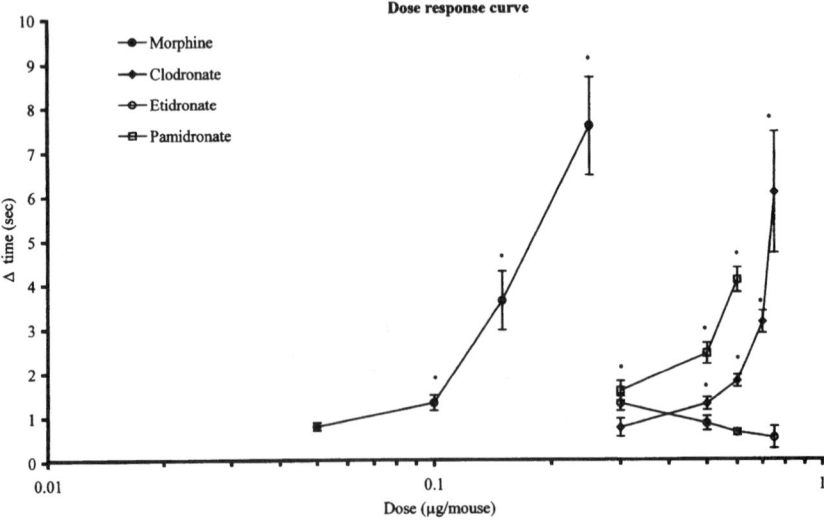

FIGURE 2.—Dose-response curves of clodronate (*solid diamond*, 50 patients), morphine (*solid circle*, 60 patients), etidronate (*open circle*, 40 patients) and pamidronate (*open square*, 30 patients) after intracerebroventricular injection in the tail-flick test. Animals were tested 30 minutes after drug administration. Each *point* represents the mean ± SEM. *Asterisk* indicates $P < .05$, compared with the difference between postdose and predose latency time of control group (0.07 ± 0.03 s). (Courtesy of Bonabello A, Galmozzi MR, Bruzzese T, et al: Analgesic effect of bisphosphonates in mice. *Pain* 91:269-275, 2001.)

Conclusion.—Clodronate and pamidronate have both central and peripheral pain-relieving effects, although the mechanism could not be verified. Based on these findings, clodronate and pamidronate may be of use for pain relief in conditions not linked to osteolytic or inflammatory bone processes.

▶ There is some variation in the ability of various bisphosphonates to provide pain relief in patients with bony metastases. Intrinsic analgesic effects of certain bisphosphates may explain some of these differences.

S. E. Abram, MD

Attenuation of μ-Opioid Tolerance and Cross-Tolerance by the Competitive N-Methyl-D-Aspartate Receptor Antagonist LY235959 Is Related to Tolerance and Cross-Tolerance Magnitude
Allen RM, Dykstra LA (Univ of North Carolina, Chapel Hill)
J Pharmacol Exp Ther 295:1012-1021, 2000   12–37

Background.—Numerous studies indicate that the coadministration of an N-methyl-D-aspartate (NMDA) receptor antagonist attenuates the development of tolerance to the μ-opioid morphine. The opioid used may influence this effect, in that the NMDA antagonist LY235959 attenuates tolerance to morphine, but not to fentanyl (also a μ-opioid). Additionally, it is unclear whether the extent of attenuation is related to the magnitude of opioid tolerance that develops. A rat model was used by the authors to compare the effects of LY235959 in the attenuation of tolerance and cross-tolerance to 3 opioids of different efficacy: morphine, etorphine (higher efficacy than morphine), and dezocine (lower efficacy than morphine).

Methods.—A warm-water tail-withdrawal protocol was used, with tail-withdrawal latencies measured at baseline, after 7 days of opioid dosing (to examine chronic tolerance), and after 1 injection of opioid (to examine cross-tolerance). Eighteen distinct groups of naïve male Sprague-Dawley rats (159 total, 6-8 animals per group) were used to compare 6 chronic treatment conditions and 3 single-dose testing conditions (ie, cross-tolerance). The 6 chronic treatment conditions consisted of etorphine (0.003 mg/kg), morphine (10 mg/kg), or dezocine (3.0 mg/kg), injected subcutaneously twice a day for 7 days, either alone or in combination with LY235959 (3.0 mg/kg). On day 8, cross-tolerance was examined by dividing the animals in each chronic treatment group into 3 subgroups which received 1 injection of etorphine, morphine, or dezocine. Dose-effect curves were plotted and compared among the 18 different test conditions.

Results.—No tolerance developed in the chronic etorphine alone group. However, cross-tolerance to morphine and dezocine did develop in this group; the potency ratios for morphine and dezocine were shifted rightward by factors of 2.2 and 3.4, respectively. The addition of LY235959 to etorphine prevented the development of cross-tolerance to morphine and dezocine (potency ratio shifts of only 1.2- and 1.2-fold, respectively). Chronic morphine caused tolerance and cross-tolerance to etorphine and dezocine; potency ratios for morphine and etorphine shifted rightward by factors of 2.9 and 2.5, respectively, while the dezocine curve flattened. The addition of LY235959 to morphine prevented morphine tolerance and cross-tolerance to etorphine and attenuated the cross-tolerance to dezocine (potency ratio shift of 4.0-fold rather than flattened).

Chronic dezocine caused the greatest degree of tolerance and cross-tolerance, and potency ratios for dezocine, etorphine, and morphine shifted rightward by factors of 9.6, 4.1, and 3.5, respectively. The addition of LY235959 to dezocine attenuated these effects, with potency ratios for dezocine, etorphine, and morphine shifting by factors of 2.8, 2.4, and 1.7, respectively.

Conclusion.—The opioid with the highest efficacy (etorphine) caused the lowest degree of tolerance and cross-tolerance, while the opioid with the lowest efficacy (dezocine) caused the greatest degree of tolerance and cross-tolerance. The magnitude of the effect of LY235959 in preventing or attenuating cross-tolerance differed according to the opioid's efficacy. Thus, with these 3 µ-opioids, both the efficacy of the opioid and the magnitude of tolerance or cross-tolerance that develops during chronic opioid administration greatly affect the ability of NMDA receptor antagonists to prevent or attenuate tolerance.

▶ This study reconfirms the previously reported finding that tolerance development is greater following drugs with lower efficacy. Paronis and Holtzman[1] showed that tolerance development to morphine, meperidine, and fentanyl was greatest after chronic meperidine administration and least following chronic fentanyl infusion. These data challenge the practice, recommended by the World Health Organization analgesic ladder, of beginning cancer pain treatment with weak opioids and progressing to strong opioids. According to the data presented by Allen and Dykstra, the use of weak opioids is most likely to result in tolerance and cross-tolerance. Co-administration of an NMDA antagonist appears to be most likely to inhibit tolerance development when weak opioids are used.

It is not clear how important a role tolerance plays in dose escalation in patients with cancer pain. There is growing evidence that most dose increases are necessitated by tumor spread and associated increases in noxious stimulation.

S. E. Abram, MD

Reference

1. Paronis CA, Holtzman SG: Development of tolerance to the analgesic activity of mu agonists after continuous infusion of morphine, meperidine or fentanyl in rats. *J Pharmacol Exp Ther* 262:1-9, 1992.

Opioid Peptide–Expressing Leukocytes: Identification, Recruitment, and Simultaneously Increasing Inhibition of Inflammatory Pain

Rittner HL, Brack A, Machelska H, et al (Freie Universität Berlin)
Anesthesiology 95:500-508, 2001   12–38

Background.—The systemic administration of opioids that act on specific opioid receptors within the CNS can provide effective relief of pain. Centrally acting opioids are effective, but they have significant side effects including nausea, vomiting, respiratory depression, and respiratory arrest. Opioid receptors are expressed not only within the CNS but also on peripheral sensory nerve terminals, and effective control of inflammatory pain can be accomplished by the interaction of opioid receptors on peripheral sensory nerve terminals with opioid peptides that are released from immune cells on stressful stimulation. Localized painful inflammation can be induced in the rat paw by intraplanar inoculation of Freund's complete adjuvant (FCA). The source of opioid peptide production was investigated by identifying and quantifying populations of opioid-containing cells during FCA-induced inflammation in the rat hind paw. The development of stress-induced local analgesia in the paw was also examined.

Methods.—Tissue samples were harvested from male Wistar rats at 2, 6, and 96 hours after injection of FCA. Cells were characterized with flow cytometry by using a monoclonal pan-opioid antibody (3E7) and antibodies against cell surface antigens, and with immunohistochemistry by using a polyclonal antibody to β-endorphin. Magnetic cell sorting was performed, and the β-endorphin content was quantified by radioimmunoassay. Pain responses were evaluated before and after cold water swim stress by paw pressure thresholds.

Results.—In the early stages of inflammation, 66% of the opioid peptide–producing leukocytes (3E7+) were HIS48+ granulocytes. However, at later stages of inflammation (96 hours), most (73%) of the 3E7+ immune cells were ED1+ monocytes or macrophages. In the 4 days after FCA inoculation, there was a nearly 6-fold increase in the number of 3E7+ cells, and a nearly 4-fold increase in the β-endorphin content in the paw. Cold water swim stress–induced analgesia increased by 160%.

Conclusions.—The inhibition of endogenous pain is proportional to the number of opioid peptide–producing cells, and there is a contribution of distinct leukocyte lineages to this function at different stages of inflammation. These mechanisms may be important for understanding pain in patients with immunosuppressive diseases such as AIDS, cancer, and diabetes, and for designing new therapies for the relief of pain in these patients.

▶ This study helps to describe the system that leads to the activation of peripheral opioid receptors. It explains the mystery of why opioid receptors exist in a milieu in which no opioids are stored or released.

S. E. Abram, MD

Opioid-Induced Hyperalgesia and Incisional Pain

Li X, Angst MS, Clark JD (Stanford Univ, Palo Alto, Calif)
Anesth Analg 93:204-209, 2001   12–39

Background.—Opioids are very useful in the treatment of many types of pain, but there are concerns regarding the long-term consequences of their use. These consequences are classified as either psychological, such as psychological dependence and addiction; or physiologic, such as analgesic tolerance and constipation. Another possible complication with opioid use is opioid-induced hyperalgesia (OIH). OIH has been observed with the use of very large doses of either intravenous or intrathecal opioids such as morphine, and in the chronic use of opioids followed by abrupt reductions in dosage. In the latter situation, the manifestation of OIH is not limited to the well-described complaints of pain from those who abuse drugs and then go through opioid withdrawal. Recently, there have been reports of spontaneous pain, allodynia, and thermal hyperalgesia in patients after reductions in dosage or abrupt cessation of opioids administered therapeutically. It was hypothesized that abrupt cessation of opioid administration at the time of hind paw incision in a rat model of incisional pain would lead to an intensified manifestation of the thermal hyperalgesia and mechanical allodynia observed after incision in control animals. The role of intrinsic opioid systems in the regulation of nociceptive thresholds was also explored.

Methods.—Rats were administered morphine, 40 mg·kg^{-1}·d^{-1}, for 6 days via subcutaneous osmotic minipumps. In the second group of experiments, a rat model of incisional pain was used to explore the development of OIH after abrupt cessation of opioids. In the final experiments, naloxone was administered chronically before incision in a rat model (20 mg·kg^{-1}·d^{-1} for 6 days) and then discontinued, and the results were compared with the acute administration of naloxone after hind paw incision.

Results.—The rats that received morphine via subcutaneous osmotic minipumps demonstrated thermal hyperalgesia and mechanical allodynia for several days after morphine administration ceased. The experiments with incisional pain in the rat model demonstrated that the effects attributable to OIH were additive with the hyperalgesia and allodynia that resulted from incision. In the final set of experiments, the chronic administration of naloxone for 6 days followed by cessation before incision led to significantly reduced hyperalgesia and allodynia. In contrast, hyperalgesia and allodynia were significantly increased when naloxone, 1 mg/kg, was administered acutely after hind paw incision.

Conclusions.—The hyperalgesia and allodynia observed in this rat model of incisional pain can be altered by the chronic administration of exogenous opioid receptor agonists and antagonists before incision. The mechanism of action may involve the alteration of intrinsic opioidergic systems that are involved in determining thermal and mechanical pain thresholds.

▶ There has been considerable progress toward elucidation of the mechanisms of opioid tolerance and hyperalgesia. Increased intracellular levels of protein kinase C are associated with nociceptor-induced spinal sensitization as well as with opioid tolerance and hyperalgesia.[1] Recent political movements that have liberalized the use of opioids for patients with chronic noncancer pain have led to the notion that all pain can be successfully managed if you just give enough opioid. This approach is clearly counterproductive for certain patients. We need to consider discontinuation of opioids for patients who receive minimal benefit from high-dose opioids. We also should consider initiation of alternative or adjunctive analgesic interventions for postoperative patients who have been receiving opioids chronically.

S. E. Abram, MD

Reference

1. Mayer DJ, Mao J, Holt J, et al: Cellular mechanisms of neuropathic pain, morphine tolerance, and their interactions. *Proc Natl Acad Sci U S A* 96:7731-7736, 1999.

Gabapentin Actions on *N*-Methyl-D-Aspartate Receptor Channels Are Protein Kinase C-Dependent
Gu Y, Huang L-YM (Univ of Texas, Galveston)
Pain 93:85-92, 2001   12–40

Background.—The analgesic gabapentin has been widely prescribed for the treatment of pain in patients with peripheral nerve injuries, diabetic neuropathy, and cancer. The mechanisms that underlie the antinociceptive actions of gabapentin have not been elucidated. The actions of gabapentin on N-methyl-D-aspartate (NMDA) receptors have been studied, since NMDA receptors have a central role in the sensitization of nociceptive neurons. The results of these studies are varied. There is evidence that the effects of gabapentin are dependent on the pain states of animals. Behavioral studies have shown that gabapentin does not affect transient responses to noxious heat or mechanical stimuli but does effectively block sustained nociceptive responses to inflammatory agents such as formalin. The effects of gabapentin on NMDA-evoked currents in single dorsal horn neurons were investigated in a rat model.

Methods.—Single dorsal horn neurons were isolated from normal rats and from rats with inflammation induced by complete Freund adjuvant injected to the hindpaw. NMDA receptor–mediated currents were examined by using the whole-cell patch clamp recording technique.

Results.—NMDA currents in normal neurons were enhanced only when protein kinase C (PKC) was added to the cells. The mechanism for this enhancement was an increase in the affinity of glycine for NMDA receptors by gabapentin. However, gabapentin enhanced NMDA responses in neurons from complete Freund adjuvant–treated rats without any addition of PKC.

Conclusions.—Endogenous PKC is elevated in inflamed tissue, so these findings suggest that gabapentin exerts its effects only on those cells affected by inflammatory injuries. Thus, the effects of gabapentin on NMDA receptors depend on the phosphorylation states of cells or receptors. These findings could indicate a new strategy for the design of drugs to alleviate pain, since a chemical that acts on the basis of the state of cells would maximize the effectiveness of antinociception with minimal side effects.

▶ We tend to think of gabapentin as being specific for neuropathic pain. Indeed, most neuropathic pain states are probably associated with elevations in PKC. However, if the drug's antinociceptive effects are dependent on elevation of PKC in spinal projection neurons, it would seem likely that gabapentin might be efficacious in other painful conditions as well. There is evidence that gabapentin should be effective for nonneuropathic pain from studies that demonstrate antinociceptive effects in the formalin test. Controlled studies of the drug's effect in chronic inflammatory states would be interesting.

S. E. Abram, MD

Miscellaneous

Effect of Preemptive Multimodal Analgesia for Arthroscopic Knee Ligament Repair

Rosaeg OP, Krepski B, Cicutti N, et al (Univ of Ottawa, Ont, Canada)
Reg Anesth Pain Med 26:125-130, 2001   12–41

Background.—Effective management of postoperative pain after arthroscopic repair of the anterior cruciate ligament (ACL) is important for improving the patient's comfort and early movement of the knee joint to facilitate same-day discharge from the hospital. This may be accomplished by the preoperative administration of analgesic medication. The preoperative administration of multiple analgesics, with different mechanisms of action, may also improve the postoperative management of pain and functional recovery. Pain scores and intravenous consumption of opioids after outpatient ACL repair were compared in patients who received a multimodal combination of drugs either preoperatively or immediately after surgery.

Methods.—Forty patients undergoing same-day arthroscopic ACL repair with a semitendinosus tendon graft were studied. The patients were randomly assigned to receive a multimodal combination of ketorolac 30 mg IV; intra-articular injection of 20 mL ropivacaine 0.25% plus morphine 2 mg and epinephrine 1:200,000; and femoral nerve block with 20 mL ropivacaine 0.25% either 15 minutes before skin incision or immediately after skin closure. Verbal pain scores were obtained from the patients in the postanesthesia care unit and again on postoperative days 1, 3, and 7, and IV patient-controlled analgesia (PCA) morphine consumption was recorded.

Results.—The group that received preoperative analgesia (preemptive group) had lower verbal pain rating scores for 2 hours after their arrival in the postanesthesia care unit. However, there were no differences between the 2 groups in pain scores on postoperative days 1, 3, and 7. The preemptive group had lower mean IV PCA morphine consumption in the postanesthesia care unit than did the group that received multimodal analgesia immediately after surgery.

Conclusions.—The preoperative administration of multimodal analgesia resulted in lower pain scores initially compared with patients who received multimodal analgesia immediately after surgery; however, by postoperative day 1, the pain scores were similar for both groups. The preemptive administration of multimodal analgesia in patients undergoing arthroscopic ACL repair did not result in a measurable, long-term advantage.

Preemptive Analgesic Effects of Ketorolac in Ankle Fracture Surgery
Norman PH, Daley MD, Lindsey RW (Univ of Texas, Houston; Baylor College of Medicine, Houston)
Anesthesiology 94:599-603, 2001   12–42

Background.—The term preemptive analgesia refers to the administration of analgesia before a painful stimulus, such as surgery, to decrease the intensity of subsequent pain. The definition of preemptive analgesia has been broadened to include treatment that prevents the development of hyperexcitability, even when it occurs postoperatively. Preemptive analgesia is a clearly demonstrable phenomenon in animal models, but there has been little evidence to support the occurrence of preemptive analgesia in human beings. The effects of ketorolac as a preemptive analgesic for patients undergoing orthopedic surgery were investigated. If it can be established that ketorolac does have preemptive effects, then the administration of this nonsteroidal anti-inflammatory drug preoperatively may be advantageous in spite of the potential for increased blood loss.

Methods.—This randomized, double-blind, controlled trial included 48 patients scheduled for surgical repair of ankle fractures. Ketorolac, 30 mg, was administered IV to 23 patients before tourniquet inflation and to 25 patients after inflation of the tourniquet. Standardized anesthesia management was used, including adequate opioid analgesia with 5 µg/kg fentanyl and 0.1 mg/kg morphine. Visual analogue scale pain scores, patient-controlled analgesia morphine consumption, the incidence of nausea and vomiting, and postoperative bleeding were measured.

Results.—Patients given ketorolac before tourniquet inflation did not experience an increase in pain postoperatively compared with their preoperative baseline. In contrast, the patients who received ketorolac after tourniquet inflation experienced significantly increased postoperative pain. However, this effect did not last; by 6 hours postoperatively, the pain scores for these patients were not significantly higher than the preoperative levels. Intergroup comparison revealed a lower visual analogue scale score at 2 and 4 hours and lower nausea scores at 6 hours in the preemptive group. The consumption of patient-controlled analgesia did not differ between the 2 groups.

Conclusions.—Intravenous ketorolac, 30 mg, appeared to have preemptive analgesic effects in patients undergoing surgical repair of ankle fractures. Postoperative pain is not perceived as more intense than preoperative pain when ketorolac is administered before tourniquet inflation.

Preemptive Bupivacaine Offers No Advantages to Postoperative Wound Infiltration in Analgesia for Outpatient Breast Biopsy

O'Hanlon DM, Colbert ST, Keane PW, et al (Univ College Hosp, Galway, Ireland)

Am J Surg 180:29-32, 2000   12–43

Background.—Adequate postoperative pain control is important for every patient but particularly so for patients undergoing ambulatory surgery. Previous reports have demonstrated that up to one third of patients experience moderate-to-severe pain postoperatively as a result of inadequate analgesia. In more than 80% of patients, on-demand intramuscular opiates fail to provide adequate pain relief. In addition, concern regarding potential adverse side effects and addiction has resulted in the underutilization of prescribed opiates. A combination of opioids, nonsteroidal anti-inflammatory drugs, and local anesthetic agents provides good pain relief and is effective for outpatient surgery. However, there are questions regarding the best schedule for administration of these agents. The preemptive administration of analgesics offers many theoretic advantages. The value of preemptive analgesia with bupivacaine in patients undergoing ambulatory breast surgery under general anesthesia was determined.

Methods.—The use of preoperative bupivacaine 0.5% (10 mL) for the relief of postoperative pain was compared with postincision administration of the same dose of bupivacaine in 74 patients in this prospective, randomized trial. Both groups had similar demographic characteristics.

Results.—There were no differences between the 2 groups in postoperative pain scores on the visual analogue scale (VAS). In the preemptive group, the visual analogue scale score at 30 minutes was 4.5, compared with 4.7 in the postincision group. There also was no significant difference in the number of patients in each group requiring additional analgesia—13 (36%) in the preemptive group compared with 18 (47%) in the postincisional group. The time to additional analgesia was similar for both groups (55.0 vs 55.3 minutes).

Conclusions.—It would appear that the use of local anesthesia with bupivacaine preoperatively does not significantly affect postoperative pain in patients undergoing ambulatory breast biopsy.

▶ Does preemptive analgesia work? I do not know, but there is much to be said for the logical planning of an analgesic regimen that is part of the anesthetic plan and carries over into the postoperative period (Abstracts 12–41, 12–42, and 12–43). Knowledge of the pharmacokinetics and dynamics of analgesic drugs may indicate that a drug should either be given preoperatively or before the surgery is concluded.

M. Wood, MD, FRCA

Preoperative Intradermal Acupuncture Reduces Postoperative Pain, Nausea and Vomiting, Analgesic Requirement, and Sympathoadrenal Responses
Kotani N, Hashimoto H, Sato Y, et al (Univ of Hirosaki, Japan; Univ of Louisville, Ky; Univ of Vienna)
Anesthesiology 95:349-356, 2001   12–44

Background.—Acupuncture offers the potential to relieve some degree of perioperative pain, relying on the placement of intradermal needles at acupoints. Objective measures have been lacking in support of acupuncture. In a group of patients undergoing upper and lower abdominal surgery, intradermal needles were inserted 2.5 cm from the spinal vertebrae and the effects on pain were determined as a function of postoperative pain scores, opioid requirements, opioid-related side effects, and adrenal responses induced by surgical stress.

Methods.—Patients were randomly assigned to either receive acupuncture (50 patients having upper abdominal surgery and 39 patients having lower abdominal surgery) or function as a control (48 patients having upper abdominal surgery and 38 having lower abdominal surgery). Those receiving acupuncture had needles inserted to the left and right of bladder meridian 18-24 (upper abdominal) and 20-26 (lower abdominal) before anesthesia was induced. Postoperatively, epidural morphine and bolus doses of intravenous morphine were given for pain control. The amount of intravenous morphine administered was measured. A 4-point verbal rating scale was used to assess incisional pain at rest and during coughing both in the recovery period and up to 4 days after surgery. The plasma concentrations of cortisol and catecholamines were evaluated to detect time-dependent changes.

Results.—No complaints of pain arose from the insertion of the acupuncture needles. All of the patients emerged from anesthesia within 10 minutes of the discontinuation of nitrous oxide and muscle relaxant antagonism. Over the first 5 days after surgery, no complications were noted, and after 1 week, over 95% of patients judged the pain management to be excellent to good. Pain relief improved significantly over time in the patients having upper abdominal surgery, with or without acupuncture, but during the period from recovery until the second day postoperatively those receiving acupuncture had significantly better pain relief than those in the control group. These findings were mirrored in patients having lower abdominal surgery. The consumption of morphine each day decreased over time in all patients, but the consumption of those having acupuncture was as much as 50% less than that in the control group. Neither respiratory depression nor other significant side effects occurred, and nausea and vomiting occurred less often among the acupuncture group, regardless of site of surgery. Significant increases in the plasma concentrations of cortisol, norepinephrine, and epinephrine were noted beginning 1 hour after upper abdominal surgery commenced; both surgical groups had increased plasma dopamine concentrations. The plasma concentration increases in epinephrine and cortisol among the control group exceeded those in the acupuncture group. No special training was required to use the acupuncture technique.

Conclusions.—Advantages to the use of acupuncture included no special training requirement, no interference with the operative process or with postoperative rest, no complications, a decrease in pain (incisional and visceral), a reduced need for analgesics, and a lessened incidence of nausea and vomiting postoperatively. The pain-induced activation of the sympathetic nervous system was also reduced with acupuncture.

▶ There are many studies that are supposed to show that complementary medicine and acupuncture are effective—but they fall short on scientific methodology. This study shows that acupuncture is effective in reducing postoperative pain in a specific clinical setting. If it is true, and the findings can be repeated, then how does it work?

M. Wood, MD, FRCA

13 Clinical Trials

An Inventory of Canadian Anesthesiology: Human Research From 1995 Through 1999
Gagnon RE, Macnab AJ, Blackstock D (Children's and Women's Health Centre of British Columbia, Vancouver, Canada)
Can J Anesth 48:452-458, 2001   13–1

Introduction.—One of the world's largest computerized databases is the Medical Literature Analysis and Retrieval System (MEDLARS), part of the National Library of Medicine in Bethesda, Maryland. As of March 2001, almost 11 million entries were included in its database. Since 1987, articles archived in MEDLARS have been catalogued with the author's affiliation address. To highlight Canadian studies in anesthesiology, the MEDLARS archive was surveyed for the years 1995 through 1999.

Methods.—Articles were sought under the headings of anesthesiology, analgesia, anesthesia, anesthetics, and analgesics. The search used field codes for address, date of publication, publication type, major heading, and subheading; only articles coded as "human" and having original research were included. When possible, Canadian counts were compared with worldwide counts. To compare the research output of anesthesiologists versus other clinical specialties as listed by the Royal College of Physicians and Surgeons of Canada, original Canadian research articles from 1988 through 1999 were counted.

Results.—There were 1842 data counts from the 5 principal categories, 22 major categories, and 421 subcategories. Canadian contributions, which ranged from 141 in 1992 to 185 in 1999, accounted for 3% of the world total in anesthesia categories annually. In Canada, from 30% to 38% of studies in each principal category involved adults aged 19 to 44. Overall, there was an equal gender distribution in the analgesic studies. The greatest sources of original research by Canadians were the *Canadian Journal of Anesthesia* (45%) and *Anesthesia and Analgesia* (18%). Affiliations cited most often were in Toronto (32%) and Montreal (15%). The most frequent topics were "pharmacology" and "therapeutic use." In general, Canadian trends were similar to world trends in terms of specific anesthetic and analgesic agents studied. This comprehensive overview o. research trends may be of value to medical students, residents, and fellows.

▶ This study is interesting because Canada has approximately 3% of the world's anesthesiologists, and produces roughly 3% of the world's anesthesia literature. The University of Toronto produced one fifth of all the Canadian studies. I believe there is that type of concentration in the United States as well. One is continually amazed at the relative importance of a few centers to medical progress. Should we only support (with research dollars) such important centers? I wonder if such centers produce the really innovative research or if, like UCSF's Boyer and Bishop, innovative research starts transformation of a medical center. While such consideration may not seem directly relevant to anesthesia or anesthesia education, they are truly important for us to educate the public about the importance of science and clinical resources to our community and to provide economic growth to the community around those centers of research.

M. F. Roizen, MD

14 Anesthesia Outside the Operating Room

Morbidity in Electroconvulsive Therapy
Tecoult E, Nathan N (CHU Dupuytren, Cédex, France)
Eur J Anaesthesiol 18:511-518, 2001   14–1

Background.—General anesthesia has been used for nearly 4 decades to provide humane conditions for the administration of electroconvulsive therapy (ECT), but there have been few studies regarding the complications associated with this practice and their implications for the anesthesiologist. Some authors have suggested that the use of general anesthesia for ECT is associated with lower standards of care than for other nonsurgical anesthetic procedures. Specific problems such as repeated exposures and the attendant risks are associated with anesthesia for ECT. Anesthesia for ECT is performed outside the operating room, there are numerous pharmacologic interactions between anesthetic agents and psychiatric medications, and convulsions are possible. Many patients cannot coherently convey their medical problems because they are elderly. Some authors have suggested that ECT is associated with a lower morbidity rate than antidepressant drugs and have suggested that ECT is unsuitable on an outpatient basis. Because ECT is commonly used in the treatment of bipolar disorders and has been suggested as a useful treatment for some forms of neurologic disease, such as Parkinson disease, the complications and morbidity of ECT were retrospectively assessed.

Methods.—Data analysis was used to review the complications that occurred in 75 patients undergoing 612 ECT procedures under propofol anesthesia.

Results.—One or more complications occurred in 51 patients (68%) during treatment. Twelve of these complications were potentially life threatening. There was 1 case each of angina pectoris and aspiration pneumopathy, 3 hypoxic episodes, and 5 severe episodes of laryngospasm causing hypoxia. Confusion for more than 2 hours after ECT occurred in 33% of patients and recurred in 13% of patients after several ECT sessions. Traumatic complications occurred in 6 patients, with 1 patient requiring surgery.

Conclusions.—The findings suggest that ECT is not a low-risk procedure. ECT was associated with a particularly high rate of respiratory complications that might have previously been overlooked. Therefore, the use of ambulatory anesthesia may not be appropriate on a regular basis for patients undergoing ECT.

▶ I have always thought that the adverse events related to ECT were underestimated. Is anesthesia for ECT associated with a lower standard of care? It is most often performed "out of the operating room," and good recovery room facilities are not always available.

M. Wood, MD, FRCA

Subject Index

A

Abdominal
hysterectomy (*see* Hysterectomy, abdominal)
pain in chronic pancreatitis, endoscopic ultrasound-guided celiac plexus block for, 341
surgery
major, in children, effect of preoperative epidural morphine on postoperative analgesia in, 332
major, ketamine/morphine after, patient-controlled, 318
major, selective postoperative inhibition of gastrointestinal opioid receptors after, 35
upper and lower, preemptive intradermal acupuncture reduces postoperative pain, nausea and vomiting, analgesic requirement, and sympathoadrenal responses in, 369

Abuse
of combinations of carisoprodol and tramadol, 352
substance, among anesthesiologists, risk of death from, 105

Academic
anesthesiology department, measurement of individual clinical productivity in, 5
health centers, graduating residents of, preparedness for clinical practice, 8

Acadesine
protective effect on lung ischemia-perfusion injury (in cat), 229

Acupuncture
preoperative intradermal, effect on postoperative pain, nausea and vomiting, analgesic requirement, and sympathoadrenal responses, 369

ADL 8-2698
effect on gastrointestinal opioid receptors, 35

Administrative
delays in discharge from postanesthesia care unit, impact on total patient care hours, statistical analysis by Monte-Carlo simulation of, 2

Age
vs. comorbidities as risk factors for complications after elective abdominal aortic reconstructive surgery, 63

Air
leak, persistent, after living donor lobectomy, 251
vs. saline for identification of epidural space, quality of labor analgesia with, 263

Airway
laryngeal mask, bronchoscopy with bronchoalveolar lavage via, in high-risk hypoxemic immunosuppressed patients, 188
pressure, continuous positive, effect on cerebral blood flow velocity in awake volunteers, 58
upper, reactivity, effect of sevoflurane and desflurane on, 43

Alcohol
-containing waterless handrub for ICU personnel, 204
withdrawal after open aortic surgery, 17

Alendronate
analgesic effects of (in mice), 359

Alpha-beta-blocker
vs. calcium channel blocker for emergence hypertension after craniotomy, 157

Alphadolone
oral, analgesic effects of, 357

Alternative medicine
use in presurgical patients, prevalence and predictors of, 28

Alveolar
fluid clearance impairment in patients with acute lung injury and ARDS, 191

Amantadine
no effect on postoperative analgesia after abdominal hysterectomy, 330

Ambulation
epidural analgesia with, effect on labor duration, 281

Amputation
transtibial, for intractable pain, 355

Analgesia
epidural
labor (*see* Labor, analgesia, epidural)
patient-controlled, with and without night-time infusion after gastrectomy, 331
intrathecal, effect on success of external cephalic version, 291

N

Author Index